Diagnosis in color

Physical Signs in Cardiology

Noble O Fowler MD
Emeritus Professor of Medicine
University of Cincinnati College of Medicine
Cincinnati, Ohio
USA

Foreword by
J Willis Hurst MD
Consultant to the Division of Cardiology
Emory University School of Medicine
Atlanta, Georgia
USA

Mosby
London · Philadelphia
St Louis · Sydney · Tokyo

Related titles published in Mosby's Diagnosis in color series:

The Nail in Clinical Diagnosis 2 ed: Beaven & Brooks
ENT Diagnosis 3 ed: Bull
Infectious Diseases 3 ed: Emond, Rowland & Welsby
Surgical Diagnosis: Greig
Medical Microbiology: Hart & Shears
Breast Diseases: Mansel & Bundred
Medical Mycology: Midgley, Clayton & Hay
Skin Signs in Clinical Medicine: Savin, Hunter & Hepburn
Pediatrics: Taylor & Raffles
Cardiology: Timmis & Brecker
Oro-Facial Diseases 2 ed: Tyldesley
Oral Medicine 2 ed: Tyldesley
Obstetrics and Gynaecology, Symonds & Macpherson
Levene's Dermatology 2 ed: White
STD & AIDS 2 ed: Wisdom & Hawkins
Physical Signs in General Medicine 2 ed: Zatouroff

Acquisitions Editor: **Jane Ryley**
Development Editor: **Jeremy Gross**
Project Manager: **Adèle Collins**
Design: **Greg Smith**
Cover Design: **Paul Phillips**
Production: **Andrea Ford**
Index: **Liza Weinkove**

Published in 1999 by Mosby, an imprint of Mosby International Limited, Lynton House, 7–12 Tavistock Square, London WC1H 9LB, UK

ISBN 0 7234 3105 1

Printed by Keslan Servicios Gráficos.

For full details of all Mosby titles, please write to Mosby International Publishers Limited, Lynton House, 7–12 Tavistock Square, London WC1H 9LB, UK.

Cataloging-in-Publication Data:
Cataloging records for this book are available from the US Library of Congress and the British Library

Foreword

In the early fifties Noble Fowler and I were young faculty members in the Department of Medicine at Emory University School of Medicine. I noted that he was a keen observer and excellent correlator. He later became the Director of Cardiology at the University of Cincinnati where he influenced more than one generation of trainees.

Observing is more than just looking. Let us look at the act from three different vantage points.

> *I once asked 100 second-year medical students what they saw in a patient with osteogenesis imperfecta. Only one student noted the blue sclera, although all of the students had seen thousands of eyes.*
>
> Lesson: We are born to see, but have to train ourselves to observe.
>
> *Helen Keller, who was deaf and blind, chided a friend who remarked that she had walked in the woods but saw nothing interesting.[1] Helen pointed out how thrilled she was to feel the 'delicate symmetry of a leaf.'*
>
> Lesson: We should use our senses to their fullest.
>
> *Louis Agassiz, the famous Harvard zoologist and teacher, asked a student to observe a fish and describe what he saw.[2] The student's first effort did not please Agassiz. After observing the fish for hundreds of hours, the student was able to describe what he saw.*
>
> Lesson: One has to be persistent in one's efforts to learn to observe.

Correlation is achieved when the observer relates an abnormality that is found in one part of the body with an abnormality that is found in another part of the body. In this book Fowler presents 65 clinical conditions which commonly involve the cardiovascular system. The diagnosis of each condition can be made, or strongly suggested, from inspection of the patient. Fowler transmits the information so well that readers will store the images in their brains and bring them into action as they inspect their patients.

J Willis Hurst MD
Emory University School of Medicine
Atlanta, Georgia

References:

1 From material prepared by the American Foundation for the Blind, 15 West 16th Street, New York, NY 10011.

2 Highet G. *The Art of Teaching*. Vintage Books, Inc. 1950: 214–216.

Preface

The goal of this book is to enable the medical practitioner to suspect a cardiovascular diagnosis by devoting a few minutes to a careful inspection of the patient. In this era of cost containment, the diagnosis or suggestion of a diagnosis can focus and limit the number and cost of often expensive diagnostic procedures. For example, xanthomata, corneal arcus, or pseudoxanthoma elasticum suggest coronary artery disease. Xanthomata or xanthelasma imply the need to evaluate the likelihood of hypercholesterolemia and its subsequent treatment. Valvular heart disease is suggested by Marfan syndrome, malar flush, relapsing polychondritis, Hurler's syndrome or the blue sclera of osteogenesis imperfecta. Disease of the aorta can be indicated or implied by ankylosing spondylitis, Marfan syndrome, chest wall mass, Turner's syndrome, or unilateral cervical venous distention. Heart muscle disease is suggested by Friedreich's ataxia, scleroderma, amyloidosis or the muscular dystrophies.

A number of the conditions illustrated in this book are associated with congenital heart disease that may be surgically corrected. Among these are Noonan's syndrome, Down syndrome, Turner's syndrome, atrial septal defect, and patent ductus arteriosus. Bilateral cervical venous distention is a clue to the diagnosis of congestive heart failure, pericardial disease, or superior mediastinal tumor. Changes in the ocular fundi may suggest severe hypertension requiring further evaluation for possible secondary causes and the required treatment. Digital and subconjunctival petechiae may be a clue to the diagnosis of infective endocarditis. Chest wall deformity may suggest cor pulmonale, atrial septal defect, or aortic aneurysm. Genetic counseling may be advisable in Noonan's syndrome, Down syndrome, Turner's syndrome, and Williams syndrome.

This book illustrates, in color, 65 clinical conditions which usually or often involve the cardiovascular system. The diagnosis of each is specifically made or strongly suggested from inspection of the patient. The accompanying text explains the background of the disorder illustrated, and indicates the genetic background and what additional tests may be needed. There are references for further reading.

This book should be especially useful to internists and family practitioners, or medical students and residents who are in training for those fields.

Noble O Fowler

Contents

Acknowledgements

Without the help of friends and colleagues, this book would not have been possible. I am especially grateful to Dr James Nordlund, Professor and Chairman of Dermatology, University of Cincinnati, who allowed me to borrow a number of color illustrations from his extensive collection (Figs 2.48, 6.12, 6.13, 7.7, 7.10, 8.1–8.4, 8.11, 8.13, 8.18, 8.48, 8.50, 8.51). Dr Brian Hoit, Associate Professor of Medicine and Director of Echocardiography, University of Cincinnati, kindly provided echocardiographic illustrations (Figs 1.45, 2.14–2.16, 2.26, 2.27, 2.33, 4.7, 4.33, 4.52, 4.53, 5.20, 5.21, 6.21, 8.16). Dr David Schwartz, Professor of Pediatrics, University of Cincinnati, furnished illustrations of several forms of congenital heart disease (Figs 1.29–1.31, 1.40, 2.2). Dr Robert Adolph, Emeritus Professor of Medicine, University of Cincinnati, allowed me to employ several useful illustrations (Figs 1.9–1.11, 1.14). Color illustrations were also provided by Dr Jacqueline Noonan, Professor of Pediatrics, University of Kentucky (Fig. 1.26), Dr Joel Sacks, Former Professor and Chairman, Department of Ophthalmology, University of Cincinnati College of Medicine (Fig. 3.9), Dr Jesse Edwards, Clinical Professor of Pathology, University of Minnesota, Minneapolis (Fig. 1.60), Dr Jerome Herman, Professor of Internal Medicine, University of Cincinnati College of Medicine (Figs 2.35–2.37), Dr Michael Criley, Professor of Medicine and Radiologic Sciences, University of California, Los Angeles (Figs 6.22, 6.26), Dr Robert Franch, Professor of Medicine (Cardiology), Department of Medicine and Radiology, Emory University School of Medicine and Hospital, Atlanta (Fig. 6.32), Dr J Van der Bel-Kahn, Former Professor of Pathology, University of Cincinnati College of Medicine (Fig. 8.33) and Dr J Willis Hurst, Professor of Medicine and Chairman Emeritus, Emory University School of Medicine, Atlanta (Figs 1.7, 6.31).

My secretary, Ms Janet Darpel, worked faithfully through many revisions to bring this work to fruition.

1 General Appearance

Marfan Syndrome

Marfan syndrome is an autosomal dominant disorder in which increased height and long, thin extremities (dolichostenomelia) are associated with abnormalities in the cardiovascular, skeletal, and ocular systems. Marfan described the skeletal features of the syndrome in 1896 but his patient did not have the ocular or cardiovascular components. It is currently accepted that the syndrome results from mutations in the FBN1 gene that encodes fibrillin-1, a protein found in elastic fiber-associated microfibrils. Its prevalence is approximately 1–2 in 20,000 people.

Clinical attention may be drawn to the possibility of Marfan syndrome in one of several ways. Tall stature (**Fig. 1.1**), or elongated extremities or fingers

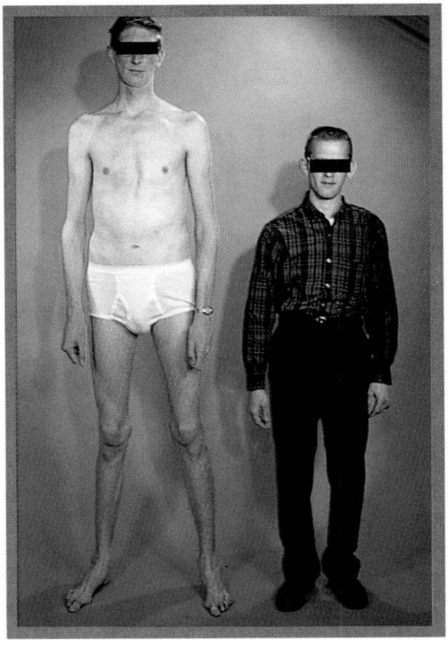

→ Fig. 1.1
Marfan syndrome. Body habitus of a patient with the syndrome (left) compared with that of a normal man of 1.78m height (right). Note the long, thin extremities and deformities of the toes. (With permission from Fowler NO. *Diagnosis of heart disease.* Springer–Verlag, 1991.)

(**Figs 1.2–1.6**), may raise the question. Ectopia lentis suggests Marfan syndrome (**Fig. 1.7**, although it also raises other possibilities (**Fig. 1.8**). Retinal detachment and myopia are common. Myxomatous degeneration of the mitral or tricuspid

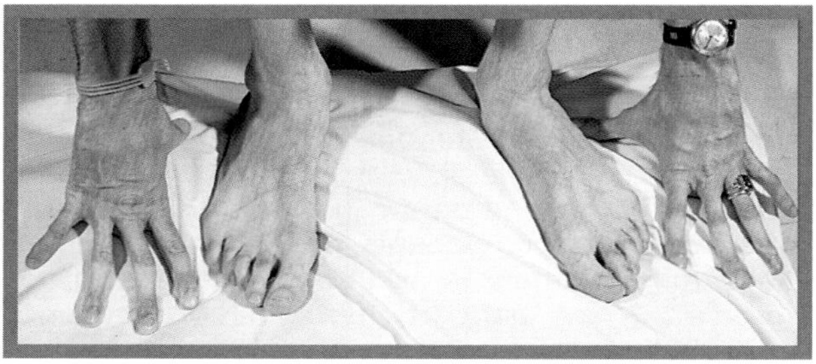

← Fig. 1.2
Marfan syndrome. Elongated fingers and toes in a patient with the syndrome.

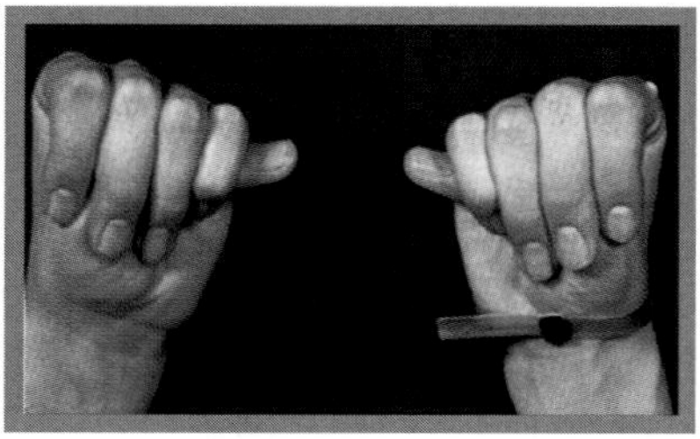

← Fig. 1.3
Marfan syndrome. 'Thumb sign' in a patient with the syndrome. The thumb protrudes beyond the ulnar border of the hand when the fingers are folded over it. (With permission from Falk, RH. *N Engl J Med* 1995, **333**:430.)

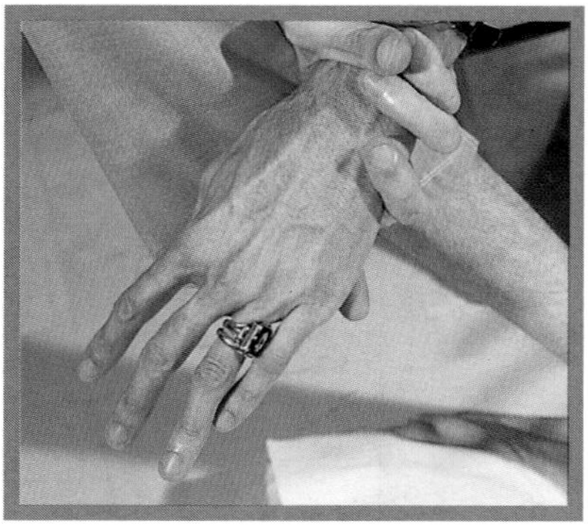

← Fig. 1.4
Marfan syndrome. Elongated fingers can more than encircle the wrist in a patient with the syndrome. The thumb and fifth finger overlap ('Walker–Murdoch wrist sign').

↓ Fig. 1.5
Marfan syndrome. Arachnodactyly or 'spider fingers' in a patient with the syndrome.

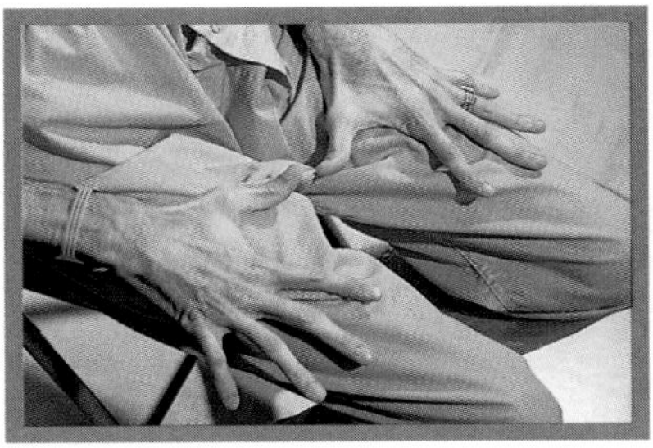

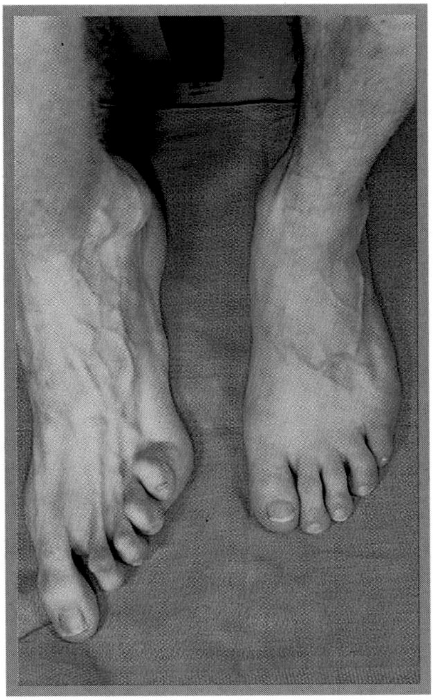

→ Fig. 1.6
Marfan syndrome. Elongated foot (left) in the syndrome, compared with a normal foot (right). Elongation of the great toe is a particular feature of the syndrome. The other toes are deformed.

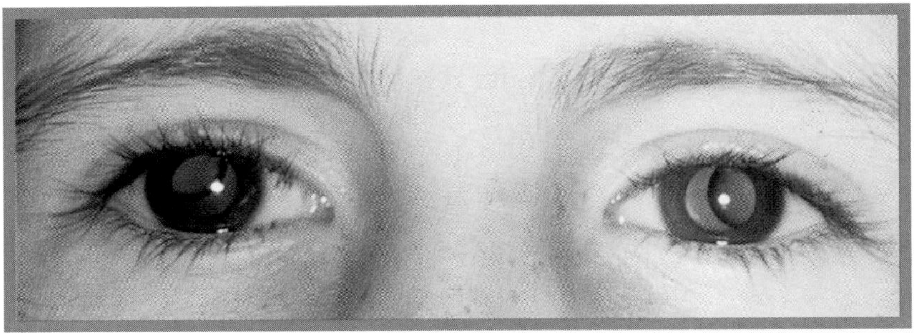

↑ Fig. 1.7
Marfan syndrome. Ectopia lentis associated with the syndrome. (With permission from Schlant RC, Alexander RW. *Hurst's the heart, arteries and veins, 8th ed.* McGraw–Hill, 1994.)

valve, with mitral or tricuspid insufficiency in a child or young adult, suggests that the diagnosis be considered (**Figs 1.9** and **1.10**). Mitral valve prolapse (**Fig. 1.11**) or calcified mitral annulus may occur. Dissecting aortic aneurysm (**Fig. 1.12**) or sinus of Valsalva aortic aneurysm (**Figs 1.13** and **1.14**), especially in a

Conditions associated with ectopia lentis
Marfan syndrome
Weill–Marchesani syndrome
Homocystinuria
Isolated autosomal recessive trait
Association with various ocular and systemic disorders
Trauma

↑ Fig. 1.8
Conditions associated with ectopia lentis.

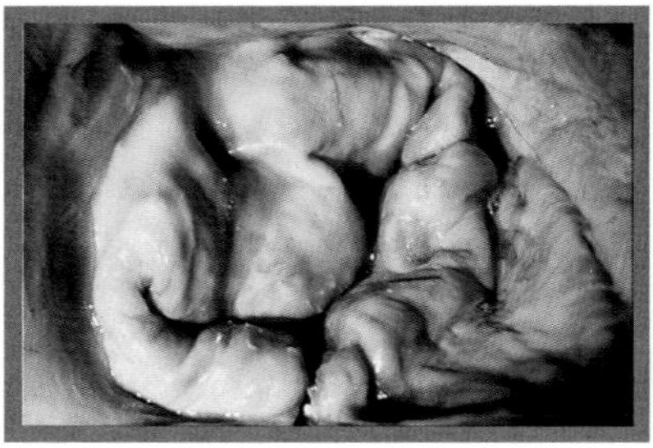

↑ Fig. 1.9
Marfan syndrome. Atrial view of a 'floppy' mitral valve with myxomatous degeneration. This valve abnormality is often seen in Marfan syndrome, and may lead to mitral prolapse and, at times, to severe mitral insufficiency.

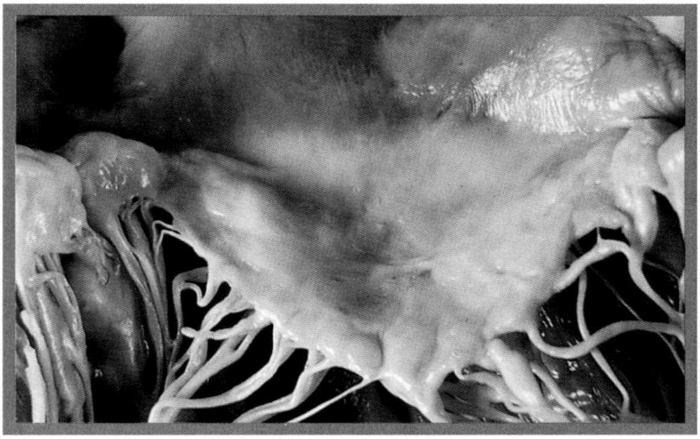

← Fig. 1.10
Marfan syndrome. A different view of a floppy mitral valve with myxomatous degeneration associated with the syndrome.

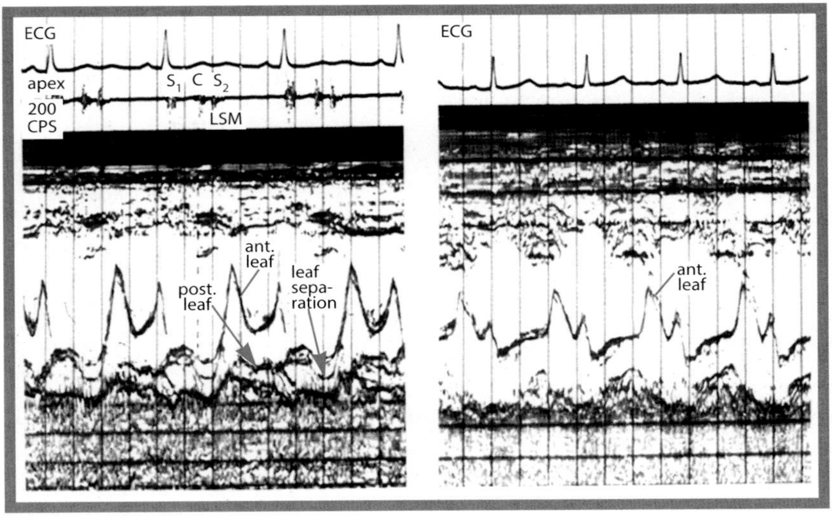

↑ Fig. 1.11
Marfan syndrome. M-Mode echocardiogram in a patient with mitral valve prolapse (sometimes called Barlow's syndrome). There is a late systolic separation of the posterior mitral leaflet from the anterior leaflet, giving rise to a late systolic click (C), followed by a late systolic murmur (LSM). S_1, first heart sound; S_2, second heart sound.

→ Fig. 1.12
Marfan syndrome. Dissecting aneurysm of the ascending aorta in a patient with the syndrome. The lower wooden probe lies in the entry intimal tear, and the upper probe lies in the exit tear The dissection extends from the entry tear along the ascending aorta to the exit tear and along the innominate artery.

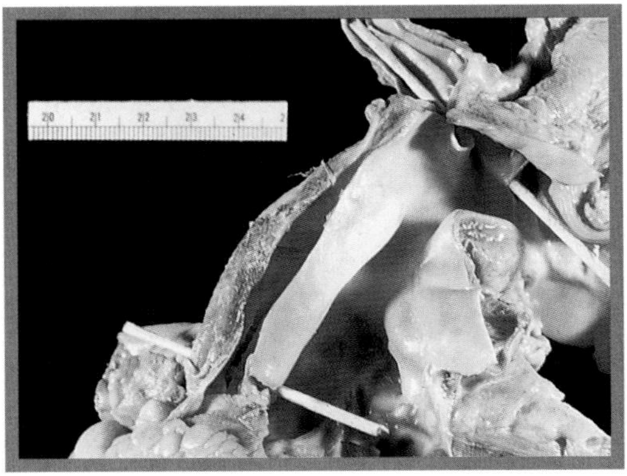

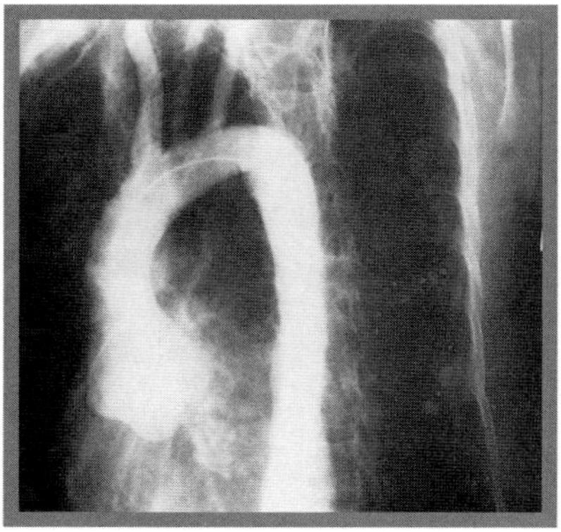

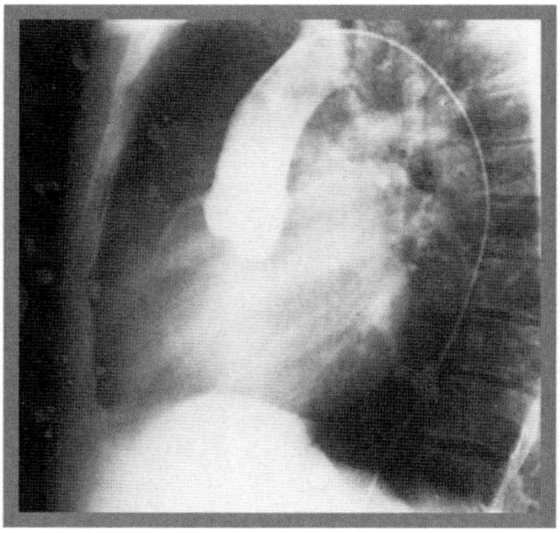

↑ Fig. 1.13a **↑ Fig. 1.13b**
Marfan syndrome. Aortogram showing (**a**) characteristic sinus of Valsalva aneurysm of the syndrome, compared with (**b**) the aortic root of normal size in a patient with mild rheumatic aortic insufficiency on the right.

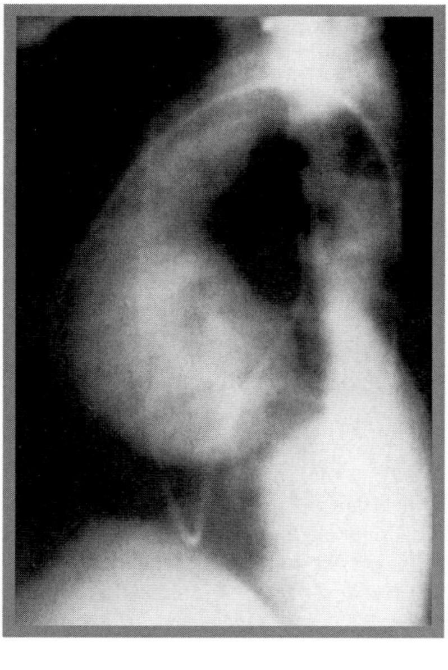

← Fig. 1.14
Lateral view of an aortogram showing an ascending aortic aneurysm in a patient with Marfan syndrome. As is typical, the sinuses of Valsalva are involved. (With permission from the American Heart Association. Silverman, ME. Marfan syndrome. *Heart disease and stroke* 1994, **3**:70.)

young adult, may be the first clinical evidence of the syndrome. Aortic root dilatation may be associated with aortic regurgitation (**Fig. 1.15**). Sixty to eighty percent of patients with Marfan syndrome show evidence of aortic root dilatation on echocardiography; the pathologic finding is that of aortic cystic medial necrosis. The presence of hyperextensible joints, such as genu recurvatum, suggests the possibility of Marfan syndrome (**Figs 1.16** and **1.17**),

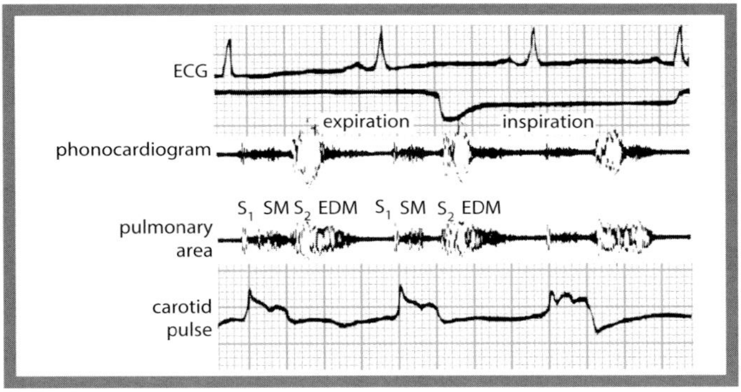

↑ Fig. 1.15
Marfan syndrome. Phonocardiogram of a murmur of aortic insufficiency in a patient with the syndrome. EDM, early diastolic murmur; SM, systolic murmur; S_1, first heart sound; S_2, second heart sound. (With permission from Fowler NO. *Diagnosis of heart disease*. Springer–Verlag, 1991.)

→ Fig. 1.16
Marfan syndrome. Genu recurvatum (hyperextensible knee) in a patient with Marfan syndrome.
(With permission Fowler NO. *Diagnosis of heart disease.* Springer–Verlag, 1991.)

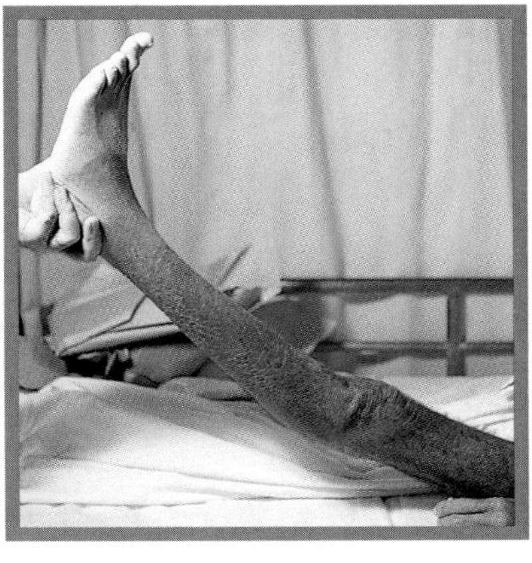

particularly if the joints can be easily dislocated (**Figs 1.18** and **1.19**); however, it should be remembered that joints may also be hypermobile in Ehlers–Danlos syndrome. The patient with Marfan syndrome may have sternal deformities

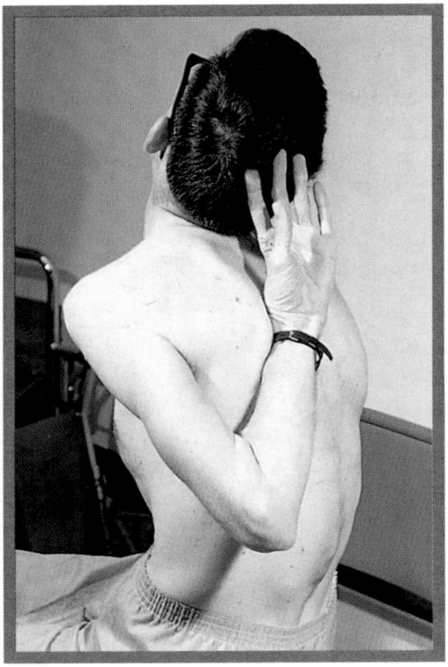

← Fig. 1.17
Marfan syndrome. Excessive mobility of the shoulder joint in a patient with the syndrome. Note arachnodactyly.

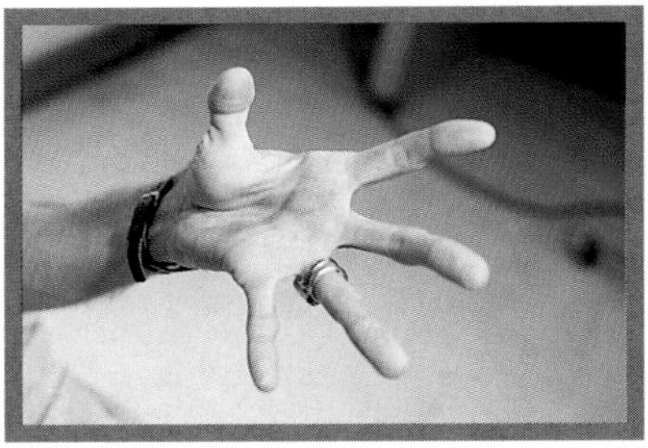

↑ Fig. 1.18
Marfan syndrome. Dislocatable thumb in a patient with the syndrome.

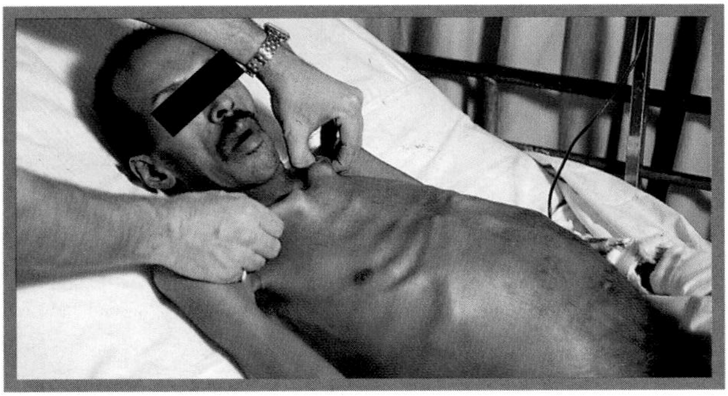

← Fig. 1.19
Marfan syndrome. Hypermobility of clavicles and sternal deformity in a patient with the syndrome. The clavicles are easily dislocated.

(**Fig. 1.20**) or kyphoscoliosis; high, arched palate (**Fig. 1.21**) and varicose veins (**Figs 1.22** and **1.23**) may also be seen. Features of Marfan syndrome may be found in asymptomatic close family members, who should be examined, because of the high penetrance of this autosomal dominant syndrome.

The clinical diagnosis of Marfan syndrome is likely when a patient has ectopia lentis, long, thin extremities, and hypermobile joints, especially if there

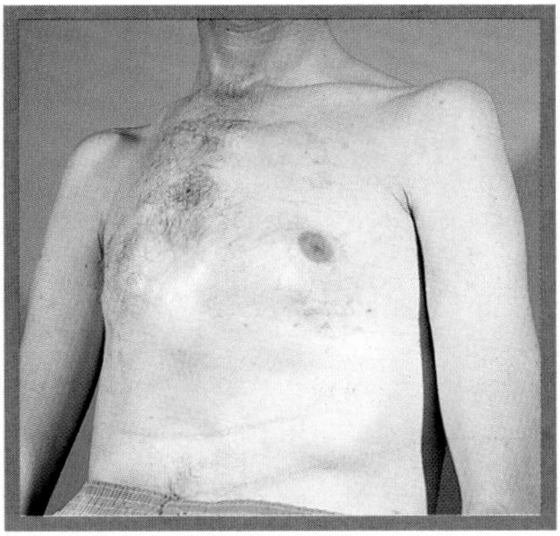

↑ Fig. 1.20
Marfan syndrome. Sternal deformity (pectus carinatum) in a patient with the syndrome.

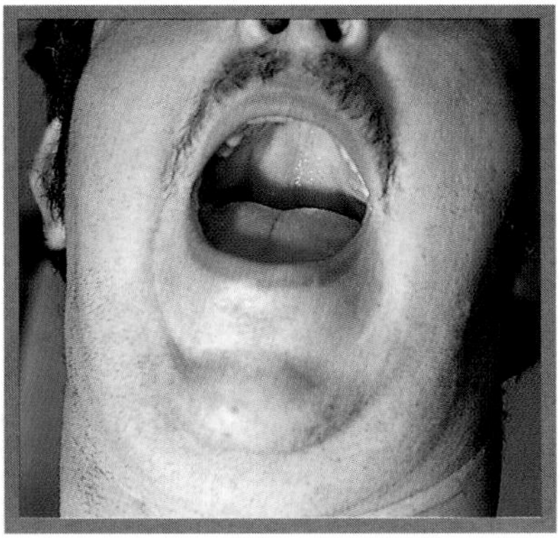

↑ Fig. 1.21
Marfan syndrome. High, arched palate in a patient with the syndrome.

→ Fig. 1.22
Marfan syndrome. Long fingers and varicose veins in a patient with the syndrome.

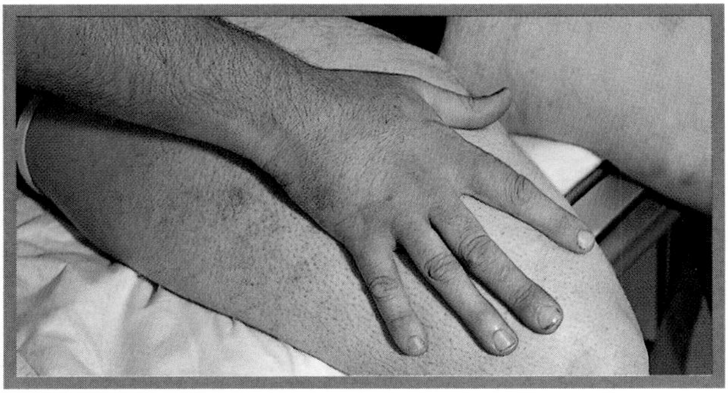

is aortic root disease and there is a positive family history of the disease. Patients with homocystinuria may have similar skeletal features but tend to have coronary and systemic venous occlusive disease; furthermore, the patient with homocystinuria may be impaired mentally, whereas the patient with Marfan syndrome is intellectually normal. Certain official criteria for the diagnosis of Marfan syndrome are recognized (**Figs 1.24** and **1.25**).

Patients with Marfan syndrome have a limited life expectancy and tend to die in youth or middle age, usually of cardiovascular complications. Close relatives of patients with the syndrome should be screened by physical examination and echocardiography; patients have often presented as young adults with acute aortic regurgitation or acute aortic dissecting aneurysm, and asymptomatic relatives of these patients have been found to have mitral prolapse or sinus of Valsalva aneurysm. Marfan syndrome is one of the leading causes of sudden death in young athletes. Eighty percent of deaths are caused by aortic rupture. In patients not treated by aortic replacement or repair,

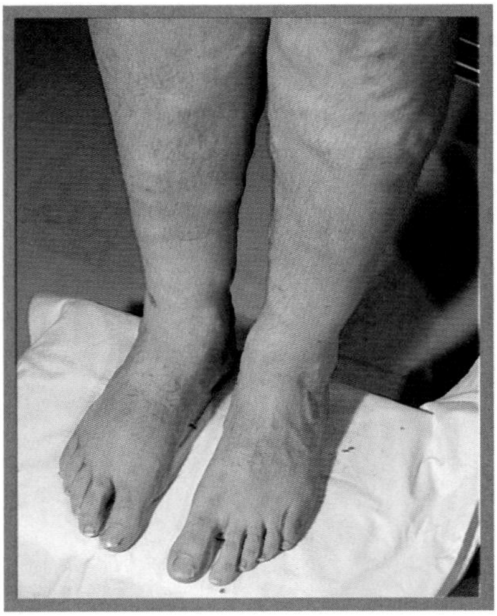

↑ Fig. 1.23
Marfan syndrome. Varicose veins and elongated great toe in a patient with the syndrome.

Systems involved in Marfan syndrome

Skeletal: anterior chest deformity, scoliosis, tall stature, arachnodactyly, dolichostenomelia

Ocular: ectopia lentis, flat cornea, myopia, retinal detachment

Cardiovascular: aortic dissection, aortic regurgitation, mitral prolapse

Pulmonary: apical bleb, spontaneous pneumothorax

Skin and integument: hernia

Central nervous system: dural ectasia, hyperactivity

↑ Fig. 1.24
Systems involved in the Marfan syndrome.

→ Fig.1.25 International criteria for Marfan syndrome.

International criteria for Marfan syndrome
Major Manifestations
Ectopia lentis Dilated ascending aorta Aortic dissection Dural ectasia
Diagnosis
Without affected first degree relative: skeletal involvement and two other systems, one major (skeletal: pectus excavatum/carinatum, arachnodactyly, scoliosis, tall stature, high arched palate, hypermobile joints) With affected first degree relative: systems involved; prefer one major; absence of homocystinuria

median survival in one study was 46.6 years. Prophylactic β-adrenergic blockade may be effective in slowing the rate of aortic dilatation and reducing the rate of development of aortic complications; replacement of the dilated ascending aorta may delay complications and prolong life.

Further reading

Beighton P, de Paepe D, Danks G, *et al.* International nosology of heritable disorders of connective tissue. Berlin 1986. *Am J Med Genet* 1988, **29**:581–594.

Finkbohner R, Johnston D, Crawford ES, Coselli J, Milewicz DM. Marfan syndrome. Long-term survival and complications after aortic aneurysm repair. *Circulation* 1995, **91**:728–733.

Godfrey M. The Marfan syndrome. In: Beighton P, ed. *McKusick's heritable disorders of connective tissue, 5th ed.* St Louis: Mosby Yearbook Inc.; 1993:51–135.

Roman MJ, Rosen SE, Kramer-Fox R, Devereux RB. Prognostic significance of the pattern of aortic root dilation in the Marfan syndrome. *J Am Coll Cardiol* 1993, **22**:1470–1476.

Shores J, Berger KR, Murphy EA, Pyeritz RE. Progression of aortic dilatation and the benefit of long-term β-adrenergic blockade in Marfan syndrome. *N Engl J Med* 1994, **330**:1335–1341.

Noonan's Syndrome

Noonan's syndrome was described by Dr Jacqueline Noonan in 1963. This autosomal dominant condition has also been called male Turner's syndrome because it shares some phenotypic features in common with Turner's syndrome. These include hypertelorism, cubitus valgus, a broad, shield-like chest with increased space between the nipples, diminished stature, webbed neck and cryptorchidism with impaired sexual development (**Figs 1.26** and **1.27**). However, Turner's syndrome is limited to females, who usually have an abnormal XO sex chromosomal pattern, whereas Noonan's syndrome may occur in either sex, and the sex chromosome pattern is normal. Unlike Turner's syndrome, the prevalence of aortic coarctation is not increased in Noonan's syndrome. Pulmonic valve stenosis or dysplasia and atrial septal defect (ASD) are commonly found. Pulmonary valve insufficiency or cardiomyopathy may occur; the latter may be either obstructive or non-obstructive. Lymphedema is common. Several other cardiac anomalies are associated with the syndrome (**Fig. 1.28**). The responsible gene has not been mapped.

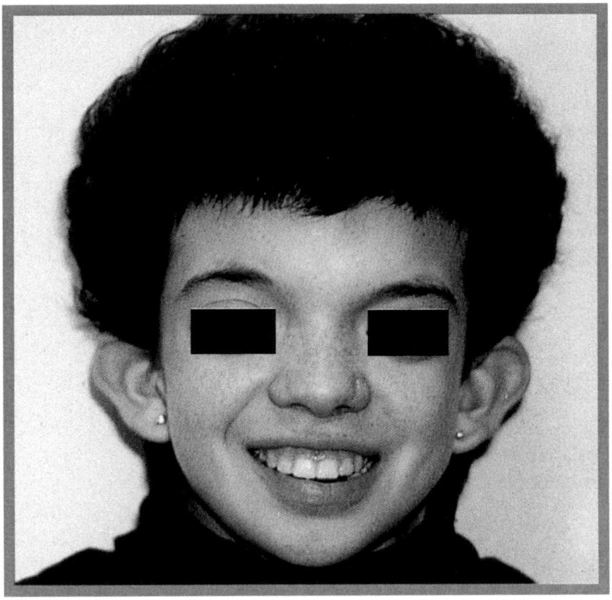

← Fig. 1.26 Noonan's syndrome. Low-set ears and hypertelorism in a patient with the syndrome.

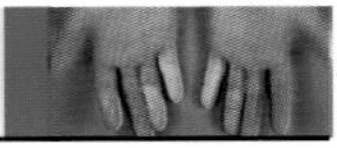

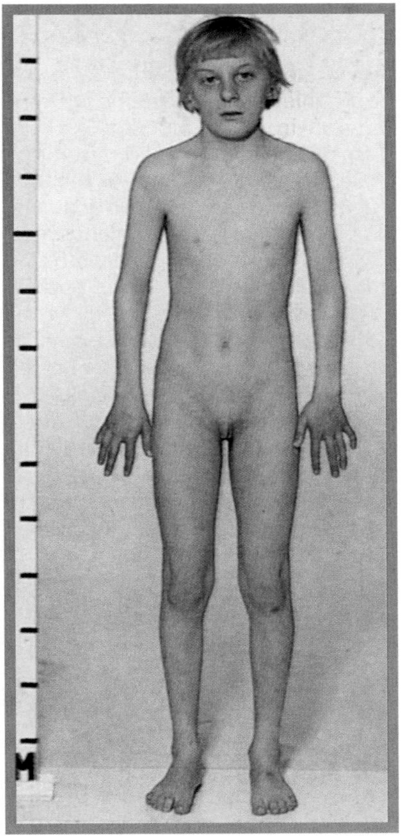

← Fig. 1.27
Noonan's syndrome. Webbing of the neck and widely spaced nipples. Somatic features similar to those of Turner's syndrome. (With permission from Hall R, Evered DC. *A colour atlas of endocrinology*. Wolfe, 1990.)

Characteristics of Noonan's syndrome

Short stature, web neck, cubitus valgus, congenital cardiac defects, mental deficiency, hypertelorism

Occurs in both sexes, normal karyotype

Autosomal dominant, gene not mapped

Pulmonary stenosis common, atrial septal defect in 33%

Other cardiovascular associations: ventricular septal defect, hypertrophic cardiomyopathy, pulmonary branch stenosis, coronary artery anomalies

Also common: testicular anomalies, mental deficiency, sternal deformity

↑ Fig. 1.28
Characteristics of Noonan's syndrome.

Further reading

Noonan JA, Ehmke DA. Associated noncardiac malformations in children with congenital heart disease. *J Pediatr* 1963, **63**:468–470.

Van der Hauwert LG, Fryns JP, Dumoulin M, Logghe N. Cardiovascular malformations in Turner's and Noonan's syndrome. *Br Heart J* 1978, **40**:500–509.

Wong CK, Cheng CH, Lau CP, Leung WH. Congenital coronary artery anomalies in Noonan's syndrome. *Am Heart J* 1990, **119**:396–400.

Turner's Syndrome

Turner's syndrome (**Fig. 1.29)** is a sex chromosome abnormality of females. Typically, there is a 45XO karyotype, but more than 50% of patients with the syndrome have a mosaic chromosomal complement—e.g., 45X/46XX. The frequency in live-born female infants is 1 in 1500–2500. It is estimated that there are approximately 50,000–75,000 females with this syndrome in the USA.

The history is that of impaired growth and failure to menstruate. The ovaries are poorly developed (streak gonads) and only 2–5% of patients menstruate; women with Turner's syndrome are usually sterile. Osteoporosis develops in women who do not receive estrogen therapy. Otitis media, scoliosis, and hip dislocation are common. Renal anomalies, including obstruction at the ureteropelvic junction with hydronephrosis, may occur. Patients should be monitored for hypothyroidism, which may develop in as many as 50% of cases. With aging, there may be progressive deafness.

The general physical findings are characteristic. The stature is diminished; the posterior hairline is low, and the neck is webbed (**Figs 1.30** and **1.31**). The mandible is small, and the pinna may be deformed. The chest is broad and shield-like, with widely spaced nipples. Lymphedema both of hands and of feet is a common finding (**Fig. 1.32**), and the nails are often hypoplastic. Inguinal hernia is common. Mental development is normal.

Turner's syndrome

XO chromosomal pattern–streak gonads

Webbed neck, shield chest, low hairline, diminished stature, amenorrhea

Cardiovascular defects in 35–50%: coarctation of the aorta, aortic dilatation, lymphedema, renal anomalies, hypertrophic cardiomyopathy, ventricular septal defect, dextrocardia, hypertension

← Fig. 1.29
Turner's syndrome.

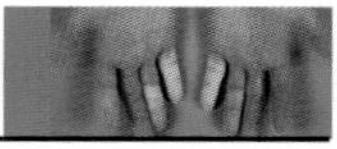

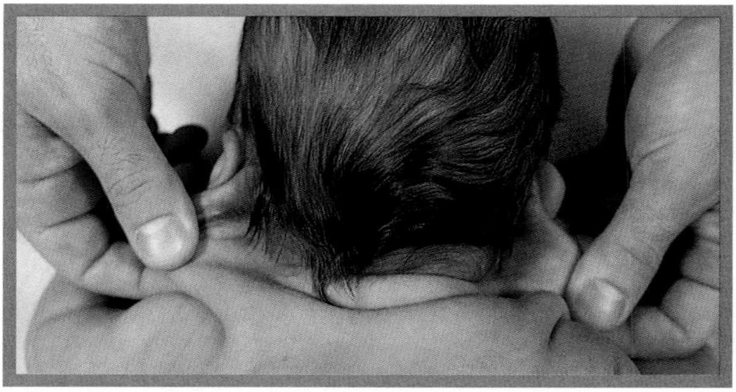

→ Fig. 1.30 Turner's syndrome. Webbed neck (rear view) in an infant with the syndrome.

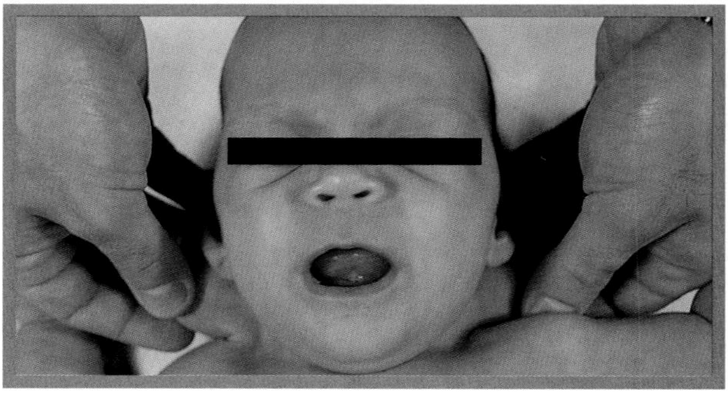

→ Fig. 1.31 Turner's syndrome. Webbed neck (front view) in an infant with the syndrome.

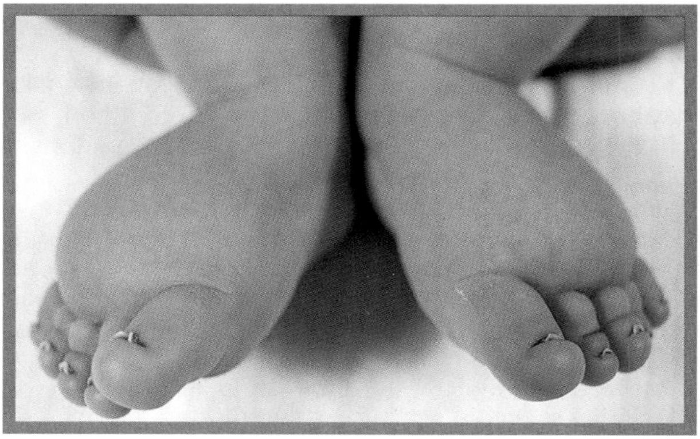

→ Fig. 1.32 Turner's syndrome. Lymphedema of feet in an infant with the syndrome.

The characteristic major cardiovascular finding is that of coarctation of the aorta, which occurs in about 20% of patients with Turner's syndrome. A bicuspid aortic valve is found in approximately 50% of patients, and aortic dilatation may develop; there is an increased risk of aortic dissection. Idiopathic hypertension is a common finding, and hypertrophic obstructive cardiomyopathy may develop. Ventricular septal defect (VSD), ASD, and aortic stenosis have been described. Partial anomalous pulmonary venous drainage without ASD is common.

The mean life expectancy is reduced in Turner's syndrome; the average age at death was 69 years in a Scandinavian study. About 50% of these patients died of cardiovascular disease and 20% of malignant disease.

Further reading

Allen DB, Hendricks SA, Levy JM. Aortic dilation in Turner syndrome. *J Pediatr* 1986, **109**:302–305.

Saenger P. Turner's syndrome. *N Engl J Med* 1996, **335**:1749–1754.

Hyperthyroidism

Hyperthyroidism, or thyrotoxicosis, may be associated with a diffuse goiter or single or multiple nodules. When associated with a diffuse goiter, it is also called Graves' disease. The disease is four to eight times more common in women than in men, and its peak incidence is in the 20–40-year age group.

The patient's history is typically that of weight loss despite good appetite, with skeletal muscular weakness, and increased frequency of bowel move-ments. Fatigue and exertional dyspnea are common, and heat intolerance may be present. Angina pectoris may occur in the absence of fixed epicardial coronary artery disease. General physical findings include exophthalmos, stare (**Fig. 1.33**), lid lag, goiter (**Fig. 1.34**), warm, moist, pink (salmon color) skin, tremor of the tongue and fingers, and occasional splenomegaly. Onycholysis (see Chapter 6) is a somewhat uncommon finding. In older patients, goiter and exophthalmos may be absent, and atrial fibrillation is more common.

Hyperthyroidism has autonomic, cardiac, and peripheral vascular effects. The velocities of myocardial systolic contraction and diastolic relaxation are increased. There is an increase in the number and affinity of myocardial β-adrenergic receptors. The echocardiogram shows an increase in the percentage of left ventricular systolic shortening, without an increase in end-diastolic dimension. Myocardial contractility is increased, as are left ventricular ejection fraction and cardiac index. There is peripheral vasodilatation, with decreased systemic vascular resistance. Total body oxygen consumption is increased.

The cardiovascular findings are reflective of the associated hyperdynamic state (**Figs 1.35** and **1.36**). There is often a cervical venous hum, which is the

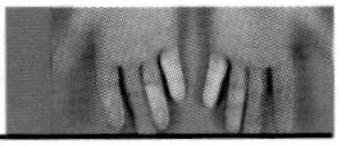

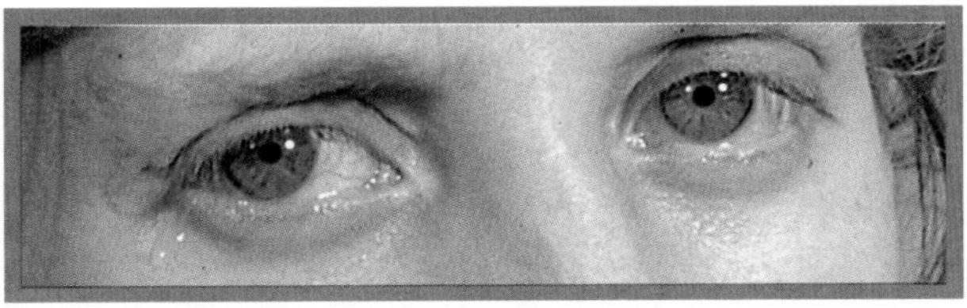

← Fig. 1.33
Hyperthyroidism. Stare without exophthalmos in a 28-year-old hyperthyroid woman.

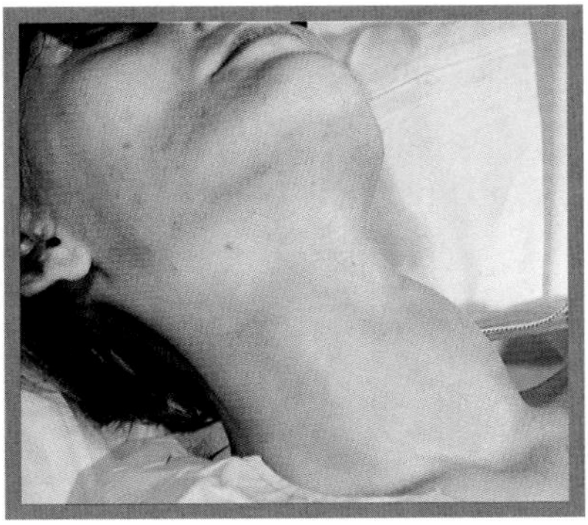

← Fig. 1.34
Hyperthyroidism. Goiter in the same patient as in Figure 1.33.

Physical signs of hyperdynamic states
Tachycardia
Increased arterial pulse pressure
Pulmonary systolic ejection murmur
S_3, S_4 heart sound gallops
Supraclavicular bruit
Cervical venous hum
Arterial pistol-shot sounds
Duroziez's murmur

↑ Fig. 1.35
Physical signs of hyperdynamic states.

Physical signs of hyperthyroidism
Unexplained sinus tachycardia (40% >100 beats/min)
Paroxysmal or sustained atrial fibrillation in 15%
Increased arterial systolic pressure
Eye signs, goiter, pink skin, tremor, onycholysis
Loud S_1; occasional S_3, S_4 gallops
Means–Lerman scratch
Cervical venous hum—'bruit de diable'
Occasional congestive heart failure without evidence of heart disease

↑ Fig. 1.36
Physical signs of hyperthyroidism.

usual reason for the 'bruit de diable' heard over the thyroid gland in thyrotoxicosis (**Fig. 1.37**). This murmur is common in normal children but in recumbent adults is very suggestive of a high cardiac output state such as hyperthyroidism. There is often sinus tachycardia: heart rates are usually 90–120 beats/min. Approximately 15–25% of patients have atrial fibrillation. The systemic arterial pulse pressure is increased; systolic pressure is increased, and diastolic pressure is decreased. The arterial pulse is somewhat bounding. The first heart sound (S_1) is increased in intensity and a third heart sound (S_3) is common; mitral stenosis may be suggested for that reason. Uncommonly, congestive heart failure may develop in the absence of underlying heart disease (**Fig. 1.38**). Congestive heart failure is more common in older patients, but may occur in children and teenagers.

Hemodynamic studies reveal an increased cardiac output, with increased cardiac rate and stroke volume (**Fig. 1.39**). The arteriovenous oxygen difference

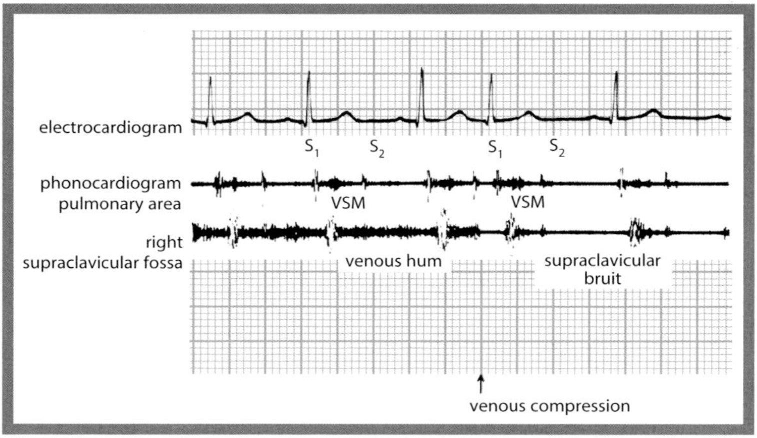

↑ Fig. 1.37
Hyperthyroidism. Phonocardiogram of cervical venous hum in an anemic 7-year-old child. This continuous murmur was easily obliterated by internal jugular venous compression, leaving an arterial supraclavicular bruit. S_1, first heart sound; S_2, second heart sound; VSM, innocent vibratory systolic murmur. All of these auscultatory findings are common in children and in hyperdynamic states such as hyperthyroidism or anemia. (With permission from Fowler NO. *Diagnosis of heart disease*. Springer–Verlag, 1991.)

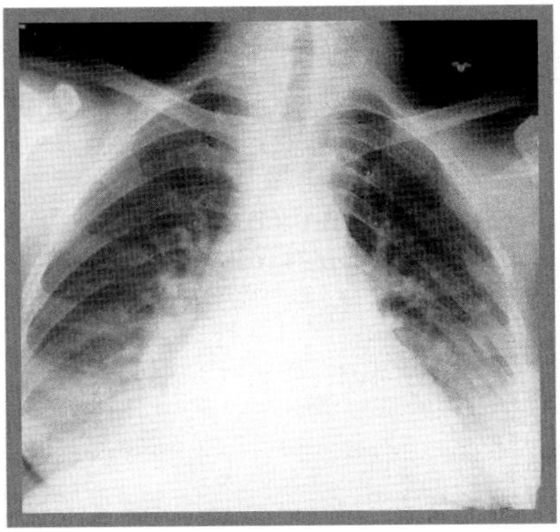

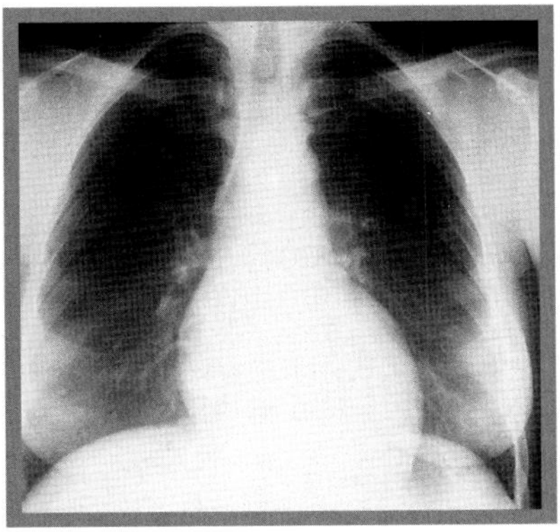

↑ Fig. 1.38a **↑ Fig. 1.38b**

Hyperthyroidism. Chest radiographs of a 17-year-old woman with hyperthyroidism, atrial fibrillation, and congestive heart failure, taken (**a**) during congestive failure, and (**b**) 11 days later, after heart failure had responded to treatment with digitalis, diuretics, and iodides. There was no evidence of underlying heart disease.

→ Fig. 1.39
Hemodynamics of hyperthyroidism.

Hemodynamics of hyperthyroidism

Cardiac index usually 5–7 liters/min/m^2

Increased total oxygen consumption of 25–75%

Usually, increased pulmonary artery blood oxygen saturation, with narrow arteriovenous oxygen difference

Usually, increased cardiac stroke volume

Decreased systemic vascular resistance; correction does not normalize hemodynamics

Increased left ventricular end-diastolic volume on echocardiogram (variable)

Normal resting ejection fraction; may fail to increase normally with exercise

Increased isovolumic systolic contraction velocity

is decreased, and the total body oxygen consumption is increased. In one patient whom we studied, the cardiac index was 8.1 liters/min/m^2 (normal value 3.1±0.4 liters/min/m^2), the systemic arteriovenous oxygen difference was 2.0ml/100ml (normal value 4.5±0.7ml/100ml), and the cardiac stroke volume was 139ml (normal value 84±17ml).

The diagnosis of thyrotoxicosis is confirmed by demonstrating increased serum tri-iodothyronine (T_3) and thyroxine (T_4) concentrations, with a decrease in serum thyroid-stimulating hormone (TSH) values. Increased free T_4 concentrations are more specific as total T_4 may be increased in non-hyperthyroid states as a result of an increase in thyroid-binding globulin. A few patients exhibit an increase in T_3 concentrations only.

Further reading

Klein I. Thyroid hormone and the cardiovascular system. *Am J Med* 1990, **88**:631–637.

Levey GS. Thyroid and the heart. *Am J Med* 1990, **88**:625.

Olshausen K, Bischoff S, Kahaly G, *et al*. Cardiac arrhythmias and heart rate in hyperthyroidism. *Am J Cardiol* 1989, **63**:930–933.

Skelton CL. The heart and hyperthyroidism. *N Engl J Med* 1982, **307**:1206–1208.

Down Syndrome

Down syndrome (**Fig. 1.40**), once known as mongolism, is usually associated with trisomy of chromosome 21. Three percent of patients have translocation of a part of chromosome 21 to another chromosome; the syndrome tends to be milder in this group. The phenotype occurs in about 1 in 600 live births. The risk of having a baby with this syndrome is lowest in young mothers and increases sharply after the age of 35 years, reaching 4% for women older than 45 years.

The physical findings are characteristic (**Figs 1.41** and **1.42**). There is an epicanthal fold; the tongue is often enlarged. The pinna is often small and low-set. The mandible is often hypoplastic. The palms show a single simian crease. The joints are hypermobile and easily dislocated. The stature is decreased. Mental development is impaired to variable degrees.

Life expectancy is impaired for several reasons. About 40% of patients have congenital heart disease. There is an increased prevalence of hematologic malignant disease and, after the fifth decade, a high prevalence of progressive dementia of the Alzheimer type.

Cardiovascular defects are found in approximately 40–50% of patients with Down syndrome (**Fig. 1.43**). The characteristic lesion is an endocardial cushion defect, resulting in either an ostium primum ASD or a common atrioventricular (A–V) canal (**Figs 1.44** and **1.45**); patients with Down syndrome are more likely to develop pulmonary hypertension than other patients with this defect.

→ Fig. 1.40
Down syndrome.

Down syndrome

One in 600 live births (4% in mothers >45 years)

Physical findings: epicanthal fold, simian crease, large tongue, short stature, mental deficiency, hypotonia, low-set ears, small mandible, Brushfield spots of iris

40–50% have congenital heart disease; also prone to duodenal atresia, hematologic malignancies

May survive into the fifth decade and later; Alzheimer's type mental deterioration may occur

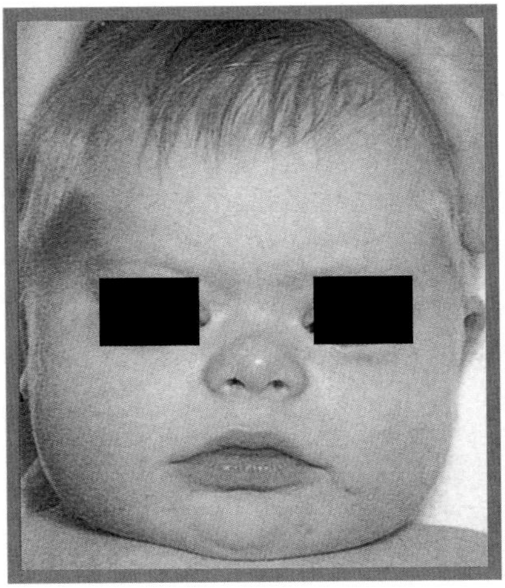

↑ Fig. 1.41
Down syndrome. Characteristic facial appearance of Down syndrome in an infant.

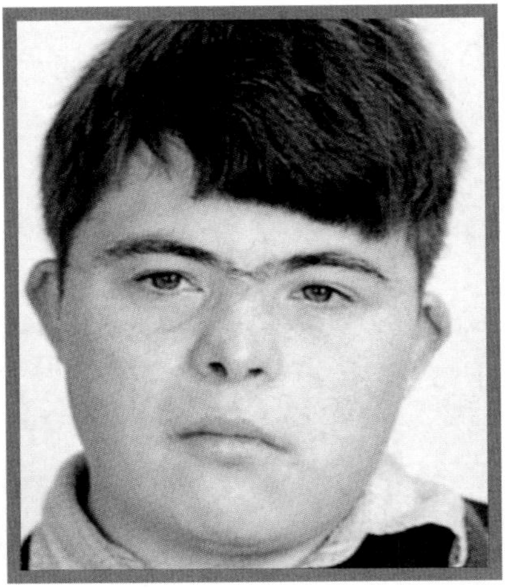

↑ Fig. 1.42
Down syndrome. Characteristic epicanthal fold and lips of Down syndrome in an adult. (With permission from Baraitser M, Winter RM. *Color atlas of congenital malformation syndromes.* Mosby–Wolfe, 1996.)

Cardiovascular defects associated with Down syndrome
Endocardial cushion defects—pulmonary hypertension more common in those with complete atrioventricular canal
Ventricular septal defect
Ostium secundum atrial septal defect
Tetralogy of Fallot
Mitral valve prolapse in 20%
Aortic and pulmonary valve fenestration
Eisenmenger's syndrome
Truncus arteriosus
Aortic coarctation

← Fig. 1.43
Cardiovascular defects associated with Down syndrome.

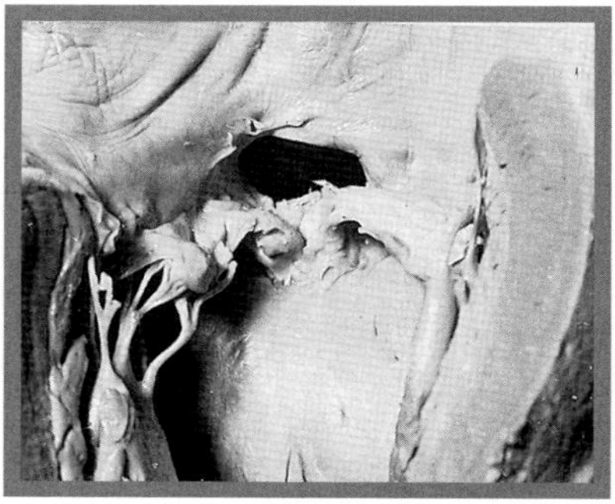

↑ Fig. 1.44
Down syndrome. Heart specimen of a patient with Down syndrome, showing ostium primum ASD just superior to the mitral valve. Note cleft in the mitral valve.

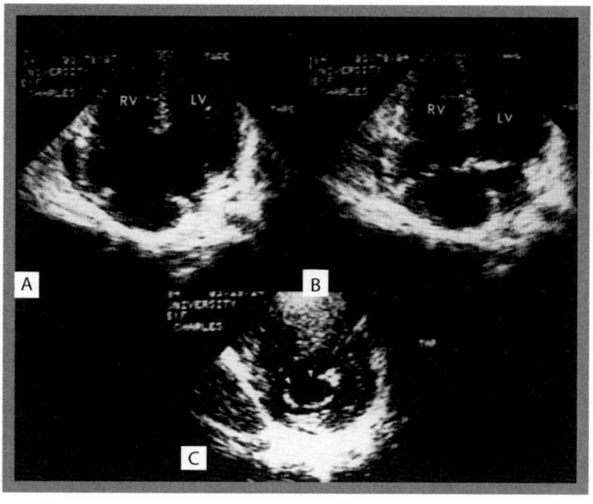

← Fig. 1.45a
Down syndrome. Echocardiogram of a patient with Down syndrome with common A–V canal. This is the characteristic cardiac lesion of this syndrome. (See Fig. 1.45b for diagram.)

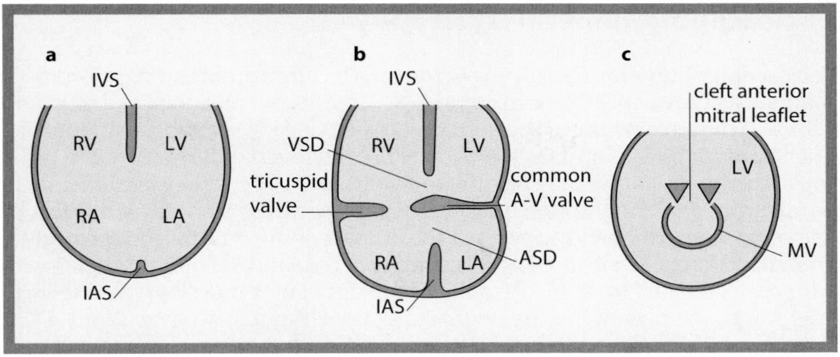

↑ Fig. 1.45b
(**a**) Apical four-chamber view of common A–V canal, showing a defect in lower interatrial septum (IAS) and upper interventricular septum (IVS). LV, left ventricle; RV, right ventricle. (**b**) Apical four-chamber view of common A–V canal, showing enlarged right ventricle and right atrium. There is a large atrial septal defect (ASD) of the ostium primum type in addition to a large interventricular septal defect (VSD). There is a common A–V valve. (**c**) Apical short-axis view of the left ventricle. The two arrowheads indicate a cleft in the anterior mitral leaflet, which is often found in association with ostium primum ASD or common A–V canal. MV, mitral valve.

However, a variety of other defects may be present (see Fig. 1.43), including VSD, patent ductus arteriosus, and tetralogy of Fallot.

In a study of institutionalized adults with Down syndrome, Goldhaber *et al.* found evidence of heart disease in 38 of 131 individuals. Thirty-seven had echocardiograms, eleven had evidence of ASD or VSD, eighteen had mitral valve prolapse, and eight had aortic regurgitation.

Reference

Goldhaber SZ, Rubin IL, Brown W, *et al.* Valvular heart disease (aortic regurgitation and mitral valve prolapse) among institutionalized adults with Down's syndrome. *Am J Cardiol* 1986, **57**:278–281.

Further reading

Clapp S, Perry BL, Farooki ZQ, *et al.* Down's syndrome, complete atrioventricular canal, and pulmonary vascular obstructive disease. *J Thorac Cardiovasc Surg* 1990, **100**:115–121.

Facioscapulohumeral Dystrophy

Facioscapulohumeral dystrophy is transmitted in an autosomal dominant manner. Its prevalence is approximately 3–10 cases per million population and clinical symptoms usually appear in the late first or early second decades of life. The shoulder girdle muscles are usually first involved, followed by the facial muscles; the hip girdle may be affected years later. There may be difficulty in whistling or drinking through a straw. The face becomes smooth, with a loss of its normal lines, dimpling appears at the corners of the mouth, and the normal lines of the forehead are lost. There is atrophy of the shoulder girdle muscles, with winged scapulae (**Fig. 1.46**). Atrophy of the upper arm muscles is also seen; in later stages the patient may be unable to sit up without assistance (**Fig. 1.47**).

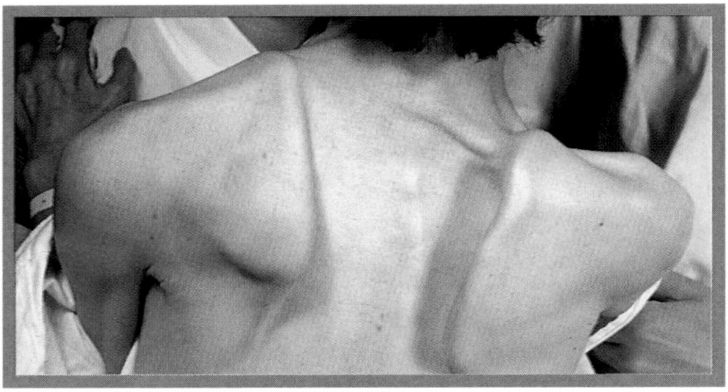

← Fig. 1.46 Facioscapulohumeral muscular dystrophy. Note pronounced winging of the scapulae.

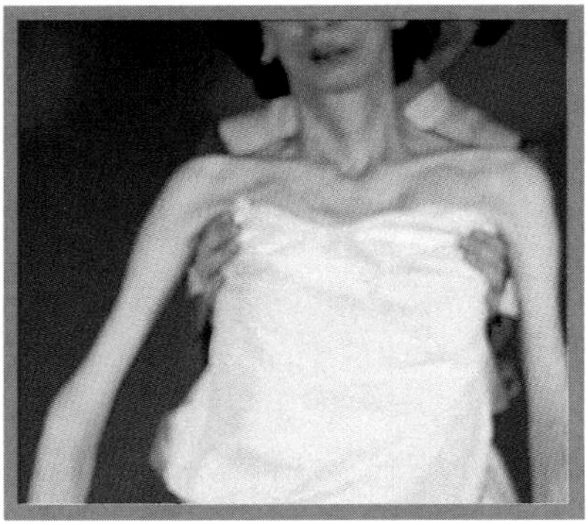

← Fig. 1.47 Facioscapulohumeral muscular dystrophy. This patient needed assistance to sit up. Note atrophy of upper arm muscles.

Stevenson *et al.* undertook a cardiographic study of 30 patients with facioscapulohumeral muscular dystrophy (13 female and 17 male) who were aged 10–78 years. The surface electrocardiogram (ECG) showed broad, bifid P waves, and electrophysiology revealed abnormal sinus node function in 10% of the group. Atrial flutter or fibrillation was easily induced. Two patients had right bundle branch block and one had left anterior fascicular block.

Facioscapulohumeral muscular dystrophy must be distinguished from Emery–Dreifuss dystrophy, in which atrial paralysis has been described. In the latter disease, one is more likely to find elbow contractures, absence of winged scapulae, and X-linked heredity. Facioscapulohumeral muscular dystrophy occurs in either sex.

Reference

Stevenson WG, Perloff JK, Weiss JN, Anderson TL. Facioscapulohumeral muscular dystrophy. Evidence for selective, genetic electrophysiologic cardiac involvement. *J Am Coll Cardiol* 1990, **15**:292–299.

Friedreich's Ataxia

Friedreich's ataxia is inherited as an autosomal recessive trait and is not genetically homogeneous. However, an associated genetic defect of chromosome 9 has been described. Its prevalence in European populations is 1 in 50,000. Friedreich's ataxia is primarily a neurologic disease affecting the cerebellum and spinal cord. There is degeneration of the spinocerebellar tracts, the pyramidal tracts, and the dorsal columns. Symptoms usually begin before the age of 20 years. There is pronounced ataxia of all four limbs and the patient may have difficulty in sitting up without support (**Fig. 1.48**). There is a loss of proprioception, deep tendon reflexes are absent, and a Babinski reflex is found (**Fig. 1.49**). Horizontal nystagmus is common. Kyphoscoliosis (**Fig. 1.50**), dysarthria, and pes cavus (**Fig. 1.51**) develop as the disease progresses, which it does inexorably and without remission. Atrophy of the lower extremities may occur (**Fig. 1.52**). There is an increased tendency to glucose intolerance. Mental retardation is uncommon.

The primary criteria for the diagnosis are gait ataxia, dysarthria, absence of deep tendon reflexes, and weakness of the lower extremities, with impaired vibration and position sense. Secondary criteria include pes cavus, Babinski reflex, and kyphoscoliosis. Cardiac involvement occurs in as many as 95% of patients studied by electrocardiography and echocardiography (**Fig. 1.53**). Electrocardiographic abnormalities were found in 92% of 75 patients studied by Child *et al.* These included S–T segment and T-wave abnormalities in 79%, right axis deviation in 40%, short PR interval in 24%, inferolateral Q waves in 14%, and left ventricular hypertrophy in 16%. Although the cardiac

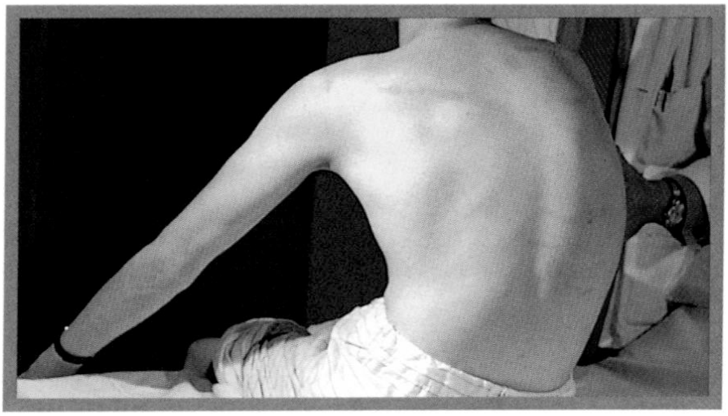

← Fig. 1.48
Friedreich's ataxia. The patient needed some assistance in sitting. Note scoliosis.

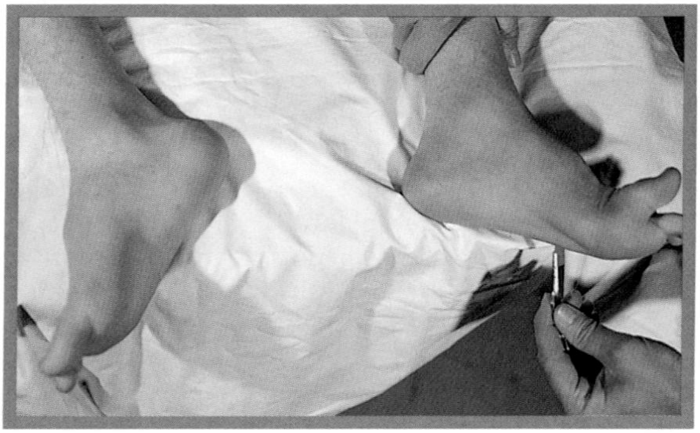

← Fig. 1.49
Friedreich's ataxia. Pes cavus and extensor plantar reflex (Babinski reflex) in a patient with Friedreich's ataxia. (With permission from Fowler NO. *Diagnosis of heart disease*. Springer–Verlag, 1991.)

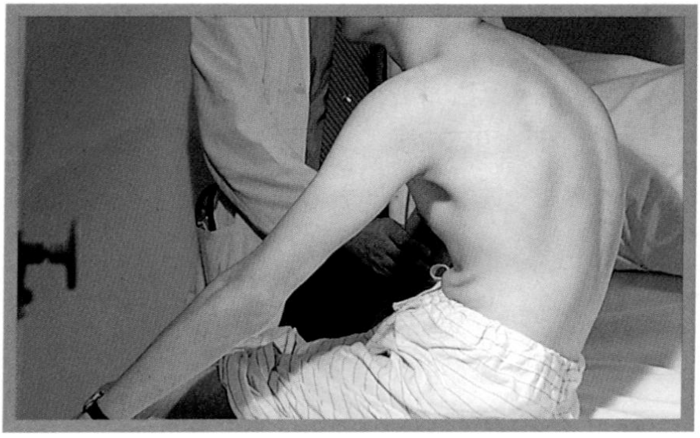

← Fig. 1.50
Friedreich's ataxia. Kyphoscoliosis in Friedreich's ataxia.

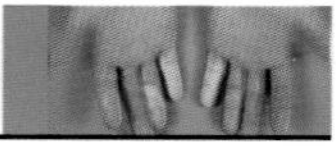

→ Fig. 1.51
Friedreich's ataxia. Pes cavus in Friedreich's ataxia.

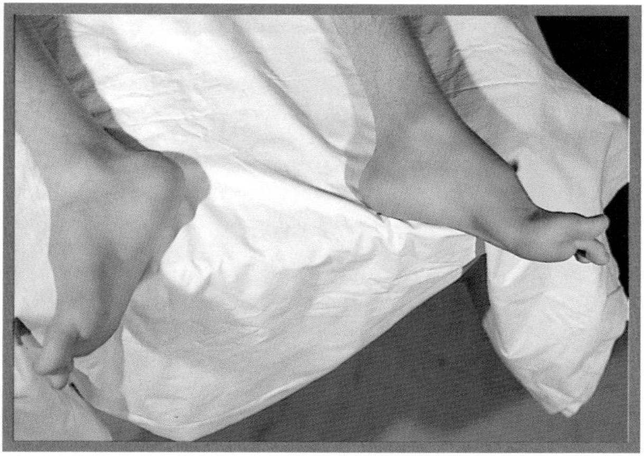

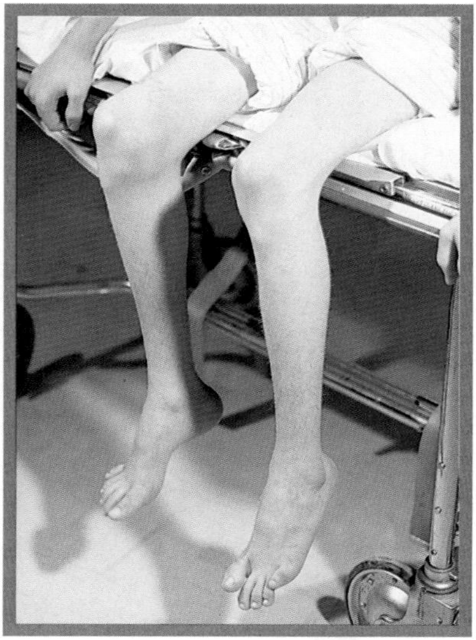

↑ Fig. 1.52
Friedreich's ataxia. Atrophy of calf muscles in Friedreich's ataxia.

Friedreich's ataxia

Autosomal recessive

Not genetically homogeneous

Neurologic: ataxia (cerebellar); absent tendon reflexes; positive Babinski sign

Musculoskeletal: scoliosis; pes cavus; muscular weakness

95% have ECG or echocardiographic abnormalities

May have cardiomyopathy, small-vessel coronary disease, cardiac cause of death

↑ Fig. 1.53
Friedreich's ataxia.

involvement is usually asymptomatic, it is often the cause of death. Congestive heart failure is unusual, except terminally.

Cardiomyopathy was found by echocardiography in 63 of 75 patients studied by Dürr *et al*. Hypertrophic cardiomyopathy is perhaps the most common echocardiographic finding. This is not always associated with asymmetric septal hypertrophy and seldom causes left ventricular outflow tract obstruction. Septal cellular disarray, characteristic of genetic hypertrophic cardiomyopathy, is not found. Dilated cardiomyopathy also is found in patients with Friedreich's ataxia but less commonly than hypertrophic cardiomyopathy (**Fig. 1.54**). Patients with dilated cardiomyopathy are prone to have atrial flutter, atrial fibrillation, and ventricular arrhythmias.

Disease of the small intramural coronary arteries has been described in Friedreich's ataxia but is not believed to be responsible for the dilated cardiomyopathy; histologic study usually demonstrates myocyte hypertrophy and interstitial fibrosis. Focal degeneration of muscle fibers is found.

Life expectancy is greatly reduced; the majority of patients with Friedreich's ataxia die between the ages of 26 and 36 years.

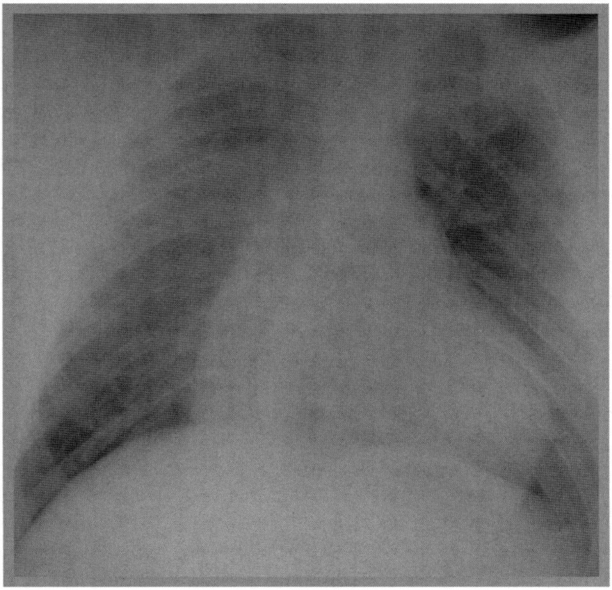

← Fig. 1.54 Friedreich's ataxia. Chest radiogram of patient with Friedreich's ataxia. Note the enlarged heart and dorsal scoliosis. This is the patient also pictured in Figs 1.48–1.52.

References

Child JS, Perloff JK, Bach PM, Wolfe AD, Perlman S, Karte RAP. Cardiac involvement in Friedreich's ataxia. A clinical study of 75 patients. *J Am Coll Cardiol* 1986, **7**:1370–1378.

Dürr A, Cossee M, Agid Y, *et al*. Clinical and genetic abnormalities in patients with Friedreich's ataxia. *N Engl J Med* 1996, **335**:1169–1175.

Further reading

Hawley RJ, Gottdiener JS. Five-year follow up of Friedreich's ataxia cardiomyopathy. *Arch Int Med* 1986, **146**:483–488.

Unverferth DV, Schmidt WR, Baker PB, Wooley CF. Morphologic and functional characteristics of the heart in Friedreich's ataxia. *Am J Med* 1987, **82**:5–10.

Cushing's Syndrome

Cushing's syndrome is one of the more common causes of secondary hypertension. It should be remembered, however, that only about 5% of instances of hypertension have a known cause (secondary); 95% are of unknown cause, or primary. Cushing's syndrome is usually caused by increased production of adrenal corticotropic hormone (ACTH). In the Mayo Clinic, among 312 patients with Cushing's syndrome, 226 had Cushing's disease caused by increased production of ACTH by the anterior pituitary gland, 34 had ectopic ACTH production by other tumors, 23 had adrenal adenoma, 18 had adrenal carcinoma, and 11 had nodular adrenal hyperplasia. Ectopic ACTH production most commonly originates from lung tumors. The possibility has also been raised that the pituitary gland is stimulated by hypothalamic centers.

The disease is three to four times as common in women as in men, and the onset of symptoms is usually in the third or fourth decade of life. Hypertension is present in 80–90% of the patients. Most patients exhibit the typical body habitus, with central obesity, slender extremities, and purplish striae of the trunk (**Fig. 1.55**). The skin is thin and easily bruised. Fatigue and weakness are common symptoms, and mood swings may occur. Women may develop masculinization, with hirsutism, amenorrhea, and deepening of the voice. Diabetes mellitus occurs in approximately 20% of patients, and osteoporosis is common. Untreated patients tend to die early from the complications of hypertension and accelerated atherosclerosis—congestive heart failure, myocardial infarction or stroke.

Laboratory tests tend to show hyperglycemia, with increased urinary excretion of 17-ketosteroids and 17-hydroxysteroids. Polycythemia or hypokalemia may be found. The diagnosis is confirmed by showing that dexamethasone 0.5mg every 6 hours for 48 hours fails to suppress plasma cortisol concentrations.

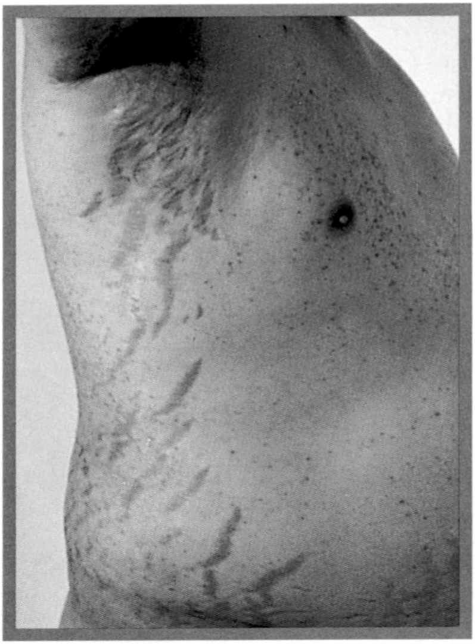

↑ Fig. 1.55a

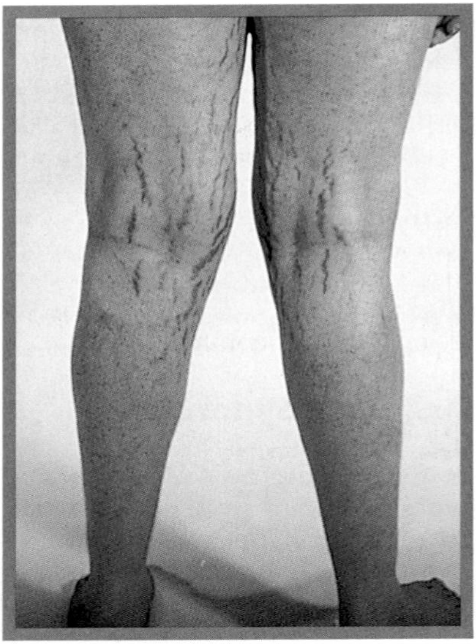

↑ Fig. 1.55b

Cushing's syndrome. Male patient showing characteristic purple striae and truncal obesity. The patient had adrenocortical hyperplasia.

Further reading

Burch WM. Cushing's disease: a review. *Arch Intern Med* 1985, **145**:1106–1111.

Carpenter PC. Diagnostic evaluation of Cushing's disease. *Endocrinol Metab Clin North Am* 1988, **17**:445–472.

Krieger DT. Physiopathology of Cushing's disease. *Endocr Rev* 1983, **4**:22–43.

Mucopolysaccharidosis

The mucopolysaccharidoses are a heterogeneous group of inborn errors of glycosaminoglycan metabolism, characterized by accumulation of mucopolysaccharides in various organs and excretion of these substances in the urine. Among them are Hunter's syndrome, Hurler's syndrome, and the rare Scheie's syndrome. The principal glycosaminoglycans that accumulate are dermatan sulfate, heparan sulfate, keratan sulfate, and chondroitin. The combined incidence of these disorders may be as high as 1 in 10,000 live births. Although seven types of mucopolysaccharidosis are described, there are certain features in common that permit clinical recognition. These include short stature (**Fig. 1.56**), hepatosplenomegaly with protuberant abdomen, corneal clouding, deafness, joint contractures, coronary artery occlusion, and cardiac valve involvement (**Fig. 1.57**). Other features that may be present include a short neck with a large head, coarse features, and flattened nasal bridge (gargoylism) (see Fig. 1.56). The hands may be short, broad, and thick. Inguinal hernias are frequent. Mental retardation is common, but not in Scheie's syndrome. Hydrocephalus may be found. Deposits of mucopolysaccharides in cardiac valves commonly cause aortic or mitral regurgitation (**Figs 1.58** and **1.59**), and aortic stenosis is also described. Cardiovascular lesions are less common in Sanfillipo's syndrome. Life expectancy is often

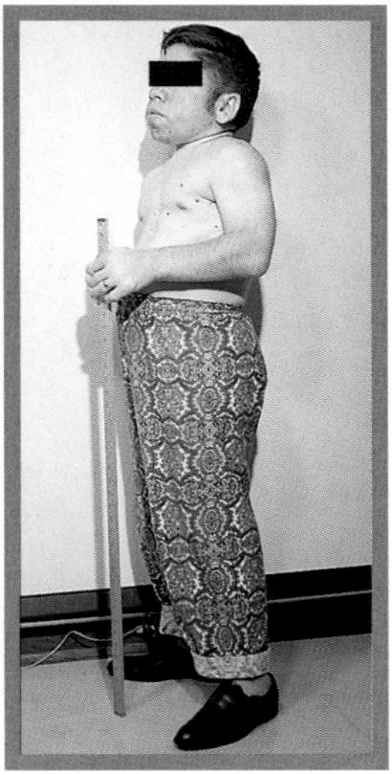

↑ Fig. 1.56
Mucopolysaccharidosis. Gargoylism in Hunter–Hurler's syndrome. Stature is diminished in this young man, who had aortic regurgitation.

Etiology and characteristics of mucopolysaccharidoses
Etiology
Inborn errors of glycosaminoglycan metabolism with deposits of mucopolysaccharides especially in fibroblasts) in various organs and excretion of these in the urine Enzyme deficiencies: iduronidase, sulfatase, galactosidase, and others Inheritance: autosomal recessive; X-linked recessive in Hunter's
Clinical Features
Large head, coarse features, flattened nasal bridge, hypertelorism, gargoylism Mental retardation (not in Scheie's syndrome), hydrocephalus, deafness Gibbus, short stature Corneal clouding (not in Hunter's syndrome) Obstructive airway disease Protuberant abdomen, hepatosplenomegaly Early death–Hunter's by 10 years (not in Scheie's)

↑ Fig. 1.57
Etiology and characteristics of mucopolysaccharidoses.

limited but may not be in milder forms. Patients with Hurler's syndrome usually die before the age of 10 years, and those with severe Hunter's syndrome before the age of 15 years. However, patients with mild Hunter's syndrome may survive into adulthood with little or no impairment, and those with Scheie's syndrome may have virtually normal longevity.

Cardiovascular lesions in mucopolysaccharidoses
Majority have multiple valvular lesions (aortic and mitral regurgitation, mitral and/or aortic stenosis)
Coronary occlusion by glycosaminoglycan and collagen
Pulmonary hypertension
Endocardial fibroelastosis, especially in type VI

← Fig. 1.58
Cardiovascular lesions in mucopolysaccharidoses.

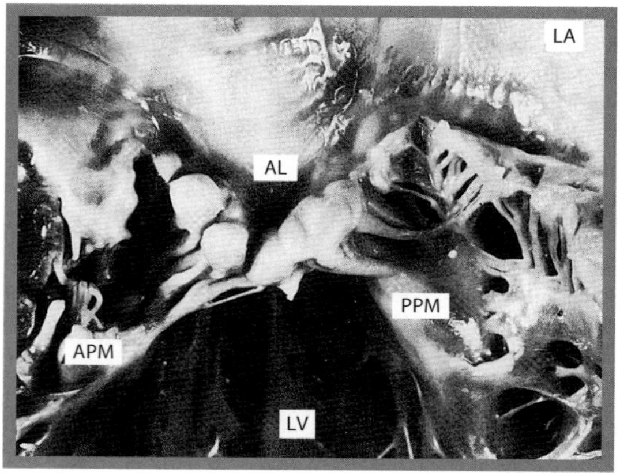

← Fig. 1.59
Hunter's syndrome. Mitral valve showing thickening of leaflets and chordae tendineae. AL, anterior leaflet of mitral valve; APM, anterior papillary muscle; LA, left atrium; LV, left ventricle; PPM, posterior papillary muscle. (With permission from Fowler NO, Kahn JM. *Am J Cardiol* 1979, **44**:148.)

Further reading

Whitley CB. The mucopolysaccharidoses. In: Beighton P, ed. *McKusick's heritable disorders of connective tissue, 5th ed.* St Louis: Mosby Yearbook Inc.; 1993:367–499.

Coarctation of the Aorta

This congenital narrowing of the aorta is usually located just beyond the left subclavian artery, in close proximity to the insertion of the ductus arteriosus. It is produced by an infolding of the posteromedial aortic wall. There is an extensive collateral circulation: the left subclavian artery communicates anteriorly with the intercostal arteries, and posteriorly with the intercostal arteries through its costocervical trunk; the transverse cervical artery, another branch of the subclavian artery, communicates with posterior intercostal arteries. Blood is thus carried to the descending thoracic aorta, bypassing the coarcted segment (**Fig. 1.60**). These collateral arteries are responsible for some of the physical and radiologic findings in aortic coarctation.

Aortic coarctation is four to five times as common in males as in females. It is one of the cardiovascular anomalies commonly found in Turner's syndrome. Mitral valve disease, VSD, patent ductus arteriosus, and bicuspid aortic valve (**Fig. 1.61**) may be found in patients with aortic coarctation. The disease usually comes to clinical attention because of hypertension or a murmur discovered in a child or young adult; coarctation of the aorta and renal disease have recently been listed as the two most common causes of hypertension in children aged 1–10 years. A minority of patients complain of cold lower extremities and claudication with exercise of the legs; about 25% show some impairment of growth of the lower extremities (**Fig. 1.62**).

Physical findings

The major finding suggesting a diagnosis of coarctation of the aorta is hypertension in the upper extremities and not in the lower. Not only is the femoral pulse impaired in amplitude but it is also delayed compared with the brachial pulse (**Fig. 1.63**). Although coarctation is the principal cause of hypertension, with bilateral impairment of the femoral pulse, other possibilities should be considered (**Fig. 1.64**). The hypertension is usually of moderate degree, and malignant hypertension is believed not to occur. The hypertension in the arms is principally produced by mechanical obstruction but impaired renal blood flow may be involved.

Murmurs may be found in patients with coarctation. Aortic insufficiency is found in 10% or so, usually in association with a bicuspid aortic valve, which has been found in 24–74% of these patients. Because the proximal aorta is dilated, a systolic ejection sound is often heard at the base of the heart. The murmur of patent ductus arteriosus, found in 5–10% of patients, may be heard.

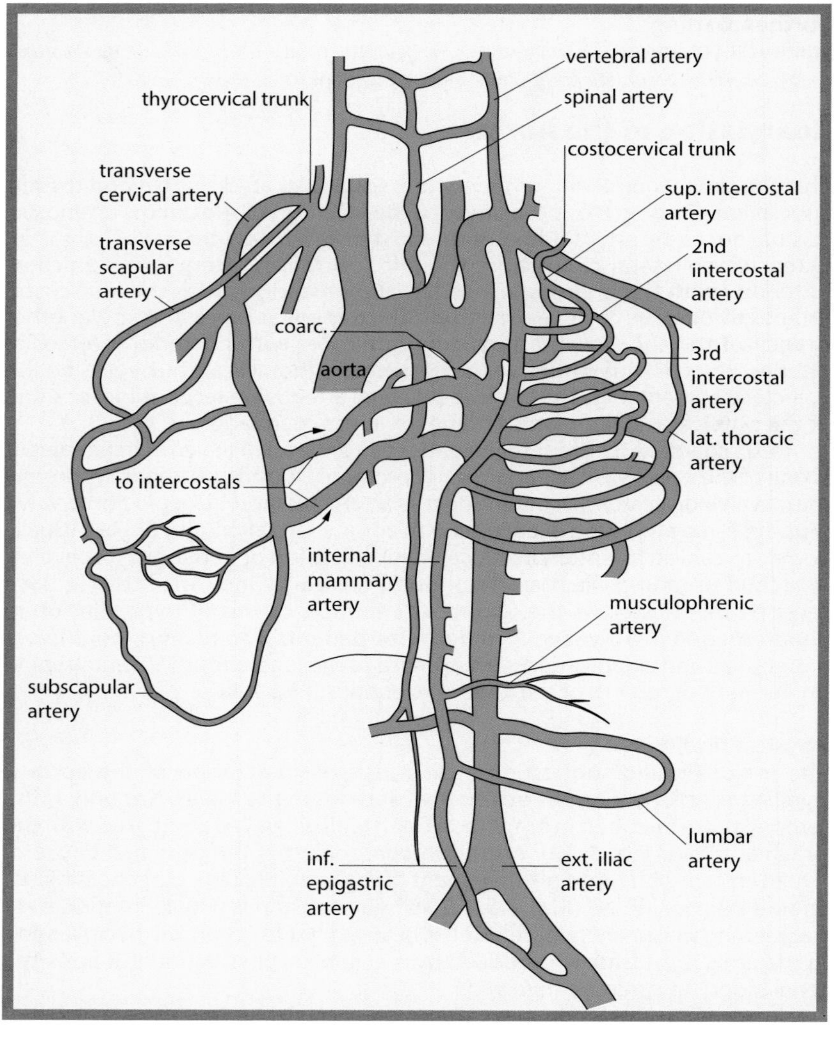

↑ Fig. 1.60

Coarctation of the aorta. Drawing of collateral circulation in aortic coarctation. (With permission from Fowler NO. *Diagnosis of heart disease*. Springer–Verlag, 1991.)

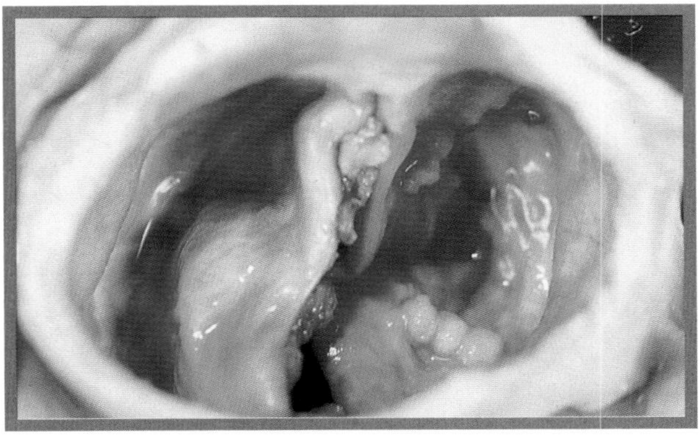

→ Fig. 1.61
Coarctation of the aorta. Congenital bicuspid aortic valve may be found in nearly 50% of patients with aortic coarctation. Compare with the normal aortic valve shown in Figure 1.75.

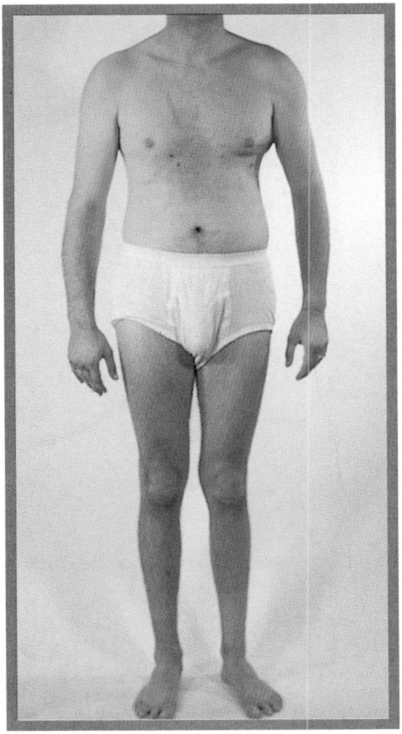

→ Fig. 1.62
Coarctation of the aorta. A patient with aortic coarctation, showing underdevelopment of the lower extremities. The operative incision in the left axilla was the result of recent surgical correction of the coarctation.

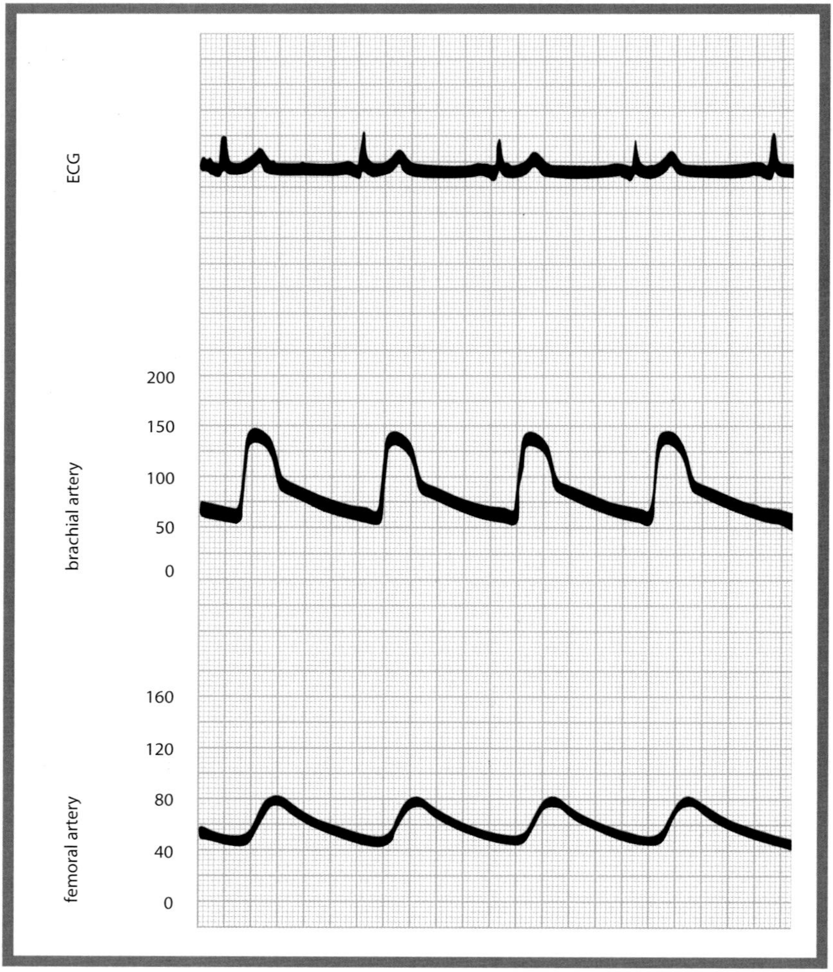

↑ Fig. 1.63
Coarctation of the aorta. Direct recording of brachial and femoral blood pressures in a patient with aortic coarctation. Note that not only is the peak femoral systolic pressure lower than the brachial pressure but also that the femoral pulse is delayed.

Brachial blood pressure greater than femoral blood pressure: possible causes
Coarctation of thoracic aorta
Coarctation of abdominal aorta
Saddle aortic embolism
Occlusive aortoiliac atherosclerosis
Dissecting aortic aneurysm
Aortitis
Traumatic aortic interruption
Pseudoxanthoma elasticum

← Fig. 1.64
Brachial blood pressure greater than femoral blood pressure: possible causes.

A few patients have murmurs of VSD, mitral stenosis or mitral insufficiency. Either a systolic or a continuous murmur may be detected over the posterior thorax. These murmurs may be related to the dilated posterior intercostal arteries or to the turbulent flow through the narrowed aortic segment itself. Especially when the patient leans forward, the dilated intercostal arteries may be seen and felt over the posterior thorax.

Radiologic findings

The chest radiogram demonstrates absence of the aortic knob in about 50% of patients with coarctation of the aorta (**Fig. 1.65**). Rib notching, produced by the dilated intercostal arteries, is a suggestive finding (**Fig. 1.66**) although it is not specific for coarctation and may also occur with superior caval obstruction, in which the intercostal veins are dilated, and with neurofibromatosis involving intercostal nerves.

A barium esophagram may show an 'E' or 'reversed 3' sign, produced by the dilated left subclavian artery or prestenotic aortic dilatation above, and the post-stenotic dilatation of the aorta below (**Fig. 1.67**).

The ECG usually shows evidence of left ventricular hypertrophy. Occasionally, there is left bundle branch block. Right ventricular hypertrophy suggests pulmonary hypertension.

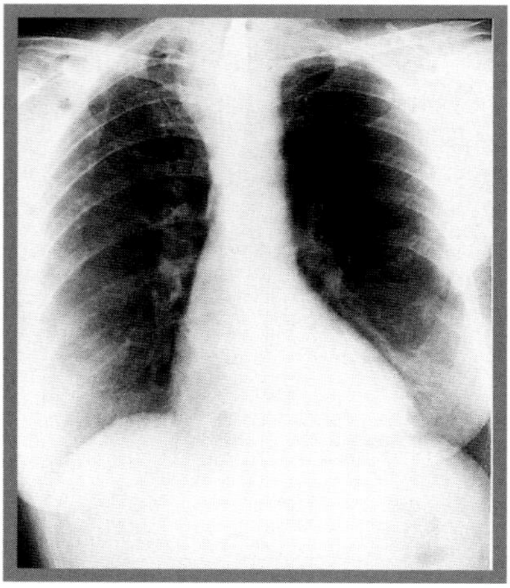

↑ Fig. 1.65
Coarctation of the aorta. Chest radiogram of a woman with aortic coarctation. Note absence of aortic knob; this radiographic sign is seen in about 50% of patients with coarctation.

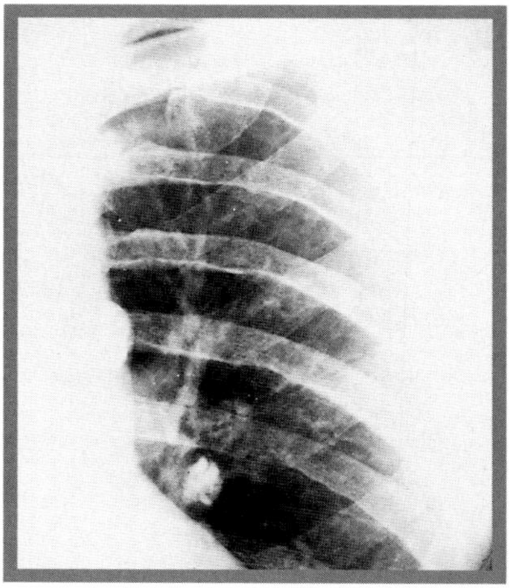

↑ Fig. 1.66
Coarctation of the aorta. Notching of lower surface of ribs four through eight in a patient with aortic coarctation.

→ Fig. 1.67
Coarctation of the aorta. Barium esophagram of a patient with aortic coarctation, showing 'E' or 'reversed 3' sign. The upper arrow indicates pressure on the esophagus by either a dilated left subclavian artery or prestenotic dilatation of the aorta. The lower arrow indicates pressure on the esophagus by post-stenotic dilatation of the aorta.

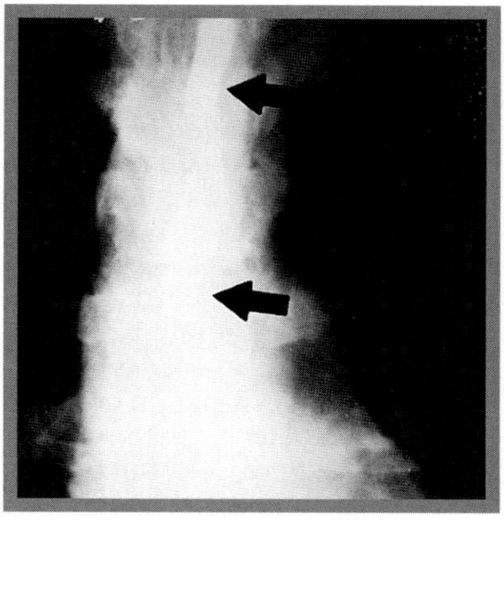

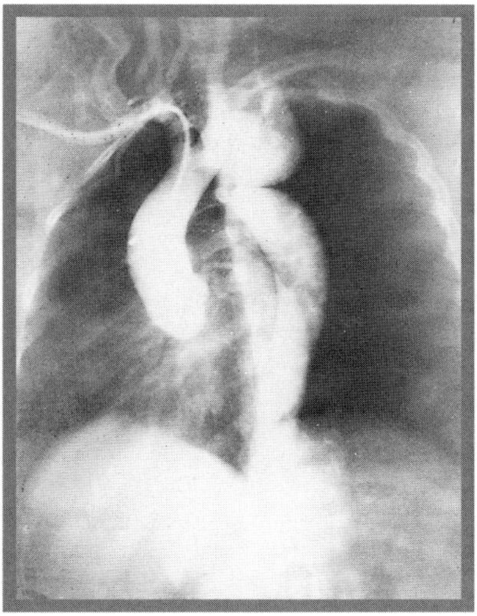

← Fig. 1.68
Coarctation of the aorta. Aortogram showing coarctation of the aorta in the usual site, just distal to the left subclavian artery. Prestenotic and post-stenotic dilatation of the aorta are seen. The left subclavian artery is dilated. (With permission from Fowler NO. *Diagnosis of heart disease*. Springer–Verlag, 1991.)

Diagnosis

The diagnosis of coarctation of the aorta is suggested when there is hypertension in the upper extremities, and lower blood pressure in the femoral arteries. The actual site and degree of the aortic narrowing may be demonstrated by aortography (**Fig. 1.68**), by aortic catheterization and pressure recording or by two-dimensional echocardiography (**Fig. 1.69**). Doppler ultrasound may be used to estimate the pressure gradient. It is important to know the site and degree of aortic narrowing, as a discrepancy between upper and lower extremity pulses may be found in pseudoxanthoma elasticum and other conditions (see Chapter 8). Magnetic resonance imaging or computerized tomography (CT) scanning may be used to demonstrate the site of narrowing in coarctation.

Clinical course

Before the advent of surgical treatment, the average age at death of patients with aortic coarctation was 35 years and 61–74% died before the age of 40 years. Congestive heart failure may develop in these patients in infancy. Various associated conditions and complications are recognized (**Fig. 1.70**). There is an association with intracranial berry aneurysm, which may rupture, with fatal intracranial bleeding. Infective endocarditis may occur. Dissecting aortic aneurysm is a risk, especially during pregnancy. The frequently associated bicuspid aortic valve may lead to either progressive aortic stenosis or aortic insufficiency.

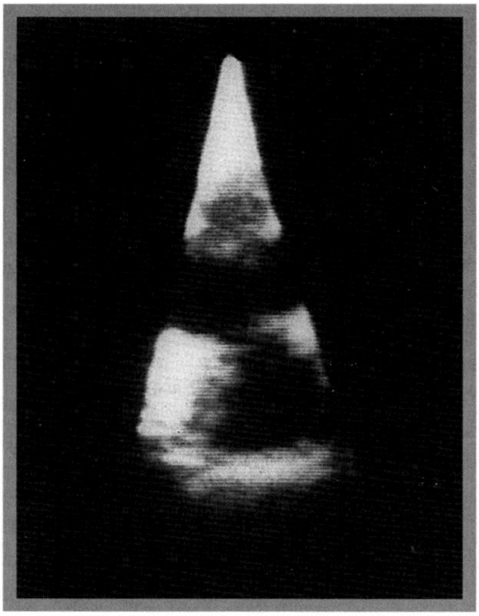

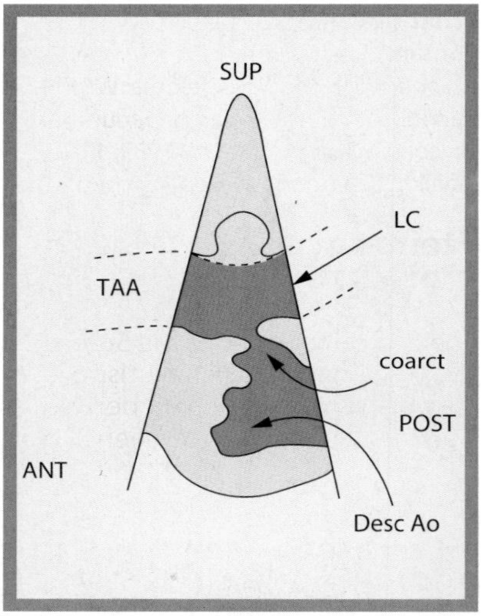

↑ Fig. 1.69a **↑ Fig. 1.69b**
Coarctation of the aorta. Two-dimensional echocardiogram showing aortic coarctation. TAA. transverse aortic arch; LC, left common carotid artery, coarct, coarctation; Desc Ao, descending aorta.

→ Fig. 1.70
Natural history of aortic coarctation.

Natural history of aortic coarctation
Hypertension
Heart failure
Dissecting aneurysm or aortic rupture
Bacterial endarteritis or endocarditis
Ruptured intracranial aneurysm
Aortic valve disease: bicuspid aortic valve; aortic regurgitation; aortic stenosis

Further reading

Fontana RS, Edwards JE. *Congenital cardiac disease: a review of 357 cases studied pathologically*. Philadelphia: WB Saunders; 1962:119.

Rao PS, Carey P. Doppler ultrasound in the prediction of pressure gradients across aortic coarctation. *Am Heart J* 1989, **118**:299–307.

Sinaiko AR. Current concepts: hypertension in children. *N Engl J Med* 1996, **335**:1963–1967.

Stein–Leventhal Syndrome (Polycystic Ovary Syndrome)

The clinical features of the Stein–Leventhal syndrome are bilateral polycystic ovaries, amenorrhea, hirsutism, and central obesity (**Fig. 1.71**). The syndrome may be associated with hypertension and diabetes mellitus, and women with polycystic ovaries have been shown to have risk factors for coronary artery

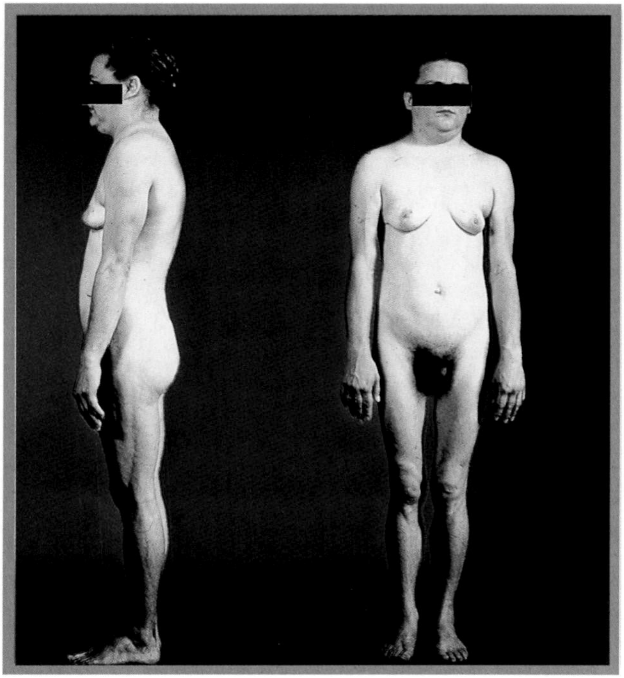

← Fig. 1.71 Stein–Leventhal syndrome. The patient was a 28-year-old woman. Note masculinization and hirsutism. The patient was infertile and had polycystic ovaries. She had sustained a massive cardiac infarction and died three years later with congestive heart failure.

disease. The 28-year-old woman patient pictured in Figure 1.71 shows the typical body habitus, with central obesity and some hirsutism. She was infertile; she had increased urinary excretion of 17-ketosteroids, and polycystic ovaries were found at surgical exploration. The diagnosis of Stein–Leventhal syndrome was made. The patient's ECG (**Fig. 1.72**), showed evidence of an anterior myocardial infarction, and she died of congestive heart failure 3 years later. Currently, the diagnosis of the Stein–Leventhal syndrome includes demonstration of polycystic ovaries by ultrasonography, and the finding of increased serum concentrations of luteinizing hormone and testosterone.

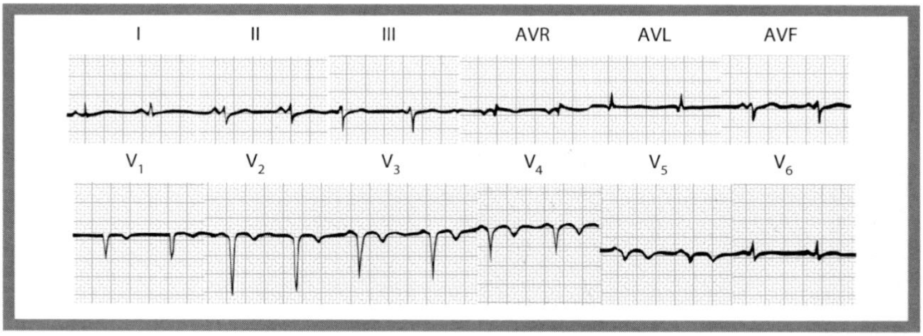

↑ Fig. 1.72

Stein–Leventhal syndrome. ECG of the patient in Figure 1.71. Note evidence of extensive anterior cardiac infarction, with Q waves and negative T waves in precordial leads V_1–V_5.

Further reading

Birdsall MA, Farquhar CM, White HD. Association between polycystic ovaries and extent of coronary artery disease in women having cardiac catheterization. *Ann Int Med* 1997, **126**:32–35.

Yen SSC. The polycystic ovary syndrome. *Clin Endocrinol* 1980, **12**:177–208.

Ankylosing Spondylitis

Criteria for the diagnosis of ankylosing spondylitis include low back pain and stiffness of more than three months' duration, pain and stiffness in the thoracic region, limited motion in the lumbar spine, limited chest expansion, evidence of iritis, and radiographic evidence of bilateral sacroiliac arthritis.

Ankylosing spondylitis, in common with Reiter's syndrome, is associated with the histocompatibility antigen, human leukocyte antigen (HLA)-B27 in approximately 80–90% of cases. The condition is from three to 10 times more common in males than in females. In the lumbar spine it leads to a loss of lumbar lordosis (**Fig. 1.73**) and a difficulty in flexing the spine and in bending over (**Fig. 1.74**). Peripheral arthritis may also appear. Urethritis, iritis, and psoriasis are of increased frequency. Aortic regurgitation may precede the radiologic signs of ankylosing spondylitis, which are characteristic, with fusion of the sacroiliac joints and calcification of the spinal ligaments (bamboo spine). In one population of patients, symptoms of arthritis developed when the patients were, on average, aged 26 years, precordial murmurs developed when they were 32, and congestive failure occurred on average at age 41 years.

The principal cardiovascular lesions in ankylosing spondylitis are aortitis and A–V block. The aortic valve ring is dilated and there is an aortitis adjacent

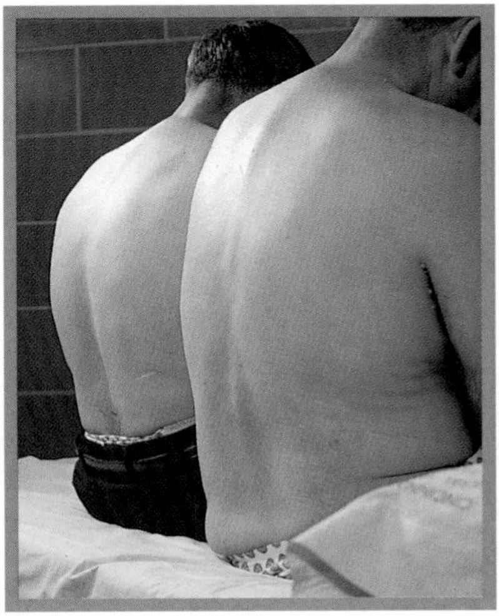

↑ **Fig. 1.73**
Ankylosing spondylitis. A patient with ankylosing spondylitis is shown on the right. Note absence of lumbar lordosis compared with that in the normal individual on the left.

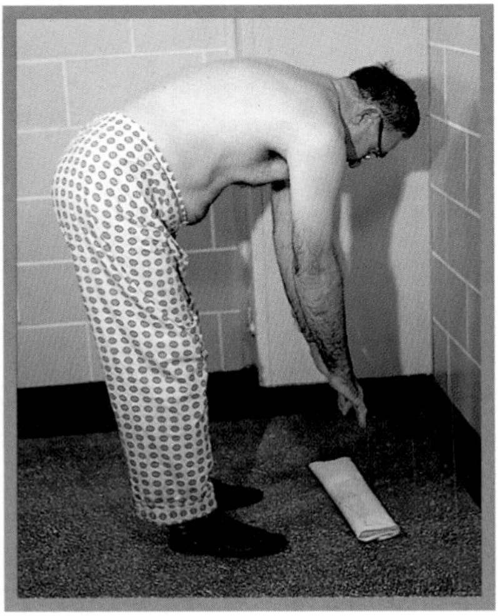

↑ **Fig. 1.74**
Ankylosing spondylitis. Limitation of flexion of the spine with ankylosing spondylitis.

to the aortic ring. The intima is puckered and the lesion resembles that of syphilitic aortitis. Unlike syphilis, in ankylosing spondylitis, fibrosis may extend below the aortic cusps into the anterior mitral leaflet. The aortic valve is thickened and fibrotic, and sags into the left ventricular cavity, producing the characteristic finding of aortic valvular insufficiency (**Figs 1.75** and **1.76**).

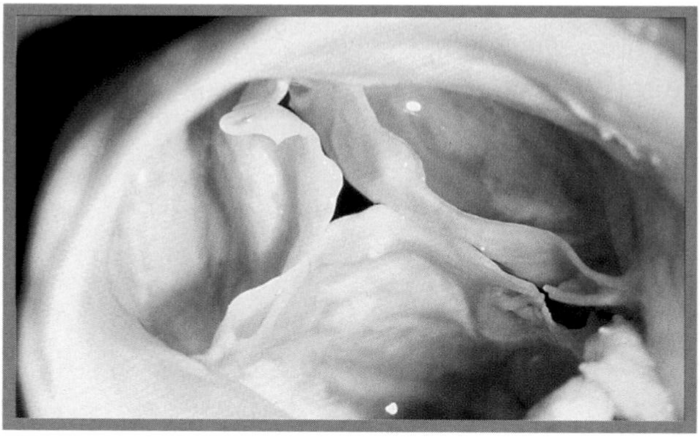

→ Fig. 1.75
Normal tricuspid aortic valve.

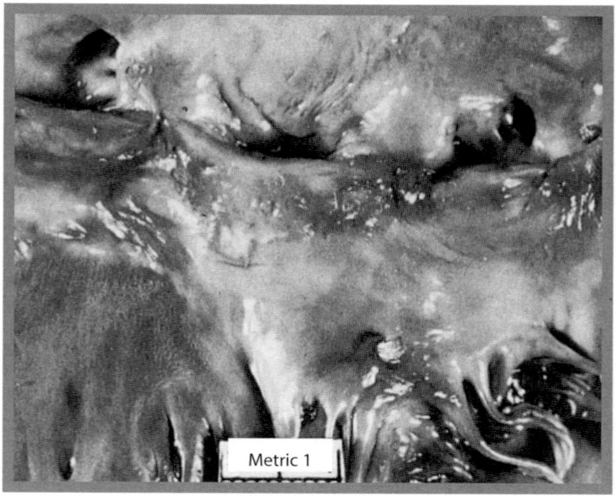

→ Fig. 1.76
Ankylosing spondylitis. Ascending aorta and aortic valve of a patient with ankylosing spondylitis. Note wrinkling of aortic intima, with deformity of the coronary orifices. The aortic cusps are thickened and separated at the commissures, causing aortic regurgitation.

Extension of the inflammatory process below the aortic valve produces a characteristic bump in the anterior mitral leaflet. Extension into the interventricular septum may produce first degree, second degree, or complete A–V block. Coronary artery ostial involvement may produce angina pectoris. Myocardial fibrosis, with cardiomyopathy and asymptomatic pericarditis, are also described. Mitral regurgitation occurs in a small percentage of patients, and mitral prolapse was found in 10% of those studied by Alves *et al.* The prevalence of aortic insufficiency increases with the duration of the disease and is about 10% after 30 years of spondylitis; it also increases if there is concurrent peripheral arthritis, and is then approximately 18% after 30 years. The average life expectancy in ankylosing spondylitis is normal when there is no aortic regurgitation, but is greatly reduced when severe aortic regurgitation is present.

References

Alves MG, Espirito-Santo J, Queirez MV, Madeira H, Macieira-Coelho E. Cardiac alterations in ankylosing spondylitis. *Angiology* 1988, **39**:567–571.

Further reading

Bergfeldt L. HLA-B27-Associated rheumatic diseases with severe cardiac bradyarrhythmias. Clinical features in 223 men with permanent pacemakers. *Am J Med* 1983, **75**:210–215.

Bulkley BH, Roberts WC. Ankylosing spondylitis and aortic regurgitation. Description of the characteristic cardiovascular lesion from study of eight necropsy patients. *Circulation* 1973, **48**:1014–1027.

Schlosstein L, Terasaki PI, Bluestone R, Pearson CM. High association of an HLA antigen, W-27, with ankylosing spondylitis. *N Engl J Med* 1973, **288**:704–706.

2 Facies

Williams Syndrome

Williams syndrome occurs in approximately 1 in 20,000 births. It is characterized by infantile hypercalcemia, mental retardation, and supravalvular aortic stenosis, often accompanied by peripheral pulmonary artery stenosis (**Fig. 2.1**), and is believed to result from submicroscopic deletion of chromosome 7q11.23. There is also an autosomal dominant variety of supravalvular aortic stenosis sometimes associated with peripheral pulmonary artery stenosis. In this latter condition, mental retardation and abnormal facies are absent. Among 22 members of one family, Ensing *et al.* described supravalvular aortic stenosis in 13, and pulmonary artery branch stenosis in four.

Patients with Williams syndrome have a characteristic facial appearance, called 'elfin facies': the face is full and the forehead is broad; there is a 'pug' nose, with a wide mouth and thick, pouting lips; the eyes are set wide apart; the chin is pointed (**Fig. 2.2**), the mandible is underdeveloped, and there is dental malocclusion (**Figs 2.3** and **2.4**). Patients with Williams syndrome exhibit some impairment of growth, and their stature is often reduced. Mental retardation is almost always present, and many of the patients are

→ Fig. 2.1 Characteristics of Williams syndrome.

Characteristics of Williams syndrome
Elfin facies, hypertelorism, pug nose, dental deformity, mental deficiency, short stature
Associated with infantile hypercalcemia
May be familial (autosomal dominant)
Associated with supravalvular aortic stenosis, peripheral pulmonary stenosis
Mitral prolapse, bicuspid aortic valve, hypertension may occur

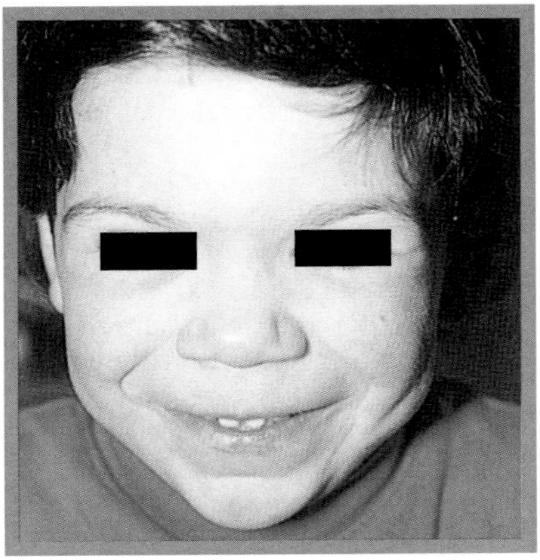

← Fig. 2.2
Williams syndrome. Typical facies in a child with Williams syndrome. Note hypertelorism (widely spaced eyes), broad forehead, and pointed chin.

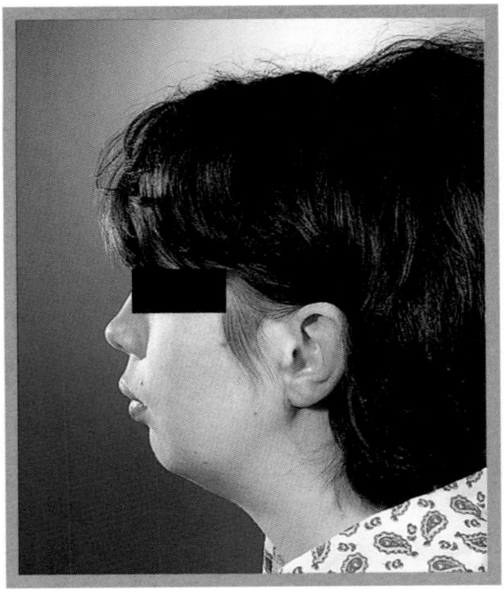

↑ Fig. 2.3
Williams syndrome. Young woman with Williams syndrome showing the characteristic malformation of the mandible. This patient had tubular narrowing of the entire ascending aorta and aortic arch.

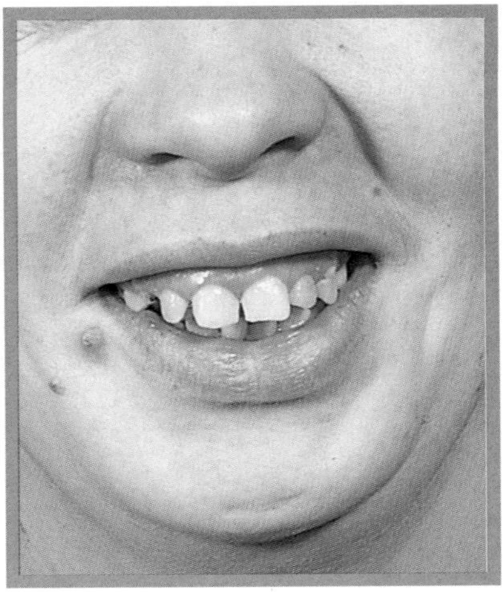

↑ Fig. 2.4
Williams syndrome. Frontal view of a patient with Williams syndrome. Note the dental malocclusion. This is the same patient as in Figure 2.3.

resident in homes for the mentally retarded. However, whereas the intelligence quotient is usually about 70 or less, there is a peculiar preservation of language skills: patients with this syndrome may be able to converse and to write well, but be unable to tie their shoelaces.

The typical cardiovascular lesions are supravalvular aortic stenosis (**Fig. 2.5**) and pulmonary arterial branch stenosis (**Figs 2.6** and **2.7**), both of which may be demonstrated by Doppler echocardiography. Supravalvular aortic stenosis may produce an aortic systolic ejection murmur that is maximal in the first right intercostal space adjacent to the sternum, rather than in the usual second right interspace as in aortic valvular stenosis; the murmur is easily heard over the

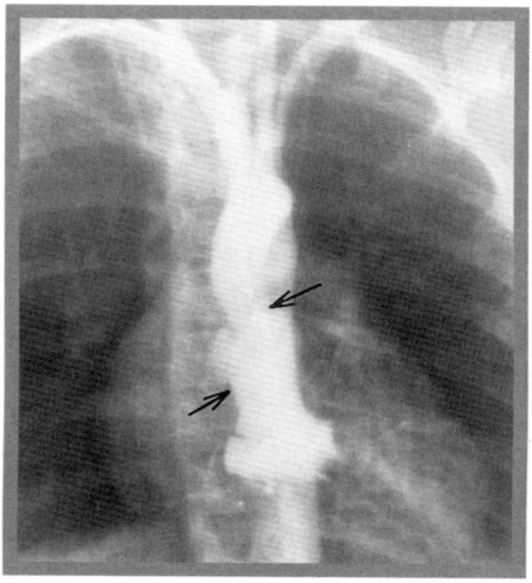

↑ Fig. 2.5
Williams syndrome. Aortogram of a patient with Williams syndrome. The upper arrow indicates the site of supravalvular aortic stenosis. The lower arrow indicates the location of the aortic valve. (With permission from Fowler NO. *Diagnosis of heart disease*. Springer–Verlag, 1991.)

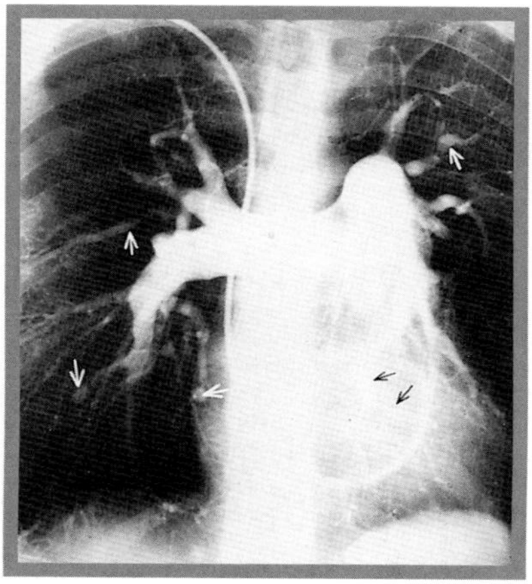

↑ Fig. 2.6
Pulmonary arteriogram of a patient with pulmonary arterial branch stenosis like that seen in Williams syndrome. Note the multiple areas of narrowing in the pulmonary artery branches, with post-stenotic dilatation (arrows). A long systolic murmur was heard over the posterior thorax and in the infraclavicular area. (With permission from Fowler NO. *Dignosis of heart disease*. Springer–Verlag, 1991.)

carotid arteries. Aortic insufficiency may be present. Pulmonary arterial branch stenosis tends to produce a systolic murmur that is louder outside the precordial area, often in the interscapular area or the axilla or infraclavicular area (see Fig. 2.7). A few patients with Williams syndrome have a bicuspid aortic valve or mitral prolapse. Surgical repair of the supravalvular aortic stenosis may be necessary.

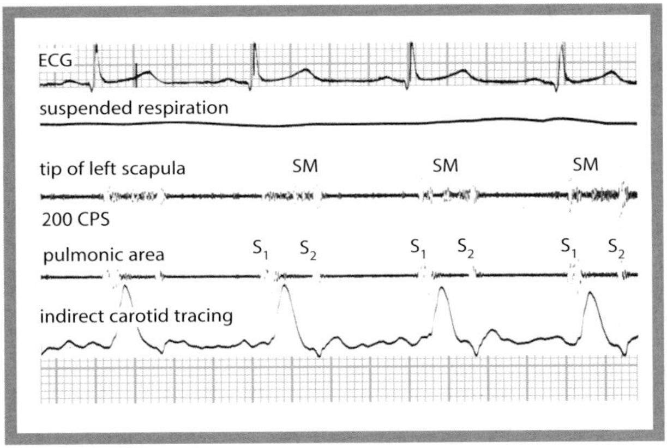

↑ Fig. 2.7
Systolic murmur of acquired pulmonary arterial stenosis in a patient with pulmonary embolism. The murmur is louder over the posterior thorax than over the precordium. The murmur is like that heard in patients with Williams syndrome and pulmonary arterial stenosis. S_1, first heart sound; S_2, second heart sound; SM, systolic murmur.

References

Ensing GJ, Schmidt MA, Hagler DJ *et al.* Spectrum of findings in a family with nonsyndromic autosomal dominant supravalvular aortic stenosis: a Doppler echocardiographic study. *J Am Coll Cardiol* 1989, **13**:413–419.

Further reading

Keating MT. Genetic approaches to cardiovascular disease. Supravalvular aortic stenosis, Williams syndrome, and long Q-T syndrome. *Circulation* 1995, **92**:142–147.

Williams JCP, Barratt-Boyes BG, Lowe JB. Supravalvular aortic stenosis. *Circulation* 1961, **24**:1311–1318.

Mitral Stenosis

Mitral stenosis is usually caused by rheumatic fever. Rarely, it is a congenital lesion or is caused by calcium infiltration associated with mitral annular calcification. Other rare causes include systemic lupus erythematosus, rheumatoid arthritis, and mucopolysaccharidosis. The condition may be simulated by left atrial myxoma (see Chapter 8). Although rheumatic fever most often occurs in young persons between the ages of 5 and 15 years, if mitral stenosis results, it is usually slowly progressive and symptoms are delayed until the third or fourth decades of life, or later. The normal mitral valve orifice has an area of 4–6cm^2; symptoms caused by mitral stenosis may appear when the valve area is reduced to 1 or 1.5cm^2/m^2 of body surface area.

The usual symptoms are those of progressive effort fatigue and dyspnea. Nocturnal dyspnea, orthopnea, and pulmonary edema may occur. At times, wheezing dyspnea may lead to a mistaken diagnosis of bronchial asthma. Chest pain is not common but may result from epicardial coronary disease or right ventricular hypertension that impairs perfusion of the right ventricle. Uncommonly, hemoptysis develops as the result of dilated bronchial veins. The onset of atrial fibrillation may be one of the first signs of the disease, and at times this arrhythmia is complicated by cerebral embolism or embolism to an extremity or coronary artery. As the disease progresses, eventually there is right heart failure with dependent edema.

Physical findings

The disease is more common in women: about 67% of cases are in women. With severe mitral stenosis there may be a malar flush (**Fig. 2.8**), and the female patient may be believed to be wearing rouge. Wood attributed this finding to peripheral vasoconstriction associated with a low cardiac output. Among severe cases, 33–50% exhibit the irregular pulse of atrial fibrillation. In advanced cases, signs of right ventricular failure, with jugular venous distention, hepatomegaly, and dependent edema may be seen. Precordial palpation discloses a palpable pulmonic valve closure in the second left intercostal space, a right ventricular parasternal lifting impulse, and, occasionally, a diastolic apical thrill. In pure mitral stenosis, the apical impulse is in the normal position inside the midclavicular line, and is of tapping quality.

Auscultation reveals a delayed-onset, rumbling diastolic murmur, loudest just inside the cardiac apex. S_1 is accentuated, and there is often a presystolic murmur when there is sinus rhythm. An opening snap of the mitral valve is usually heard, when the valve is not calcified (**Fig. 2.9**). The murmur is usually increased by the left lateral decubitus position, by exercise, and by the inhalation of amyl nitrite. The diastolic apical rumbling murmur associated with severe aortic regurgitation (Austin Flint murmur) is not associated with an opening snap, and is decreased by amyl nitrite inhalation. With significant mitral stenosis, an S_3 gallop is not to be expected.

In mitral stenosis, the earliest finding on the chest radiogram is that of left atrial enlargement. When pulmonary hypertension ensues, the pulmonary artery segment becomes enlarged (**Fig. 2.10**). Mitral valve calcification may be seen. The ECG tends to show evidence of left atrial enlargement when there is sinus rhythm (**Fig. 2.11**). In more severe symptomatic mitral stenosis, 33–50% of patients exhibit atrial fibrillation (**Fig. 2.12**). When there is pulmonary hypertension, right axis deviation and electrocardiographic evidence of right ventricular hypertrophy are likely (see Fig. 2.12).

Echocardiography is extremely useful in evaluating patients with mitral stenosis. With this technique, for example, left atrial myxoma can be excluded as a cause of an apical diastolic murmur. The severity of mitral stenosis can be quantified by planimetry of the mitral valve in the parasternal short-axis view or by the pressure half-time technique when Doppler methods are used. Disease of other valves—aortic or tricuspid—can be evaluated. Thus the delayed apical diastolic murmur of mitral stenosis can be distinguished from

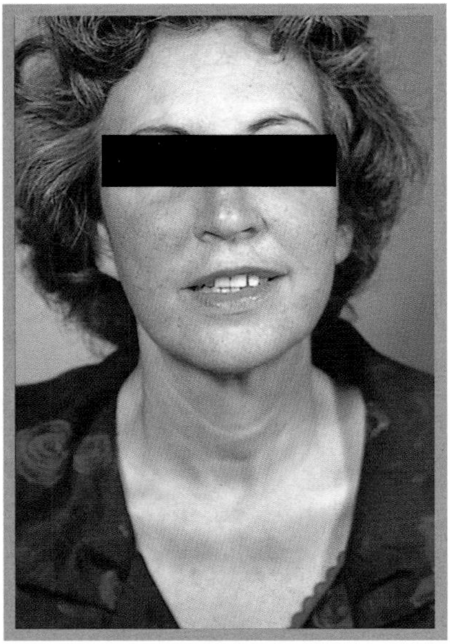

← Fig. 2.8
Mitral stenosis. Malar flush of mitral stenosis. This pinkish-purple discoloration has been attributed to vasoconstriction associated with the low cardiac output of severe mitral stenosis.

the Austin Flint murmur of aortic regurgitation. Right ventricular systolic pressure and pulmonary arterial systolic pressure can be estimated; left ventricular systolic function can be measured. M-mode echocardiography estimates left atrial size and demonstrates mitral stenosis, but not its severity (**Fig. 2.13**), whereas two-dimensional echocardiography enables one to demonstrate left atrial size, right ventricular dimensions, and mitral valve thickening with impaired opening (**Figs 2.14–2.16**).

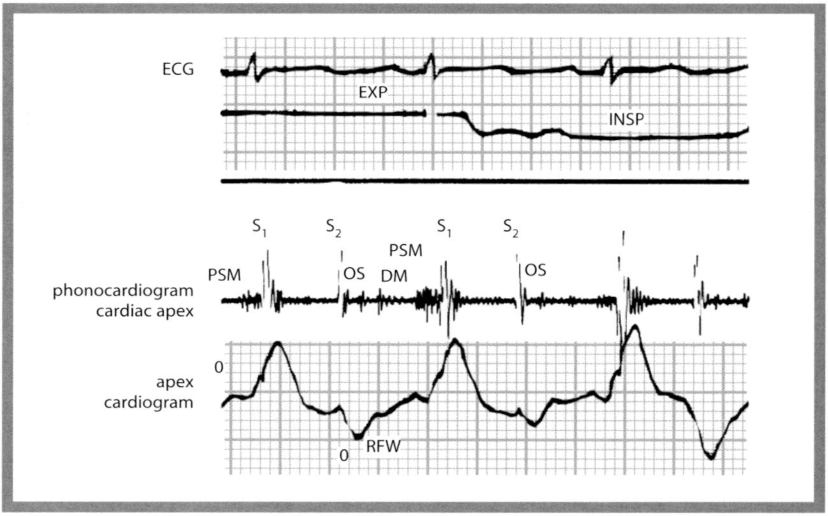

↑ Fig. 2.9
Mitral stenosis. Phonocardiogram of a patient with the typical auscultatory findings of mitral stenosis. A, A wave of apex cardiogram, a reflection of atrial systole; DM, diastolic murmur; ESS, reflection of left ventricular systolic thrust in the apex cardiogram; O, diastolic nadir and approximate time of mitral valve opening; OS, opening snap of the mitral valve; PSM, presystolic murmur; RFW, rapid filling wave; S_1, first heart sound; S_2, second heart sound. The presystolic murmur follows just after the A wave of the apex cardiogram and just precedes the first heart sound (S_1). The opening snap (OS) occurs approximately 0.08 seconds after the second heart sound (S_2). (With permission from Fowler NO. *Diagnosis of heart disease*. Springer–Verlag, 1991.)

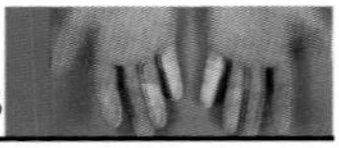

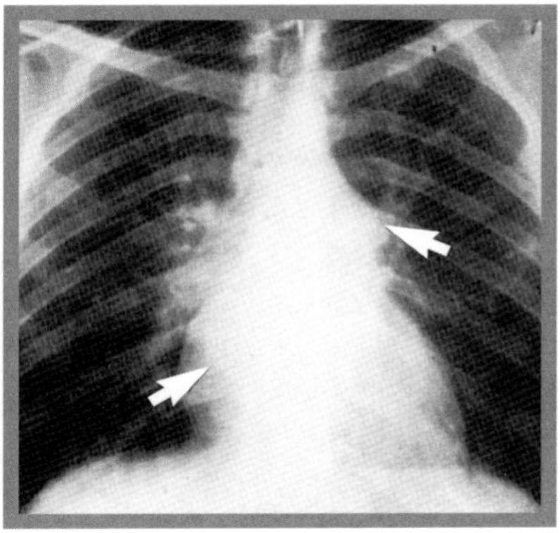

← Fig. 2.10
Mitral stenosis. Typical chest radiogram of a patient with mitral stenosis. The lower arrow on the observer's left indicates the enlarged left atrium, seen through the right heart border. The upper lobe pulmonary vessels are prominent. The pulmonary arterial segment is enlarged (upper arrow on observer's right).

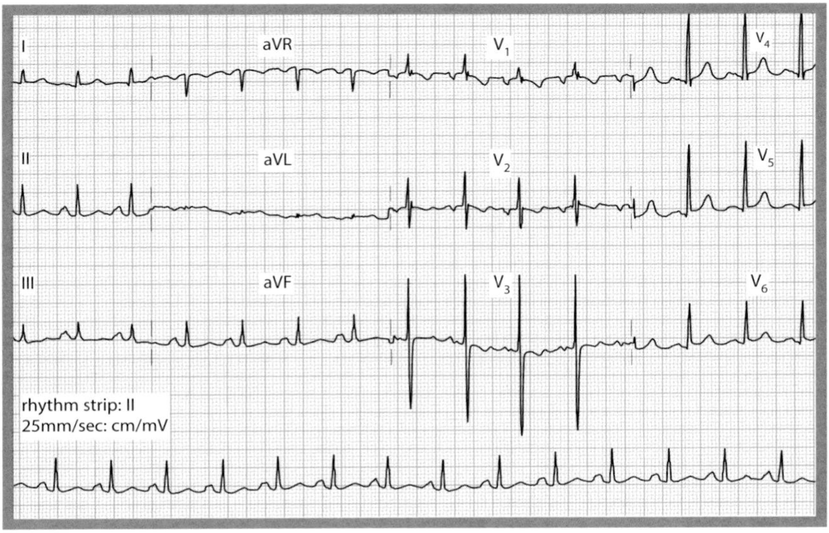

↑ Fig. 2.11
Mitral stenosis. Typical electrocardiogram of a patient with severe mitral stenosis and pulmonary hypertension. The prominent negative component of the P wave in lead V_1 is consistent with left atrial enlargement. The RsR′ wave in lead V_1 is consistent with right ventricular hypertrophy.

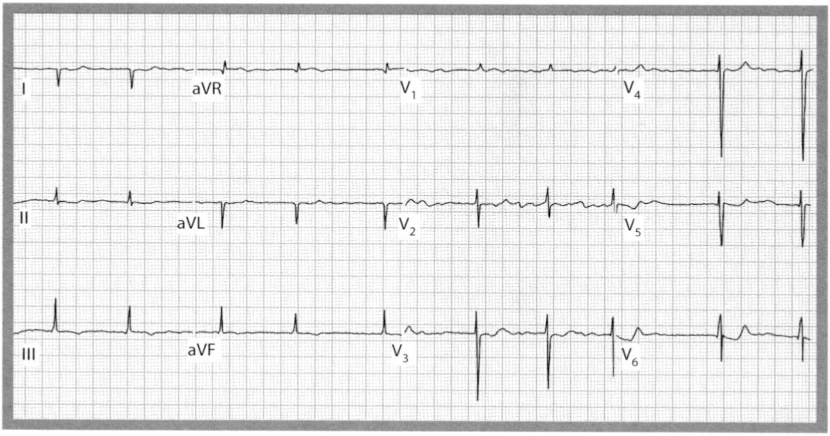

↑ Fig. 2.12
Mitral stenosis. Typical electrocardiogram of a patient with severe mitral stenosis. The combination of right axis deviation of the QRS complex and atrial fibrillation is very suggestive of mitral stenosis, but is occasionally seen in atrial septal defect, cor pulmonale, or constrictive pericarditis.

→ Fig. 2.13
Mitral stenosis. The M-mode echocardiogram before operation (left) shows a reduced E–F slope of the anterior mitral leaflet (AML) and lack of the normal posterior diastolic movement of the posterior mitral leaflet (PML). After mitral commissurotomy (right), the E–F slope of the anterior mitral leaflet is more nearly normal.

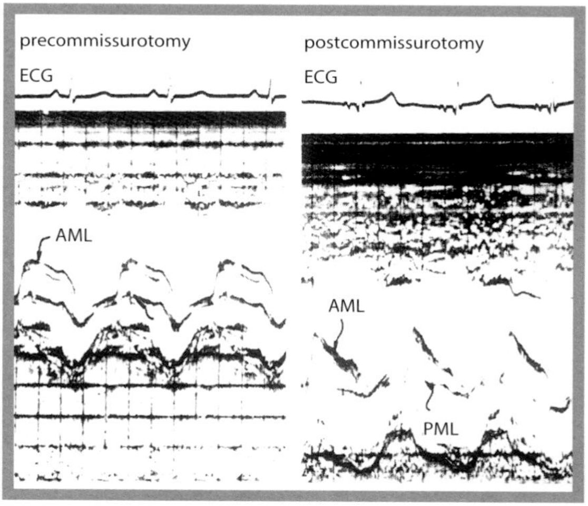

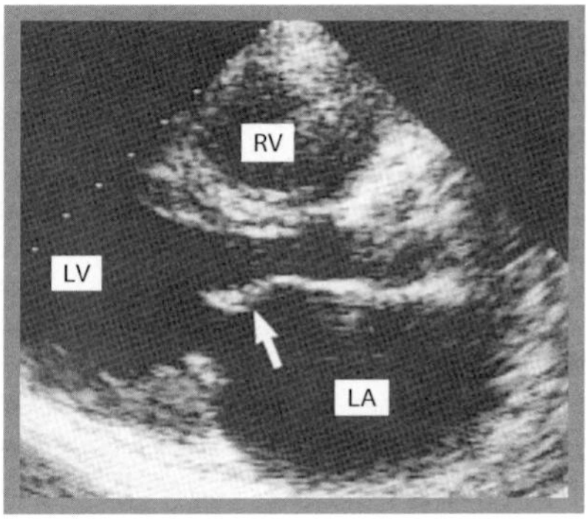

← Fig. 2.14
Mitral stenosis. Two-dimensional transthoracic echocardiogram, parasternal long-axis view. The left atrium (LA) and the right ventricle (RV) are enlarged. The anterior leaflet of the mitral valve (arrow) is thickened and has a hockey-stick appearance. LV, left ventricle.

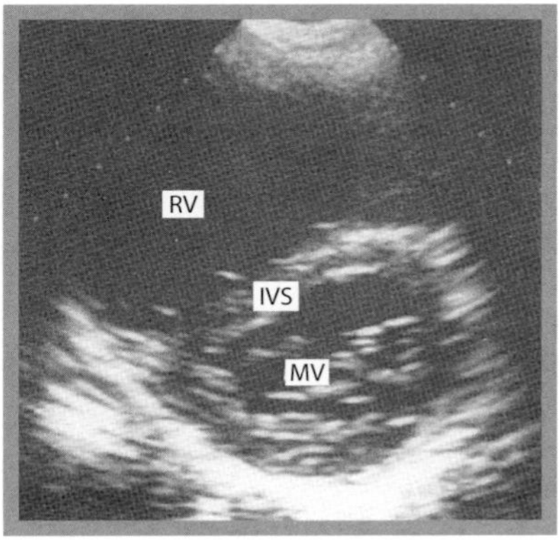

← Fig. 2.15
Mitral stenosis. Two-dimensional transthoracic echocardiogram, apical short-axis view. The right ventricle (RV) is enlarged and the mitral valve (MV) is thickened. IVS, interventricular septum.

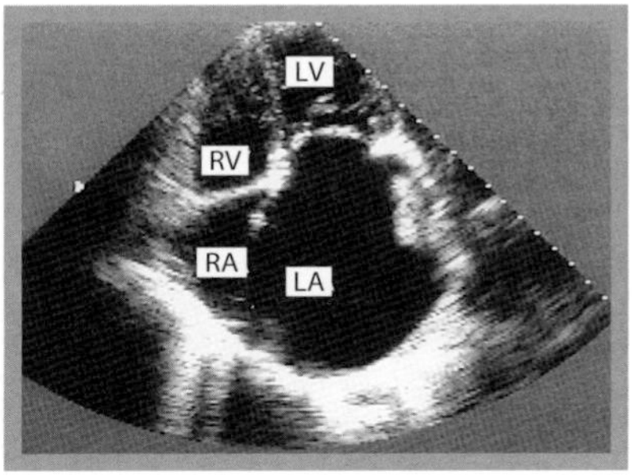

← Fig. 2.16
Mitral stenosis. Two-dimensional transthoracic echocardiogram, apical four-chamber view. The left atrium (LA) and right ventricle (RV) are enlarged. The mitral valve is thickened. LV, left ventricle; RA, right atrium.

Mitral stenosis can be demonstrated and its severity evaluated by combined right and left heart catheterization. Severe mitral stenosis is usually associated with a left atrial diastolic pressure that exceeds the left ventricular diastolic pressure by 10mmHg or more (**Fig. 2.17**). The pressure gradient depends not only upon the cardiac output but also on the mitral valve area and the diastolic filling period. The area of the mitral valve orifice can be estimated by using the Gorlin formula.

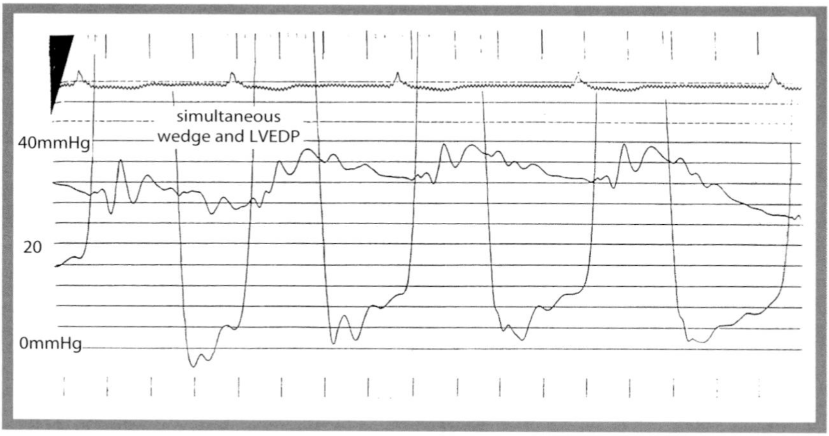

↑ Fig. 2.17
Mitral stenosis. Simultaneous recording of pulmonary atrial wedge pressure and left ventricular pressure. At end-diastole, the pulmonary wedge pressure exceeds the left ventricular end-diastolic pressure by an average of 23mmHg. Normally, this difference should not exceed a few mmHg. The mitral stenosis is severe.

Further reading

Assey ME, Usher BW, Hendrix GH. Valvular heart disease: use of invasive and non-invasive techniques in clinical decision making. Part 2: Mitral valve disease. *Mod Concepts Cardiovasc Dis* 1989, **58**:61–66.

Gorlin R, Gorlin SE. Hydraulic formula for calculation of the area of stenotic mitral valve, other cardiac valves, and central circulatory shunts. *Am Heart J* 1951, **41**:1–29.

Wood P. An appreciation of mitral stenosis. *BMJ* 1954, **1**:1051–1063.

Primary Pulmonary Hypertension

Primary or idiopathic pulmonary hypertension (PPH) is a condition in which there is a sustained increase in pulmonary arterial pressure without demonstrable cause. In particular, there should be no evidence of lung disease, connective tissue disease, congenital heart disease, left-sided heart disease, or pulmonary embolism. The National Institutes of Health (NIH) registry required a mean pulmonary artery pressure at rest of more than 25mmHg to be considered for this diagnosis (normal range 12–17mmHg). The disease is relatively rare, with a prevalence of 1–2 cases per million population. It occurs with particular frequency in women in the third and fourth decades of life. In the NIH registry, the ratio of female to male patients was 1.7:1.

In considering the diagnosis of PPH, there are several associations to be kept in mind. Approximately 0.5–2% of patients with human immunodeficiency virus (HIV) infection or portal hypertension have pulmonary vascular disease. The illicit use of intravenous drugs, especially if they are impure, may lead to pulmonary hypertension; the use of appetite-suppressant drugs such as amphetamines, aminorex, fenfluramine, and dexfenfluramine increases the risk of PPH by 6.3–20 times. Ingestion of toxic rapeseed oil also may be associated with pulmonary hypertension. Familial pulmonary hypertension accounted for 6% of cases of PPH in the NIH registry, and pulmonary hypertension may occur in hereditary hemorrhagic telangiectasia.

Histopathologic studies may reveal various lesions of the pulmonary arteries. These include medial hypertrophy of small arteries, intimal fibrosis, plexiform lesions, thrombotic lesions, and veno-occlusive disease. Plexiform lesions have been reported in 28–71% of patients. None of these changes is specific for PPH, and may be found in secondary pulmonary hypertension.

History

Dyspnea is the most common complaint, occurring as an early symptom in about 60% of patients with PPH (**Fig. 2.18**) and in 90% or more at the time of presentation. Fatigue, angina, and exertional syncope are also common symptoms. Raynaud's syndrome is reported in approximately 10% of patients. Eventually, right ventricular failure may develop. The average time from onset of symptoms to diagnosis is 2 years. Median survival from the time of diagnosis is reported to be 3 years, but some patients survive 10 years or more.

Physical findings

A few patients have a malar flush similar to that seen in mitral stenosis (**Fig. 2.19**). The NIH registry study reported the characteristic physical findings (**Fig. 2.20**): right ventricular enlargement, loud pulmonic component of the second heart sound (P_2), right ventricular S_3 or S_4 gallops, and increased systemic venous

→ Fig. 2.18
NIH study of primary pulmonary hypertension. Data from 187 patients at 32 centers, between 1981 and 1985.

NIH study of primary pulmonary hypertension	
Female:male ratio	1.7:1
Age	
Average (years)	36
Range	1–81
% of patients >60years	9
Symptoms (% of patients)	
Dyspnea	60
Fatigue	19
Syncope or near-syncope	13
Raynaud's phenomenon	10
Family history (% of patients)	6

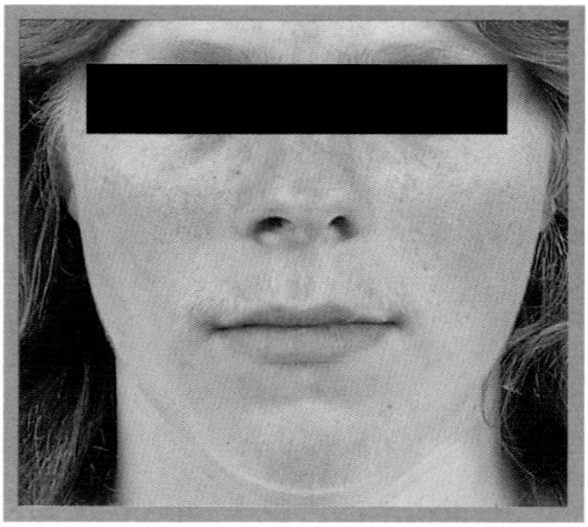

↑ Fig. 2.19
Primary pulmonary hypertension. Malar flush in an 18-year-old man with severe primary pulmonary hypertension. The patient died of this disease within a year. The flush resembles that seen in mitral stenosis.

Primary pulmonary hypertension	
Physical findings	**% of cases**
Jugular venous pressure >5mmHg	73
P_2 palpable	50
P_2 increased	88
Right-sided S_3	38
Right-sided S_4	57
Left-sided S_3 or S_4	0
Digital clubbing	5

↑ Fig. 2.20
Primary pulmonary hypertension. Physical findings in NIH registry patients.

pressure are common findings and tricuspid insufficiency is frequently observed. Atrial fibrillation was not reported and digital clubbing was uncommon.

Chest radiogram

As a rule, the lung fields are clear. In the NIH registry study, an enlarged pulmonary artery shadow was seen in 90% of patients, and the hilar vessels were enlarged in 79% (**Figs 2.21** and **2.22**). There is peripheral vascular pruning.

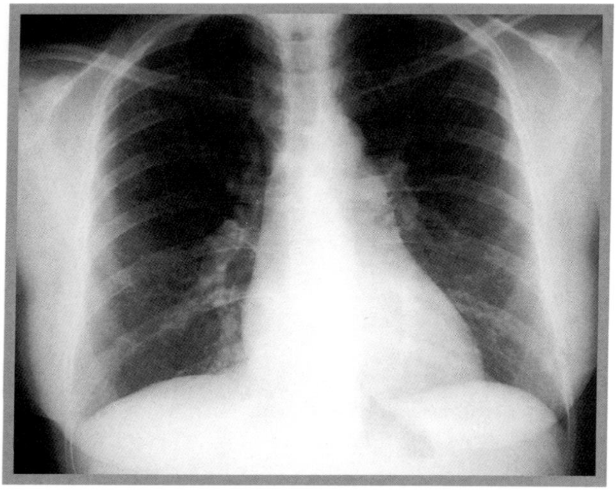

← Fig. 2.21 Primary pulmonary hypertension. Chest radiogram of a 42-year-old woman with PPH. Note prominent pulmonary artery segment, with pruning of the peripheral pulmonary vasculature.

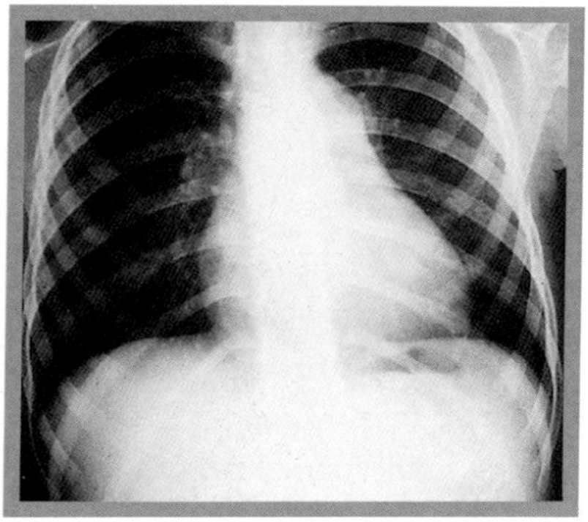

← Fig. 2.22 Primary pulmonary hypertension. Chest radiogram of a 7-year-old child with PPH. The pulmonary artery segment is enlarged and the lung fields are clear.

Electrocardiogram

Electrocardiographic evidence of right ventricular hypertrophy was found in 79% of patients reported in the NIH registry (**Figs 2.23** and **2.24**). All patients had normal sinus rhythm. Other ECG findings may include right axis deviation of the QRS complex, peaked P waves of increased amplitude in leads II and III, and prominent S waves in the left precordial leads.

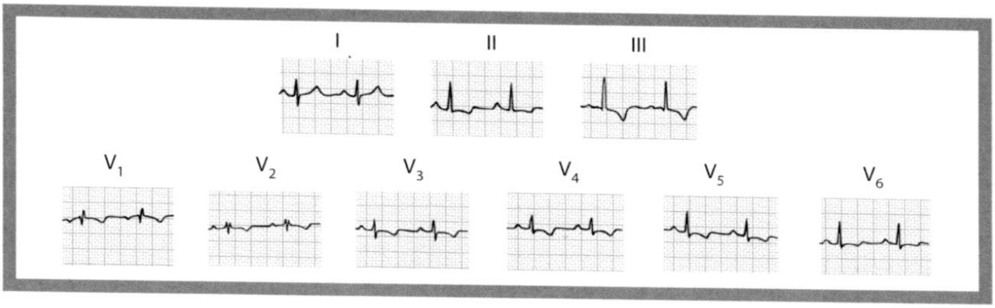

↑ Fig. 2.23

Primary pulmonary hypertension. ECG of a 38-year-old woman with PPH. The rSR' pattern in lead V_1 and the rightward QRS axis are consistent with right ventricular hypertrophy.

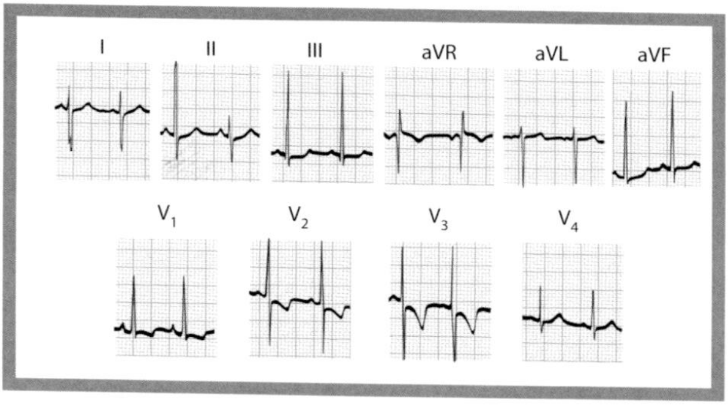

↑ Fig. 2.24

Primary pulmonary hypertension. ECG of a 7-year-old child with PPH. This is the same patient as in Figure 2.22. The pattern of right ventricular hypertrophy is seen in lead V_1. There is also pronounced right axis deviation of the QRS complex.

Echocardiogram

The echocardiogram is useful in the diagnosis of PPH. It demonstrates right ventricular and right atrial enlargement, and can be used to estimate pulmonary artery systolic pressure (**Figs 2.25–2.27**). Reversal of the interventricular septal curvature is usually seen. Echocardiography also serves to exclude left ventricular dysfunction or mitral valve disease as a cause of pulmonary hypertension, and to exclude congenital heart disease.

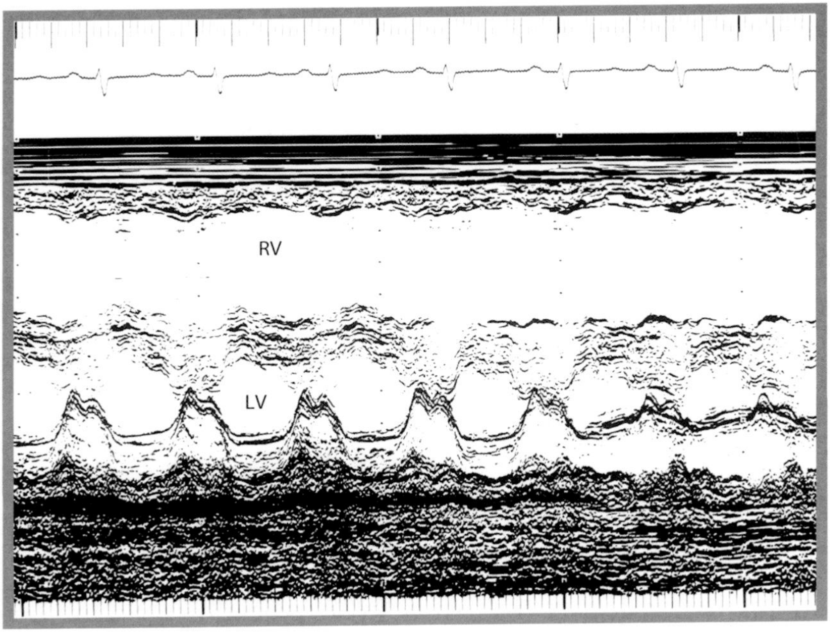

↑ Fig. 2.25
M-mode echocardiogram of a drug addict. The patient acquired pulmonary hypertension by intravenous injection of drugs contaminated by particulate matter. The pulmonary arterial pressure was 90/38mmHg. The echocardiographic findings are like those of 'pure' primary pulmonary hypertension. The right ventricle (RV) is greatly enlarged, especially in comparison with the left ventricle (LV).

Diagnosis

The diagnosis of PPH can usually be made or suspected on the basis of the history, physical findings, and diagnostic procedures described above. However, congenital intracardiac shunts, especially ASD, may be difficult to exclude. Chronic thromboembolic pulmonary hypertension is also difficult to exclude, as many patients with this disease lack a history of acute pulmonary embolism and the clinical findings in the two conditions are similar. In addition

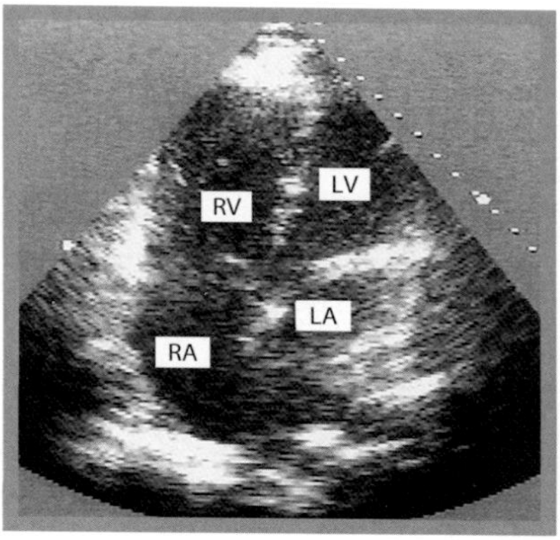

→ Fig. 2.26
Primary pulmonary hypertension. Two-dimensional transthoracic echocardiogram, apical four-chamber view. The right ventricle (RV) and right atrium (RA) are greatly enlarged, especially in comparison with the left ventricle (LV) and the left atrium (LA).

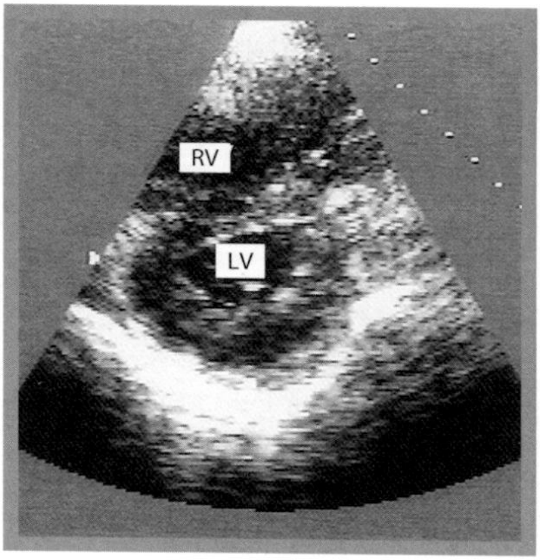

→ Fig. 2.27
Primary pulmonary hypertension. Transthoracic two-dimensional echocardiogram, apical short-axis view. The right ventricle (RV) is considerably enlarged, but the left ventricle (LV) is of normal size.

to the criteria described above, the NIH registry required for the diagnosis a right heart catheterization demonstrating a pulmonary arterial mean pressure exceeding 25mmHg, a normal pulmonary arterial wedge pressure of 12mmHg or less, and the absence of congenital shunt lesions; pulmonary function was required to be relatively normal. However, it is common to find a reduction in lung volume of up to 20%, mild hypoxia, and reduction in diffusing capacity. Thromboembolic pulmonary hypertension may be excluded by either pulmonary arteriogram or V/Q pulmonary radioisotopic scanning. Several conditions associated with pulmonary hypertension are excluded from the NIH registry of primary pulmonary hypertension (**Fig. 2.28**).

Primary pulmonary hypertension: exclusions from the NIH registry
Obstructive or interstitial lung disease
Congenital right-to-left shunts
Lung disease with hypoxemia and hypercapnia
Left ventricular myocardial disease or mitral or aortic valve disease with pulmonary wedge pressure >12mmHg
Connective tissue disease
Pulmonary thromboembolism
Pulmonary arterial branch stenosis
Parasitic lung disease
Intravenous drug abuse

← Fig. 2.28
Primary pulmonary hypertension: exclusions from the NIH registry.

Further reading

Rich S, Dantzker DR, Ayres S, *et al*. Primary pulmonary hypertension. A national prospective study. *Ann Int Med* 1987, **107**:216–223.

Rich S. Primary pulmonary hypertension. *Progr Cardiovasc Dis* 1988, **31**:205–238.

Rubin LJ. Primary pulmonary hypertension. *N Engl J Med* 1997, **336**:111–117.

Carcinoid Syndrome

The carcinoid syndrome occurs in about 4% of patients with carcinoid tumors. The malignant carcinoid syndrome includes metastatic carcinoid tumor, diarrhea, wheezing, and cutaneous flushing. The syndrome often includes carcinoid heart disease, characterized by fibrous lesions on the mural endocardium of the right heart chambers and thickening of the tricuspid or pulmonic valves (**Fig. 2.29**). At times, the endocardium of the left heart and the aortic or mitral valves are involved.

The primary site of the carcinoid tumor is most often the ileum; other sites include the jejunum, the stomach, the cecum, and, occasionally, a bronchus or a Meckel's diverticulum. More than 50% of patients with the carcinoid syndrome have hepatic metastases. Ross & Roberts reported autopsy studies of 36 patients with carcinoid syndrome. Only one of them did not have hepatic metastases. Twenty-one (57%) had carcinoid heart disease. Of these 21, all had right heart valvular or endocardial involvement, or both (**Fig. 2.30**). Seven also had mitral valve involvement; none had isolated mitral valve involvement. Carcinoid lesions are fibrous white plaques located on valvular and mural endocardium; the valve leaflets are thickened, rigid, and reduced in area. The lesions are believed to be produced by a direct effect of vasoactive substances on the endocardium.

→ Fig. 2.29 Carcinoid syndrome.

Carcinoid syndrome

Consists of cutaneous flushing, bronchospasm, diarrhea, endocardial plaque

Usually associated with hepatic metastases from a primary carcinoid tumor in appendix, ileum, stomach, duodenum, bronchus

Associated with increased circulating serotonin, bradykinin, other humoral substances

Endocardial plaques contain smooth muscle cells, collagen, acid mucopolysaccharides

Approximately 67% have cardiac abnormalities; tricuspid insufficiency and pulmonic stenosis most common

A high cardiac output state may occur

Physical findings

The clinical picture in carcinoid syndrome is characterized by cutaneous flushing (**Fig. 2.31**), bronchospasm with wheezing, and watery diarrhea. Involvement of the pulmonary valve may lead to combined pulmonic stenosis and regurgitation (**Fig. 2.32**); involvement of the tricuspid valve may produce tricuspid regurgitation, tricuspid stenosis, or both. Eventually, congestive heart failure develops, with fatigue, dyspnea, and dependent edema.

The ECG commonly shows low QRS voltage, right atrial enlargement, and either right bundle branch block or right ventricular hypertrophy. Echocardiography is useful in demonstrating tricuspid and pulmonary valve involvement, and may also show thickening of the mural endocardium of the

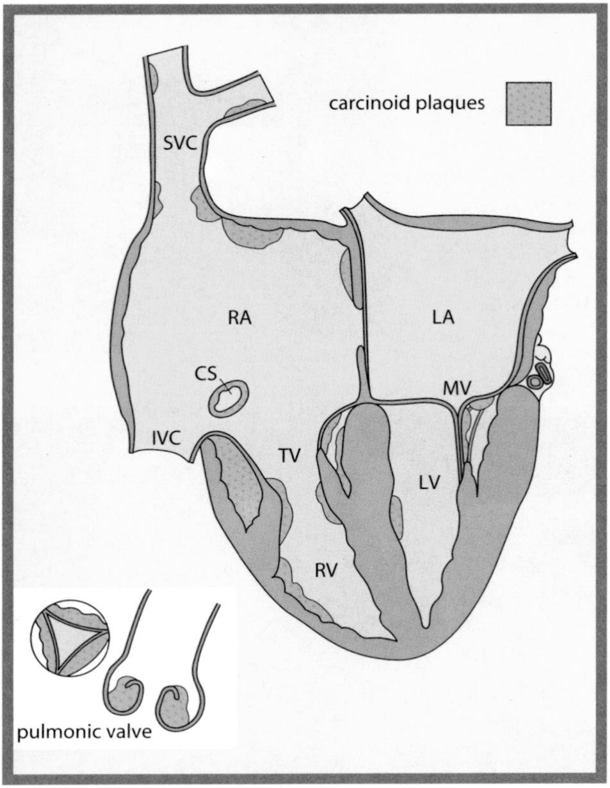

← Fig. 2.30 Carcinoid syndrome. Diagram of the heart, showing distribution of cardiac plaque lesions. CS, ostium of coronary sinus; IVC, inferior vena cava; LA, left atrium; LV, left ventricle; MV, mitral valve; RA, right atrium; RV, right ventricle; SVC, superior vena cava; TV, tricuspid valve. (With permission from Ross EM, Roberts WC. *Am J of Med* 1995, **79**:339–354.

right heart (**Fig. 2.33**). Cardiac catheterization typically shows evidence of tricuspid valvular stenosis and regurgitation. Pulmonary valvular stenosis and regurgitation are also commonly demonstrated.

Diagnostically, a history of cutaneous flushing, wheezing, and watery diarrhea suggests the possibility of carcinoid syndrome. Clinical evidence of tricuspid or pulmonic valve stenosis or insufficiency in a patient with the carcinoid syndrome

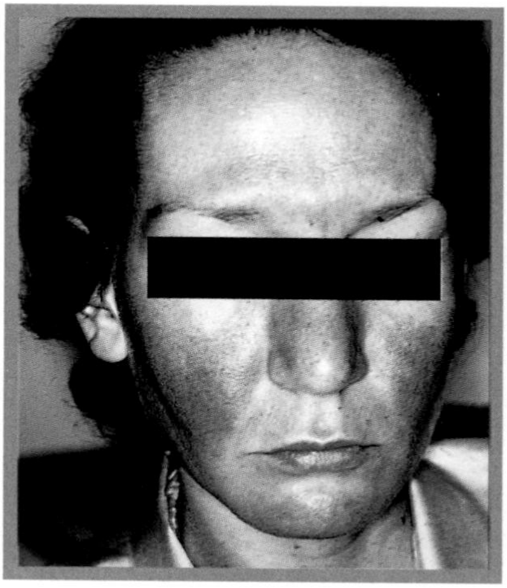

→ Fig. 2.31
Carcinoid syndrome. Typical cutaneous flush in a patient with carcinoid syndrome.

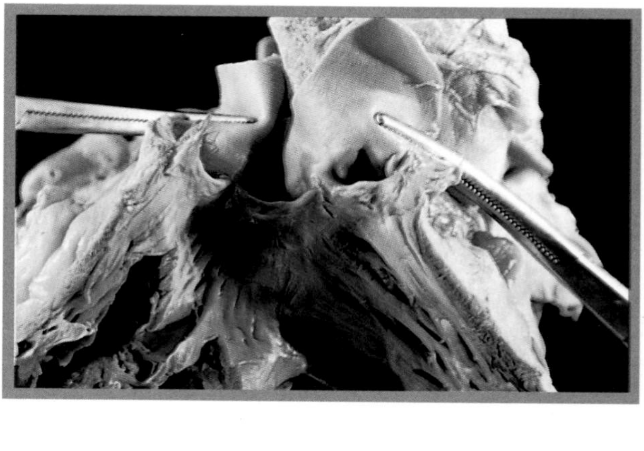

→ Fig. 2.32
Carcinoid syndrome. Diffuse thickening of the pulmonary valve cusps in a patient with a carcinoid tumor.

provides evidence for the diagnosis of carcinoid heart disease. CT scan of the liver will demonstrate evidence of hepatic metastases, which are nearly always present in carcinoid heart disease. The diagnosis is further confirmed by the finding of an increased 24-hour urine excretion of 5-hydroxyindoleacetic acid (**Fig. 2.34**).

The prognosis in carcinoid syndrome is poor, with an average survival of 38 months from the onset of systemic symptoms. The average survival in patients with clinical evidence of carcinoid heart disease is 11 months. Some improvement in symptoms and survival has been reported with the use of the somatostatin analog, sandostatin. Hepatic dearterialization has also been reported to be effective. In patients with severe right heart failure, tricuspid or pulmonary valve replacement or repair may be considered.

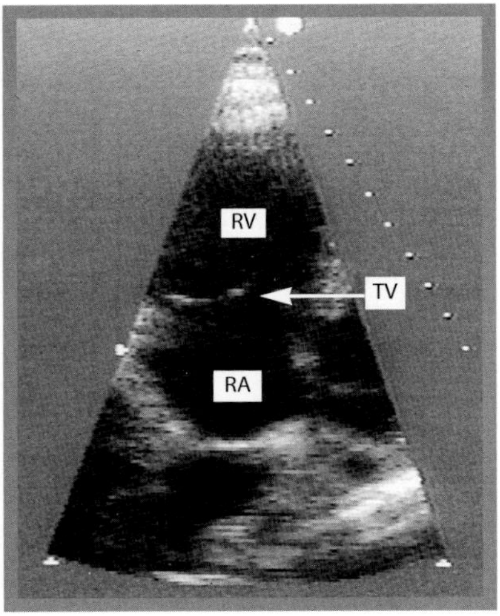

← Fig. 2.33
Carcinoid syndrome. Transthoracic two-dimensional echocardiogram of a patient with tricuspid insufficiency. The right atrium (RA) and right ventricle (RV) are greatly enlarged. The arrow indicates the tricuspid valve (TV).

Reference

Ross EM, Roberts WC. The carcinoid syndrome: comparison of 21 necropsy subjects with carcinoid heart disease to 15 necropsy subjects without carcinoid heart disease. *Am J Med* 1985, **79**:339–354.

Further reading

Anderson AS, Krauss D, Korcarz C, Lang RM. Images in cardiovascular medicine. Carcinoid heart disease. *Circulation* 1996, **93**:187–188.

Connolly HM, Nishimura RA, Smith HC *et al.* Outcome of cardiac surgery for carcinoid heart disease. *J Am Coll Cardiol* 1995, **25**:410–416.

→ Fig. 2.34 Carcinoid syndrome. Data from a study of 30 patients. (Himelman RB and Schiller NB. *Am J Cardiol* 1989, **63**:347.)

Carcinoid syndrome
A study of 30 patients

Patients with one or more symptoms (flushing, diarrhea, wheezing, dependent edema, telangiectasia)	30
Primary tumors	
ileum	17
bronchus	2
jejunum	1
rectum	1
Meckel's	1
unknown gastrointestinal site	8
Metastases	
multiple hepatic	26
single metastasis	4
Echocardiographic evidence of heart disease	17
Valve thickening*	
tricuspid	16
pulmonary	8
mitral	5
Mild or moderate pericardial effusion without tamponade	9
5-Hydroxyindoleacetic acid (5HIAA) concentrations	
Patients with heart disease who had 24-hour urine 5HIAA >100mg	16/17†
Patients without heart disease who had 24-hour urine 5HIAA <100mg	11/13†

*Pulmonary and tricuspid stenoses were mild
†17 patients diagnosed had heart disease; 13 had no heart disease

Relapsing Polychondritis

Relapsing polychondritis most commonly affects middle-aged men. It is a disease of unknown etiology, characterized by multiorgan cartilage inflammation; saddle nose is another feature of the disease. According to Michet, the diagnostic criteria are met by evidence of inflammation of cartilage at two of the following three sites: nasal, auricular, or laryngotracheal. Alternatively, there is inflammation in one of these three sites and at least two other manifestations: ocular inflammation, hearing loss, vestibular dysfunction or seronegative arthritis. Ocular inflammation may take the form of conjunctivitis, keratitis, uveitis or episcleritis. Inflammation of the auricular cartilage can be improved by treatment with adrenal corticosteroids (**Figs 2.35–2.37**).

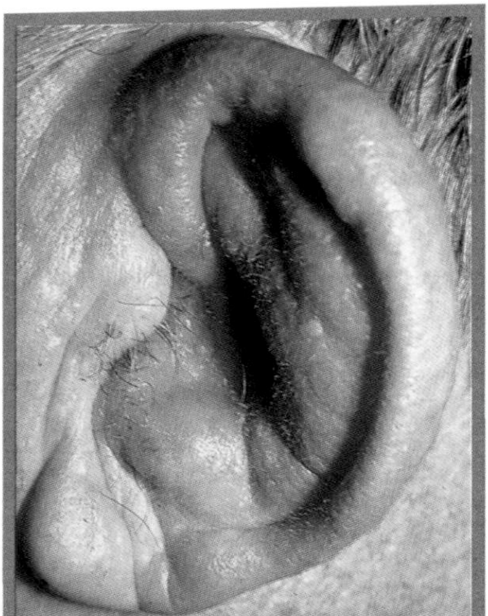

↑ Fig. 2.35
Relapsing polychondritis. The ear is swollen and reddish in color as a result of inflammation of the auricular cartilage.

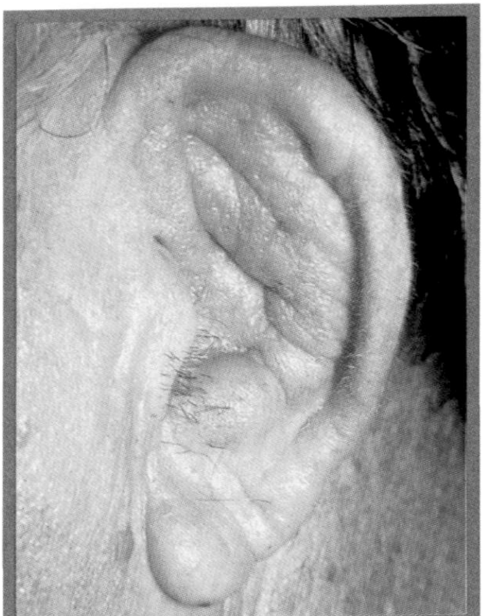

↑ Fig. 2.36
Relapsing polychondritis. The same patient as in Figure 2.35. The auricular inflammation is greatly improved after four days of immunosuppressive therapy.

Vasculitis is reported in 11–56% of cases according to Michet, but was found in only 6% of those in a Mayo Clinic study (**Fig. 2.38**). Fifteen percent or fewer have aortitis, which may lead to the aortic arch syndrome, thoracic or abdominal aortic aneurysm, or to aortic insufficiency resulting from aortic ring involvement.

→ Fig. 2.37
Relapsing polychondritis. Histologic picture of biopsy of the auricular cartilage of the patient in Figure 2.35, showing inflamed cartilage.

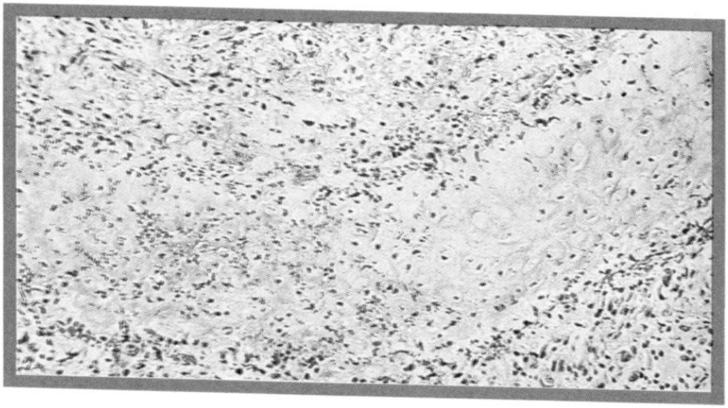

→ Fig. 2.38
Relapsing polychondritis. Data from 112 patients studied at the Mayo Clinic.

Relapsing polychondritis

Physical findings	% of cases
Auricular chondritis	85
Nasal chondritis	54
Arthritis	52
Ocular (scleritis)	51
Laryngotracheal symptoms (stricture 23%)	48
Fever	39
Saddle nose	29
Cardiovascular	
vasculitis	6
aortic regurgitation	4
aortic aneurysm (2 dissecting)	4
mitral regurgitation	2

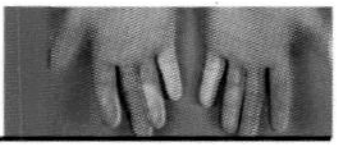

Histopathologic study of the aorta shows cystic degeneration of collagen, elastic fiber destruction, and decreased acid mucopolysaccharides. Vandecker & Panadis described aortic regurgitation in 4–6% and mitral regurgitation in 2–3% of patients with relapsing polychondritis. Myxomatous degeneration with prolapse of the aortic and mitral valves may occur, and infective endocarditis has been reported. The valvular insufficiency may be severe enough to require replacement of the aortic or mitral valve, or both; in one study, 11 of 31 reported patients exhibiting aortic regurgitation had required surgical replacement of the aortic valve. A–V block, pericarditis, and myocarditis have also been described in association with this condition (**Fig. 2.39**).

As many as 30% of these patients have other rheumatic diseases. Necrotizing glomerulonephritis has been reported. Cutaneous lesions are common, including vasculitis, erythema multiforme, erythema nodosum, and subcutaneous nodules.

The prognosis is poor, with a 5-year survival averaging only 45%. Death is most commonly caused by respiratory disease; cardiovascular disease is the second most common cause.

Manifestations of relapsing polychondritis
Vasculitis with recurrent inflammation of auricular, nasal or laryngotracheal cartilages
Seronegative arthritis
May produce aortic or mitral regurgitation, or both
Dissecting aortic aneurysm has been reported
Complete atrioventricular block has been described
Pericarditis may occur

← Fig. 2.39 Manifestations of relapsing polychondritis. Influence of at least one cartilage site is always present; incidence of other manifestations is variable.

References

Michet CJ. Vasculitis and relapsing polychondritis. *Rheum Dis Clin N Am* 1990, **16**:441–444.

Vandecker W, Panadis IP. Relapsing polychondritis and cardiac valvular involvement. *Ann Int Med* 1988, **109**:340–341.

Further reading

Balsa-Oriado A, Garcia-Fernandez P, Roldan I. Cardiac involvement in relapsing polychondritis. *Int J Cardiol* 1987, **14**:381–382.

Myxedema (Hypothyroidism)

The prevalence of hypothyroidism in one community survey was about 1%; in elderly inpatients it was about 2%. Hypothyroidism is cause by decreased secretion of thriiodothyronine (T_3) and thyroxine (T_4), and may be either primary or secondary. Primary hypothyroidism results usually from destruction of the thyroid gland by previous thyroiditis, surgical removal of part of the thyroid gland, or radioiodine therapy for thyrotoxicosis. Amiodarone therapy is another potential cause of hypothyroidism. Secondary hypothyroidism is much less common and results from decreased secretion of thyroid stimulating hormone (TSH), which may be due to either anterior pituitary or hypothalamic disease. Myxedema is a more advanced form of hypothyroidism and is associated with increased capillary permeability and leakage of protein-containing fluid into subcutaneous tissues, pericardium, pleural spaces, peritoneal cavity, and myocardium. Hypothyroidism is twice as common in women as in men, and its peak incidence occurs in those between 30 and 60 years of age.

The primary clinical features of hypothyroidism include non-pitting edema of the skin and subcutaneous tissues (**Fig. 2.40**), enlargement of the tongue (**Fig. 2.41**), cold intolerance, sluggishness of mentation, and a low-pitched, husky voice. The skin is dry. There may be impairment of vision and hearing, and loss of scalp hair and the outer eyebrows. Menstrual irregularity may occur.

Neurologic features include sluggish speech and mentation and, at times, mental depression. A characteristic feature is a slow relaxation phase of the deep tendon reflexes, especially the biceps jerk. In extreme cases, hypothermia and coma may develop.

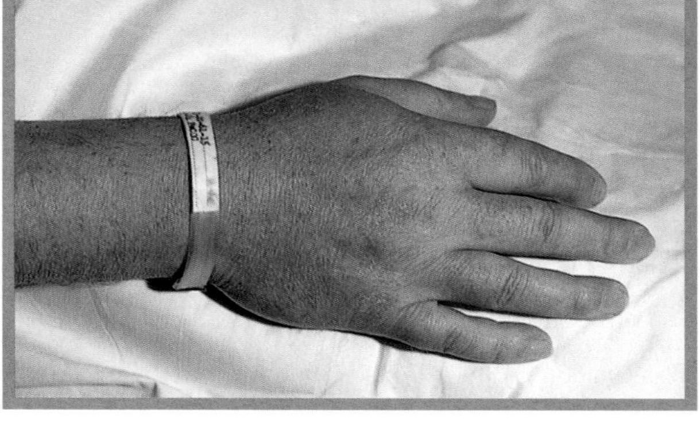

→ Fig. 2.40
Myxedema. Non-pitting edema of the hand in a patient with myxedema.

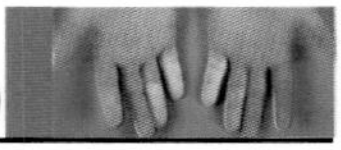

Cardiovascular features

Sinus bradycardia is usually present. Pericardial effusion is common when the clinical features of myxedema are present (**Fig. 2.42**), and occurs in about 33% of patients. Uncommonly, there is cardiac tamponade. Isovolumic ventricular relaxation time is prolonged, and, in experimental animals, myocardial contractility is reduced.

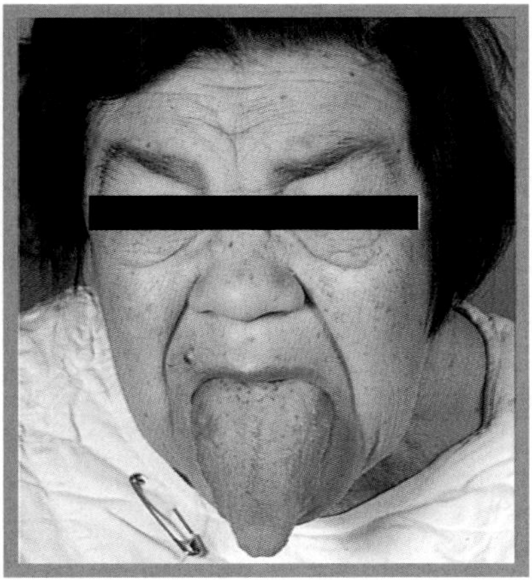

← Fig. 2.41
Myxedema. Large tongue, puffy features, and coarse hair in a patient with myxedema.

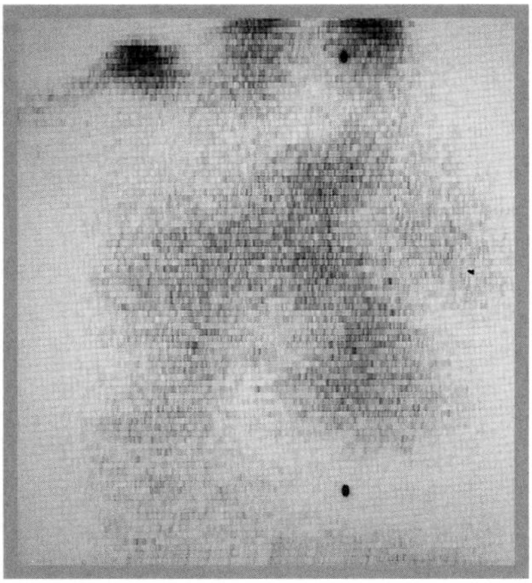

← Fig. 2.42
Myxedema. Cardiac blood pool radioisotope scan, showing evidence of pericardial effusion in a patient with myxedema. The marker in the lower center of the Figure lies in the halo produced by the large pericardial effusion surrounding the central cardiac blood pool.

Cardiomyopathy may occur, but clinical evidence of cardiac dysfunction is usually due to complicating hypertension or coronary artery disease, rather than to myxedema *per se*. Hypertension is of increased frequency in hypothyroidism but not in overt myxedema. In the typical patient, hemodynamic studies demonstrate a decreased cardiac output and stroke volume. However, in the absence of myocardial involvement, the decrease is proportional to the decrease in total body oxygen consumption (up to 40% less than normal); thus the arterio–venous oxygen difference is normal. In the absence of myocardial involvement or tamponade, right and left ventricular filling pressures are normal.

Characteristically, the ECG demonstrates sinus bradycardia, with low voltage of the P, QRS, and T complexes (**Fig. 2.43**). The PR, QRS, and QT intervals may be prolonged. Occasionally there are negative T waves. These changes are usually reversed within 3 weeks of the commencement of thyroid replacement therapy.

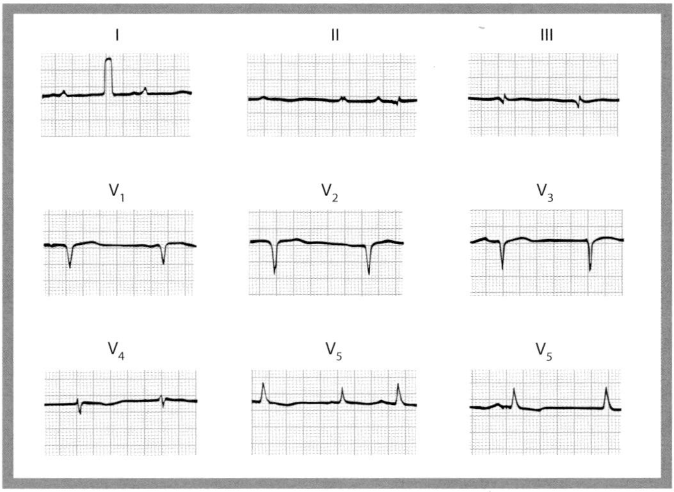

↑ Fig. 2.43
Myxedema. ECG of same patient as in Figure 2.41. The sinus bradycardia, low-voltage QRS complexes in the limb leads, and ST and T wave changes are typical of myxedema. Note also occasional atrial premature systoles. At autopsy, there was no evidence of myocardial infarction.

Diagnosis

Various clinical features are suggestive of a diagnosis of myxedema (**Fig. 2.44**). The diagnosis is confirmed by the finding of low circulating concentrations of T_4. The serum TSH concentration is increased, unless hypothyroidism is due to the secondary form characterized by decreased TSH production by the anterior pituitary or hypothalamus.

→ Fig. 2.44 Clinical features of myxedema.

Clinical features of myxedema
Coarse features with partial loss of scalp and eyebrow hair
Macroglossia
Low-pitched, husky voice
Non-pitting edema with dry skin (no axillary sweat)
Slow relaxation phase of biceps reflex
Ascites and pleural effusion
Cardiac features: cardiomyopathy, bradycardia, pericardial effusion in up to 33% of cases (tamponade uncommon)
ECG features: sinus bradycardia; low voltage; T wave changes

Further reading

Bastenie PA, Bonnyns M, Vanhaelst L. Natural history of primary myxedema. *Am J Med* 1985, **79**:91–100.

Smolar EN, Rubin JE, Avramides A, Carter AC. Case report. Cardiac tamponade in primary myxedema and review of the literature. *Am J Med Sci* 1976, **272**:345–352.

Zimmerman J, Yaholom J, Bar-on H. Clinical spectrum of pericardial effusion as the presenting feature of hypothyroidism. *Am Heart J* 1983, **106**:770–771.

Myotonic Muscular Dystrophy

Myotonic muscular dystrophy (Steinert's disease) is an autosomal dominant disease of skeletal muscle that also affects the heart, the smooth muscle of the gastrointestinal tract, the lungs, the endocrine system, the bony thorax, the eyes, and the skin. The responsible gene has been linked to chromosome 19q13.2–13.3. The disease is characteristically of variable severity; symptoms usually appear when the patient is aged between 20 and 50 years. Reported series show an approximately equal distribution between the two sexes.

The facial appearance of patients is characteristic. There is a lack of expression, with premature graying and frontal baldness (**Fig. 2.45**). Cataracts, ptosis, and retinal degeneration are common. In the infantile form, there is retraction of the upper lip with a 'Cupid's bow' appearance. Muscular weakness and wasting may occur; testicular atrophy and infertility are also seen. Characteristically, patients experience difficulty in relaxing the hand grip, and it is possible to demonstrate a myotonic response on percussion of the tongue and thenar eminences.

The cardiovascular effects are principally upon the conducting system, not upon the myocardium. Congestive heart failure is unusual. Evidence of heart disease on clinical examination is uncommon; however, atrial and ventricular tachyarrhythmias may occur, and about 4% of patients die suddenly, some with complete A–V block. At autopsy, the myocardium usually appears normal; occasionally, there is focal or diffuse fatty infiltration or fibrosis.

Perloff *et al.* studied 25 patients (11 men and 14 women) aged 21–40 years who had myotonic muscular dystrophy. Twenty-three had a family history of the disease. Twenty had increased serum creatine kinase concentrations. At electrocardiography, 10 showed a prolonged QRS interval, 10 showed a prolonged PR interval, eight revealed left anterior hemiblock, and seven showed sinus bradycardia. One had atrial flutter, which is said to be an

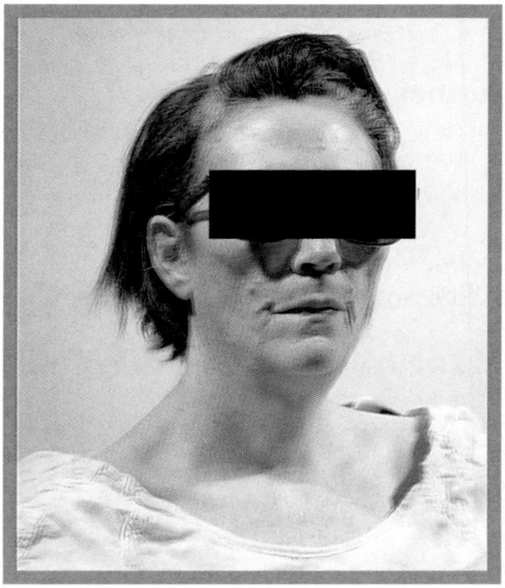

→ Fig. 2.45
Myotonic muscular dystrophy. Front view showing frontal balding of a woman with myotonic muscular dystrophy.

arrhythmia that is characteristic of this condition (**Fig. 2.46**). Echocardiograms showed normal left ventricular function, and chest radiograms were normal. Electrophysiologic studies revealed normal atrial–His (A–H) intervals in 24 of the 25 patients and prolonged His–ventricular (H–V) intervals in 14; 20 had evidence of His–Purkinje disease. In another study, 17 of 46 patients had mitral valve prolapse; this was not found in the study by Perloff's group.

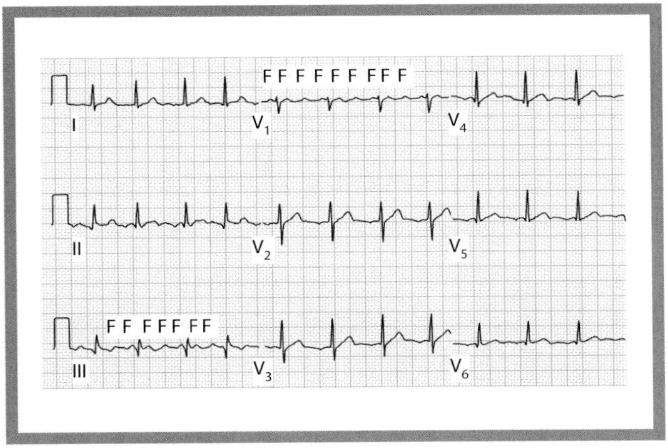

↑ Fig. 2.46
Myotonic muscular dystrophy. ECG of a 36-year-old man with myotonic muscular dystrophy, showing atrial flutter, a characteristic arrhythmia. The flutter waves are indicated by F.

References

Perloff JK, Stevenson WG, Roberts NK, Cabeen W, Weiss J. Cardiac involvement in myotonic muscular dystrophy (Steinert's disease): a prospective study of 25 patients. *Am J Cardiol* 1984, **54**:1074–1081.

Further reading

Moorman JR, Coleman RE, Packer DL, *et al.* Cardiac involvement in myotonic muscular dystrophy. *Medicine* 1985, **64**:371–381.

Tamura K, Tsusi H, Matsui Y, *et al.* Sustained ventricular tachycardias associated with myotonic dystrophy. *Clin Cardiol* 1996, **19**:674–677.

Kearns–Sayre Syndrome

Kearns–Sayre syndrome is classified as a mitochondrial myopathy characterized by progressive external ophthalmoplegia (**Fig. 2.47**), pigmentary retinopathy, and abnormality of specialized conducting fibers within the heart.

In addition to this triad, clinical manifestations may include short stature, kyphoscoliosis, pes cavus, hirsutism, and sexual immaturity. Cardiac manifestations usually take the form of Stokes–Adams seizures or sudden death. As a rule, heart block develops after the discovery of retinitis and ophthalmoplegia, but, occasionally, syncope is the presenting symptom.

Petty *et al.* studied a large series of 66 patients with Kearns–Sayre syndrome, 35 females and 31 males. Sixty-one percent presented before the age of 20 years; the age range was from birth to 68 years. Ptosis was the most common presenting feature and was present in 39. Twenty-four had retinal pigmentation at presentation; typically it was of a 'salt and pepper' distribution. Fatigue was a complaint in 28 of the patients and 18 had proximal limb weakness. Twenty-seven had cerebellar ataxia, 13 had dementia, and 17 eventually had neural deafness. Among 35 who underwent CT scan, the brain

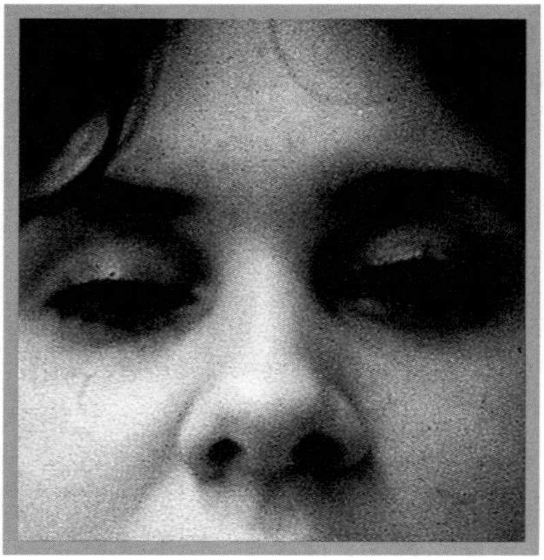

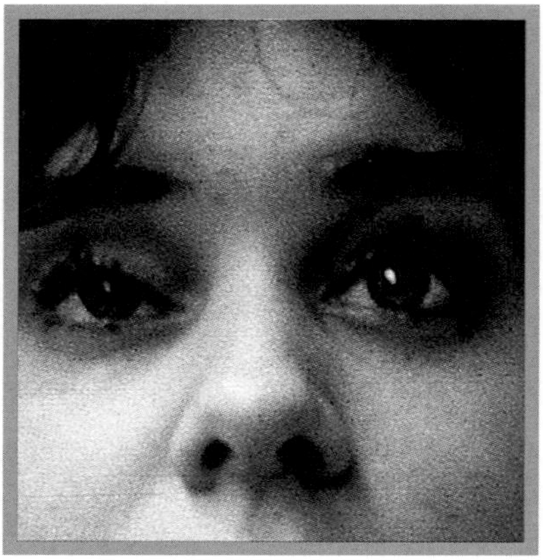

↑ Fig. 2.47a **↑ Fig. 2.47b**

Kearns–Sayre syndrome. Photograph of an 18-year-old woman, showing ptosis of the right eyelid (**a**), which persists on upward gaze (**b**). She also had pigmentary retinopathy and her ECG showed bifascicular block. (With permission from Perloff JK. Cardiac manifestations of neuromuscular disease. In *Atlas of heart disease*, **2**: *Cardiomyopathies, myocarditis, and pericardial disease*, ed. Abelmann WH. Philadelphia: Current Medicine, 1995.)

was normal in 17, but 18 had cerebral atrophy, with additional cerebellar atrophy in 12.

Cardiovascular abnormalities are usually confined to the conducting system, although two patients with dilated cardiomyopathy have been reported, one of whom received a cardiac transplantation. In this patient, the histopathology of the heart revealed abnormal mitochondria with normal myofibrils.

In a study of 19 cases, electrocardiographic abnormalities were common. Thirteen had a combination of left axis deviation and right bundle branch block; two of these had complete heart block. Three had left axis deviation alone.

Reference

Petty RKH, Harding AE, Morgan-Hughes JA. The clinical features of mitochondrial myopathy. *Brain* 1986, **109**:915–938.

Further reading

Akaike M, Kawai H, Yokoi K. Cardiac dysfunction in patients with progressive external ophthalmoplegia. *Clin Cardiol* 1997, **20**:239–243.

Channer KS, Channer JL, Campbell MJ, Reef JR. Cardiomyopathy in the Kearns–Sayre syndrome. *Br Heart J* 1988, **59**:486–490.

Roberts NK, Perloff JK, Kark RAP. Cardiac conduction in the Kearns–Sayre syndrome (a neuromuscular disorder associated with progressive external ophthalmoplegia and pigmentary retinopathy). *Am J Cardiol* 1979, **44**:1396–1400.

Disseminated Lupus Erythematosus

Disseminated lupus erythematosus is a systemic disease, with circulating antibodies against cellular nuclei and phospholipids. The basic anatomic lesion is a diffuse microvasculitis. Clinically, the disease affects many organs and systems, including kidneys, brain, cardiovascular system, lungs, blood, and joints. The disease is much more common in the female sex.

The diagnosis may be suggested by a characteristic red rash in the areas of the body exposed to sunlight; exposure to sunlight tends to aggravate the disease. There is a characteristic butterfly rash of the face (**Fig. 2.48**). A similar rash may be found on the back of the hands and the V-shaped area encompassing the neck and the upper chest. Unlike discoid lupus, the skin lesions do not lead to scarring. The characteristic skin rash is found in 33–67% of patients.

As many as 76% of patients with disseminated lupus erythematosus develop arthritis and 10% develop deformities of the hands, including Jaccoud's arthropathy.

The kidney is affected in some 75% of patients, including focal proliferative, diffuse proliferative, or membranous glomerulonephritis. Renal failure is a common cause of death.

Neuropsychiatric symptoms are common: 20% of patients may have an organic brain syndrome; 10% may have a psychosis. Epileptiform seizures, occurring in 15%, may be an early symptom, especially in children.

Pulmonary involvement may lead to alveolar hemorrhage, interstitial lung disease, and pulmonary hypertension resembling primary pulmonary hypertension.

Hematologic abnormalities are common. As many as 25% of patients have autoimmune thrombocytopenia. Hemolytic anemia and leukopenia also occur.

Cardiovascular features

The heart almost always shows evidence of involvement at autopsy, but clinical heart disease is less common. The cardiovascular findings are various (**Fig. 2.49**). Pericarditis is found at autopsy in 67% of patients, but occurred clinically in 19–48% of reported series; acute pericarditis may be the presenting symptom of the disease. Pericarditis may be due to complicating renal failure or infection, in addition to lupus *per se*. Cardiac tamponade may occur, and constrictive pericarditis has been reported, but is rare. Myocarditis is recognized in about 10% of patients; the presenting clinical feature may be arrhythmia or congestive heart failure.

Valvular heart disease has been commonly reported. The characteristic Libman–Sacks lesion is that of verrucous vegetations that occur on both

→ Fig. 2.48
Disseminated lupus erythematosus. This patient has the typical reddish facial rash. Xanthelasma can also be seen on the eyelids.

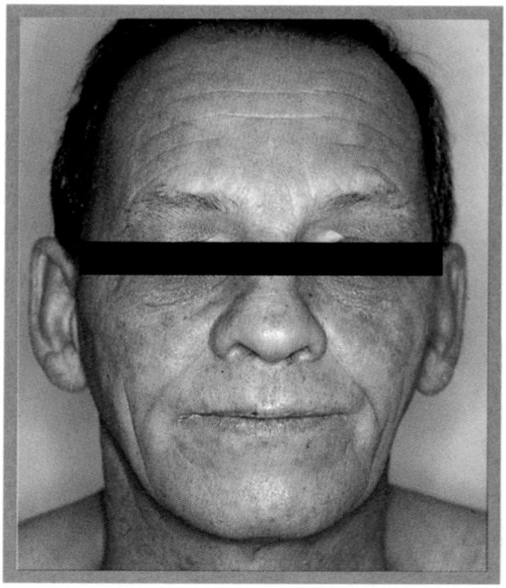

valvular and endocardial surfaces, especially in the valve pockets and on the ventricular aspect of the posterior leaflet of the mitral valve. Prospective echocardiographic studies showed typical verrucous vegetations in 9% of 74 patients in one study, although some valvular abnormality was found in 61% of 69 patients in a study by Roldan *et al.* About 1–2% of patients have clinically significant valve disease; uncommonly, valve replacement is required. The valvular involvement is more likely to lead to valvular insufficiency than to stenosis, but aortic stenosis, insufficiency, or both, and mitral stenosis, insufficiency, or both, have been reported. Tricuspid valve involvement is less common (**Fig. 2.50**).

Coronary artery disease has been recently appreciated as a significant cause of morbidity and mortality in systemic lupus erythematosus, and the coronary disease etiology is believed to be multifactorial. Hyperlipidemia and hypertension as a result of renal disease are common in patients with lupus.

Cardiac involvement in systemic lupus erythematosus

- A diffuse microvasculitis; heart usually involved
- Clinical pericarditis in about 33% of cases; presenting symptom of lupus in 6%
- Cardiac tamponade and constrictive pericarditis are uncommon, but may occur
- Myocarditis with left ventricular dysfunction is common, but congestive failure is uncommon
- More than 50% have aortic or mitral valve thickening, vegetations, or both (Libman–Sacks lesions) on echocardiogram
- Valvular lesions may lead to ischemic stroke
- A few patients develop severe mitral or aortic regurgitation requiring valve replacement
- Newborns of mothers with lupus may have complete atrioventricular block
- Antiphospholipid antibodies may lead to recurrent arterial or venous thrombosis, including coronary artery disease

← Fig. 2.49 Cardiac involvement in systemic lupus erythematosus.

Glucocorticoid therapy may induce dyslipoproteinemia. Autopsy studies of patients who died of lupus have shown a high incidence of coronary disease in those treated with costicosteroids for more than 2–3 years. Circulating immune complexes may promote intracellular accumulation of cholesterol.

Patients with systemic lupus may develop a secondary antiphospholipid antibody syndrome, with livedo reticularis and venous and arterial occlusive disease, including coronary artery disease. This syndrome may cause fetal death in pregnant women with lupus, especially in the second trimester. Babies of mothers with systemic lupus may have congenital complete A–V block.

An American Rheumatism Association subcommittee listed 11 criteria for the diagnosis of systemic lupus erythematosus: malar rash, discoid rash, photosensitivity, oral ulcers, arthritis, serositis, renal disorder, neurologic disorder, hematologic disorder, immunologic disorder, and antinuclear antibody in the absence of drugs known to produce a lupus-like syndrome. The presence of four of these 11 criteria was considered sufficient for the diagnosis.

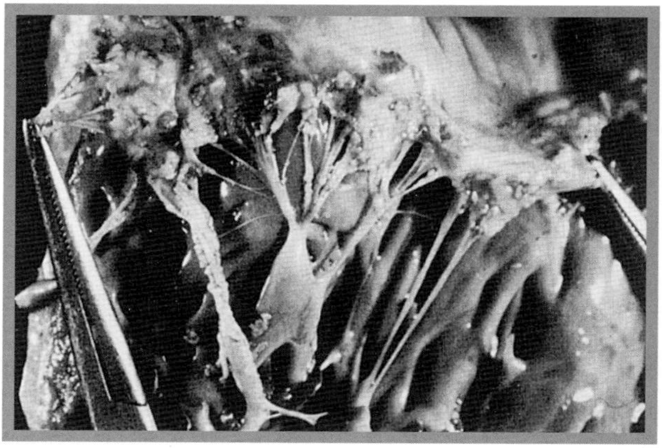

→ Fig. 2.50 Disseminated lupus erythematosus. Heart specimen showing thickening of the tricuspid valve leaflets; verrucous vegetations are seen on the leaflets and chordae tendineae.

Reference

Roldan CA, Shively BK, Crawford MH. An echocardiographic study of valvular heart disease associated with systemic lupus erythematosus. *N Engl J Med* 1996, **335**:1424–1430.

Further reading

Boumpas DT, Austin HA III, Fessler BJ, *et al.* Systemic lupus erythematosus: emerging concepts. Part 1. *Ann Int Med* 1995, **122**:940–950.

Stevens MB. Lupus carditis. *N Engl J Med* 1988, **319**:861–862.

Tan EM, Cohen AS, Fries JF, *et al.* The 1982 revised criteria for the classification of systemic lupus erythematosus. *Arthritis Rheum* 1982, **25**:1271–1277.

Pigmentation Caused by Amiodarone

Amiodarone is an antiarrhythmic agent that is generally recommended only for life-threatening cardiac arrhythmias. Common adverse effects include hepatotoxicity, interstitial pneumonitis, visual disturbances, changes in thyroid function, and neuropathy. Approximately 10–15% of patients develop adverse dermatologic reactions after long-term therapy. Photosensitivity is the most common reaction, occurring in about 10% of treated patients. One occasional effect of prolonged treatment, which is of cosmetic importance only, is that it may cause a blue-gray pigmentation (**Fig. 2.51**); in one report, this occurred in fewer than 1% of patients. The pigmentation usually occurs in areas of skin that are exposed to the sun, and is slowly and occasionally reversible upon discontinuation of the drug.

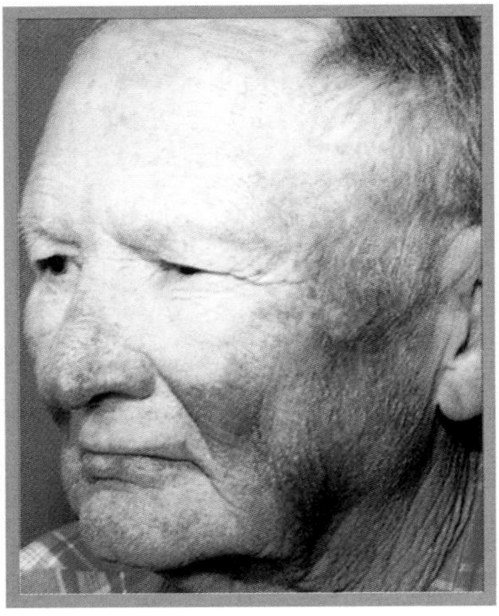

← Fig. 2.51
Pigmentation caused by amiodarone. Blue-gray pigmentation of lips, cheeks, and nose in a man who had received oral amiodarone therapy for 6 years. (With permission from the Massachusetts Medical Society. *New England Journal of Medicine* 1997, **37**:1814.)

3 Eyes

Corneal Arcus

Corneal arcus or corneal annulus is a sign that may be suggestive of hypercholesterolemia, especially in patients younger than 50 years (**Fig. 3.1**). In younger patients, it has been called arcus juvenalis. It may form a triad in type II hyperlipidemia, along with tendinous xanthomata and xanthelasma. In older patients, it may be called annulus senilis, and has little specificity. However, there may be a correlation between the width of the corneal annulus and the serum cholesterol concentration in older patients.

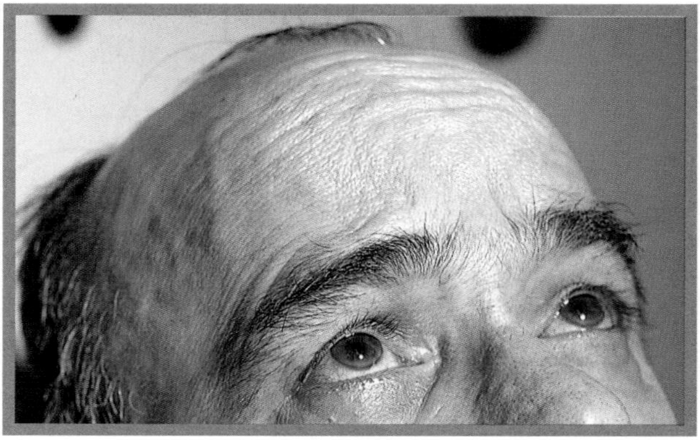

→ Fig. 3.1
Corneal arcus. Corneal arcus in a 49-year-old man who had a myocardial infarction at the age of 45 years. (With permission from Fowler NO. *Diagnosis of heart disease.* Springer–Verlag, 1991.)

Osteogenesis Imperfecta

Osteogenesis imperfecta is a rare disease, and an even more rare cause of valvular heart disease. It is an autosomal dominant genetic disease of connective tissue, also known as 'brittle bone disease'. All forms of the disease are caused by mutations of either of the two chains that form type J collagen, the principal structural protein of the extracellular matrix of bone, skin, and tendon. The disease varies a great deal in severity, from forms that are lethal in the prenatal period to those that are mild and may even elude clinical detection. Four forms have been described by Marini & Gerber: type I is mild and is associated with blue sclerae, hearing loss, short stature, and prepubertal bone fragility; type II is perinatally lethal; type III is associated with severe bone fragility, skull deformity and extremely short stature, but blue sclerae are absent; type IV is moderately severe and is associated with preambulatory fractures and blue sclerae in infancy.

Active adults with osteogenesis imperfecta usually have a history of deafness and prepubertal fractures of long bones, and belong to type I. Blue sclerae are a prominent finding in these patients (**Fig. 3.2**) but they also have several other causes (**Fig. 3.3**). Valvular heart disease with myxomatous degeneration of the mitral or aortic valves may be present (**Fig. 3.4**); less

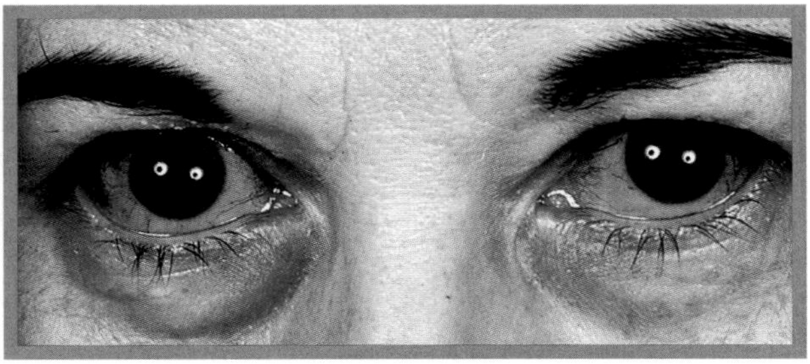

← Fig. 3.2
Osteogenesis imperfecta. Blue sclerae in a patient with osteogenesis imperfecta and severe mitral regurgitation.

Causes of blue sclerae

- Osteogenesis imperfecta
- Pseudoxanthoma elasticum (Autosomal Dominant type II–Marfanoid features)
- Marfan's syndrome
- Fragilitas oculi
- Ehlers–Danlos syndrome (skin hyperextensibility, hypermobile joints, connective tissue fragility)

↑ Fig. 3.3
Causes of blue sclerae.

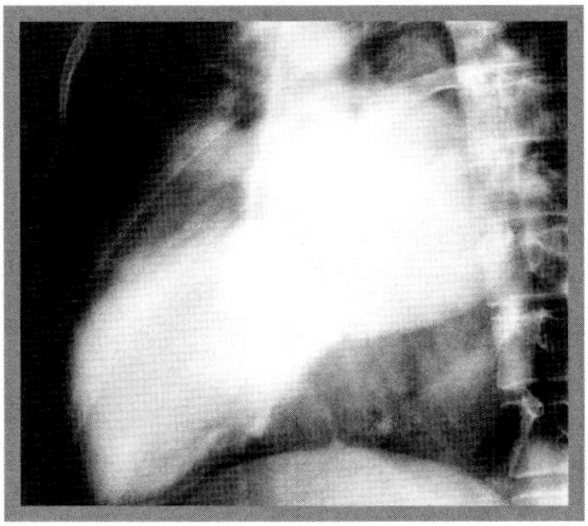

↑ Fig. 3.4
Osteogenesis imperfecta. Left ventriculogram showing severe mitral regurgitation in the patient in Figure 3.2.

commonly, the tricuspid valve is affected. Aortic root dilatation is fairly common but clinical valvular disease is relatively uncommon (**Fig. 3.5**). Between 1965 and 1993, 20 cases of osteogenesis imperfecta with severe valvular incompetence had been reported in persons aged 19–61 years. Aneurysms of the sinuses of Valsalva or ascending aorta have also been reported.

→ Fig. 3.5 Osteogenesis imperfecta.

Osteogenesis imperfecta

Qualitative defect in type I procollagen synthetase

Cardiac involvement: aortic regurgitation, mitral regurgitation

Aortic root dilatation

Echocardiographic study of 109 patients:
- aortic root dilatation in 12%
- aortic insufficiency in 2/109
- aortic stenosis in 1/109
- mitral prolapse in 1/109

Aortic and/or mitral valve replacement have been reported

Reference

Marini JC, Gerber NL. Osteogenesis imperfecta. Rehabilitation and prospects for gene therapy. *JAMA* 1997, **277**:746–750.

Further reading

Hortop J, Tsipouras P, Hanley JA, Maron BJ, Shapiro JR. Cardiovascular involvement in osteogenesis imperfecta. *Circulation* 1986, **73**:54–61.

Stein D, Kloster FE. Valvular heart disease in osteogenesis imperfecta. *Am Heart J* 1977, **94**:637–641.

Thibault GE. The heart of the matter. Clinical problem solving. *N Engl J Med* 1993, **329**:1406–1409.

Ocular Fundi

Cholesterol emboli

Cholesterol emboli involving the retinal arteries usually arise from the ascending aorta, aortic arch, or the carotid arteries; their source is an atherosclerotic plaque, and an aortic source can be demonstrated by echocardiography. Those found in the retinal artery branches are often needle-shaped, and may cause transient visual field defects (**Fig. 3.6**). Cholesterol emboli may damage the arterial wall and cause a perivascular exudate.The retinal photograph of cholesterol emboli shown in Figure 3.6 was taken in a 56-year-old woman who had severe hypertension and later died of cerebral hemorrhage.

Malignant hypertension

Ophthalmoscopic examination of the retina in hypertensive patients characteristically shows evidence of arterial vasoconstriction, with arterial narrowing, increased light reflex, and silver- and copper-wiring. When the arterial pressure increases rapidly or when hypertension is severe, retinal hemorrhages, exudates, and papilledema may appear (**Fig. 3.7**); in such

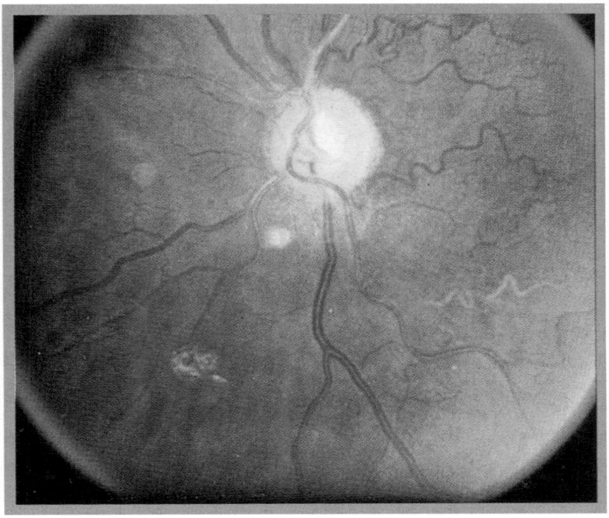

← Fig. 3.6
Ocular fundi: cholesterol emboli. Plaque emboli with obliteration of retinal artery branches, in a 56-year-old woman.

cases, there is an increased likelihood of secondary hypertension. Renal disease is common, and there is a risk of cerebral hemorrhage, hypertensive encephalopathy, or pulmonary edema, or any of these.

Increased intracranial pressure

Retinal photography may reveal a patient without malignant hypertension to have papilledema caused by increased intracranial pressure (**Fig. 3.8**). This finding may occur in patients with brain tumor, brain abscess, intracranial hemorrhage, or meningitis. It also may occur with pseudotumor cerebri. It must be distinguished from optic neuritis and retinal venous outflow obstruction.

Calcific retinal embolus in aortic stenosis

An unusual symptom of calcific aortic stenosis is the abrupt loss of all or part of the visual field in one eye, caused by a calcific embolus (**Fig. 3.9**). Four cases of calcific retinal embolus in patients with aortic stenosis were reported by Brockmeier *et al.*

Calcific aortic stenosis may be of congenital or rheumatic origin, or may occur on a congenital bicuspid aortic valve. However, in the elderly, it is most

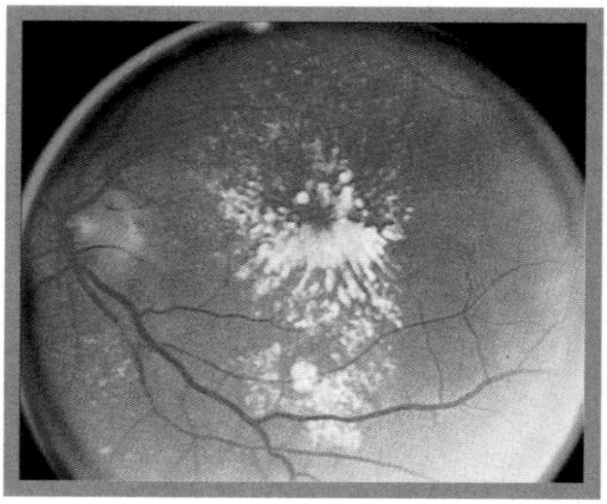

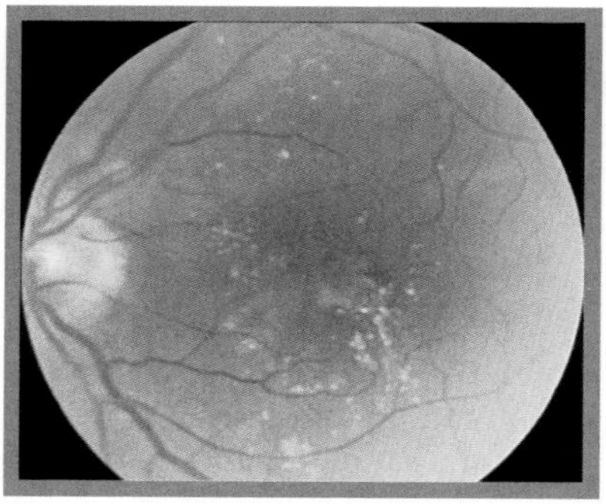

↑ Fig. 3.7a **↑ Fig. 3.7b**

Malignant hypertension: ocular fundi. Serial retinal photographs in a 43-year-old woman with malignant hypertension. (**a**) This photograph shows papilledema and extensive retinal exudate. (**b**) A retinal photograph taken 6 months later, after treatment, showing improvement in the exudate, but persistent papilledema.

often caused by calcific degeneration of a tricuspid aortic valve (**Figs 3.10** and **3.11**). The common symptoms of severe aortic stenosis (aortic valve area less than 0.8cm^2) are angina, syncope, and effort dyspnea. Retinal embolism is a rare complication, and may occur in patients without other symptoms of aortic stenosis.

Sudden loss of vision in one eye may be due to embolus, thrombosis, or spasm of a retinal artery. An embolus may arise from the left atrium, the mitral valve, a left ventricular mural thrombus, a cardiac myxoma, or from vegetations of infective or marantic endocarditis. Aortic stenosis may be suspected as the cause of a retinal embolus when the characteristic ejection systolic murmur is found in the second right intercostal space, adjacent to the sternum (**Fig. 3.12**). The murmur often radiates to the carotid arteries and the cardiac apex, and may have a rough or grunting quality. The degree of the aortic stenosis can be established by left heart catheterization (**Fig. 3.13**).

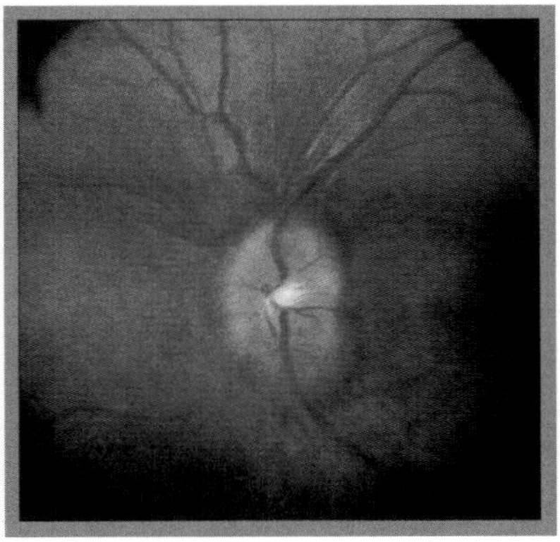

↑ Fig. 3.8
Increased intracranial pressure: ocular fundi. Papilledema in a 42-year-old man with increased intracranial pressure who did not have malignant hypertension. Note absence of exudate.

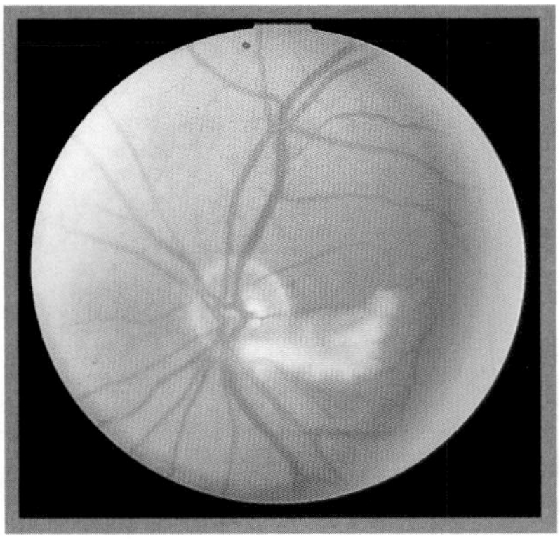

↑ Fig. 3.9
Aortic stenosis: ocular fundi. Calcific retinal embolus in a patient with calcific aortic stenosis. There is a wedge-shaped infarction of the nerve fiber layer of the retina. The arteriolar occlusion is probably at the disc margin, obscured by edema. (With permission from Brockmeier LB, *et al. Am Heart J* 1981, **101**:32–37.)

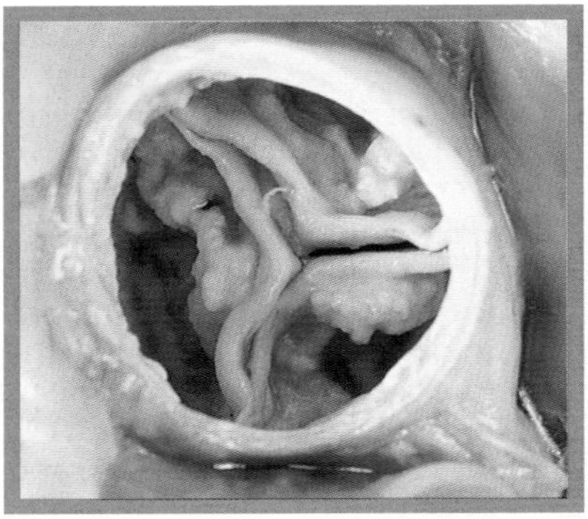

↑ Fig. 3.10
Aortic stenosis. Typical degenerative calcific aortic stenosis in a tricuspid aortic valve. Compare with Figure 3.11.

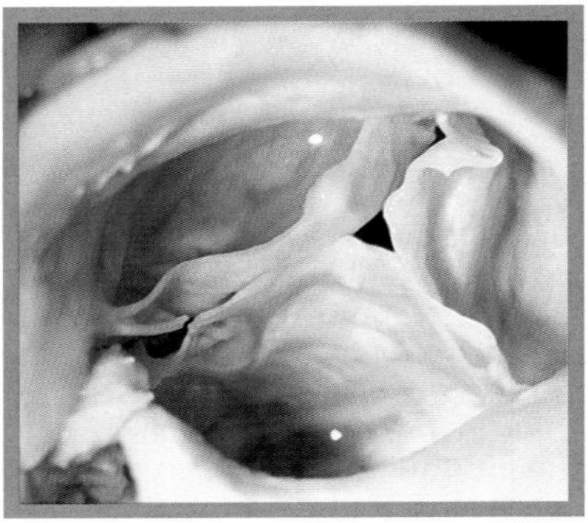

↑ Fig. 3.11
Aortic stenosis. Relatively normal aortic valve, showing thin translucent cusps without calcium deposits.

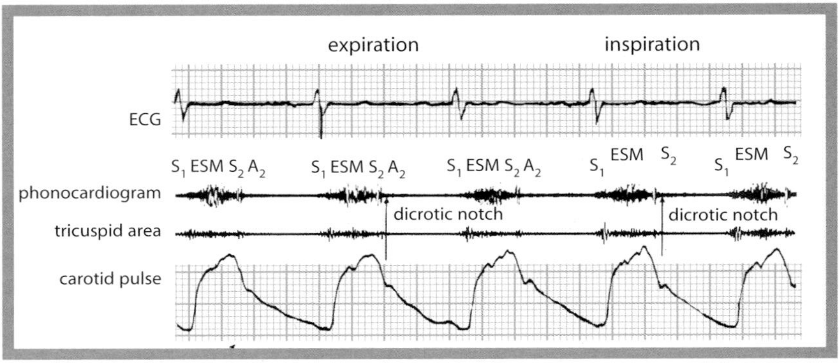

↑ Fig. 3.12
Aortic stenosis. Phonocardiogram and carotid artery pulse record of a patient with severe calcific aortic stenosis. There is a delayed carotid upstroke with an anacrotic notch. The delay in the aortic component (A_2) of the second heart sound (S_2) causes S_2 to become single in inspiration; hence, there is reversed or paradoxical splitting of S_2. ESM, ejection systolic murmur; P_2, pulmonic component of S_2; S_1, first heart sound. (With permission from Fowler NO. *Diagnosis of heart disease*. Springer–Verlag, 1991.)

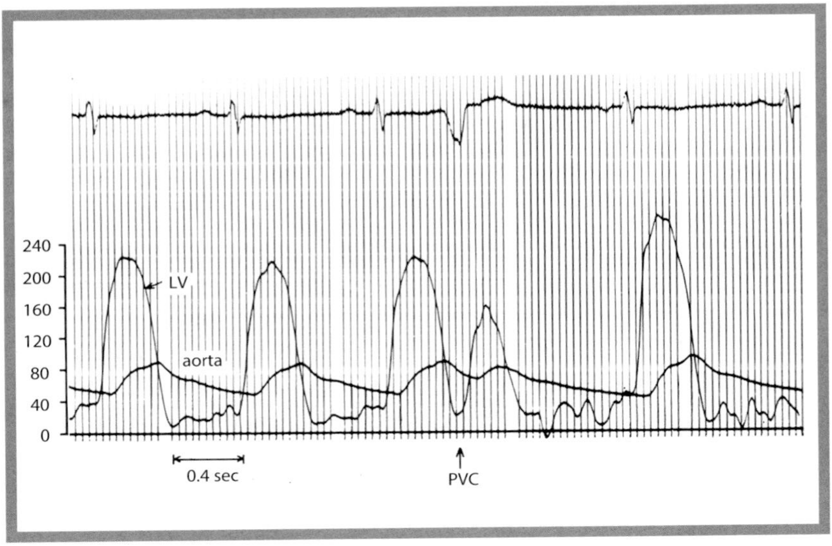

↑ Fig. 3.13
Aortic stenosis. Simultaneous left ventricular and aortic pressure recordings in a 49-year-old man with severe calcific aortic stenosis. The peak left ventricular (LV) systolic pressure is 220mmHg; peak aortic pressure is 90mmHg. At thoracotomy, the aortic valve orifice was only 3–4mm in diameter. PVC, premature ventricular contraction. (With permission from Fowler NO. *Diagnosis of heart disease*. Springer–Verlag, 1991.)

Reference

Brockmeier LB, Adolph RJ, Gustin BW, Holmes JC, Sacks JG. Calcium emboli to the retinal artery in aortic stenosis. *Am Heart J* 1981, **101**:32–37.

Angioid streaks

Angioid streaks represent tears in Bruch's membrane of the retina (see Fig. 8.35) and are associated with pseudoxanthoma elasticum. However, they are not pathognomonic for pseudoxanthoma elasticum, but may be found also in Ehlers–Danlos syndrome, acromegaly, Paget's disease, diabetes mellitus, neurofibromatosis, sicklecell anemia, hemochromatosis, and tuberous sclerosis. Nevertheless, when angioid streaks are found in a young person with premature vascular disease, the diagnosis of pseudoxanthoma elasticum should be suspected (**Fig. 3.14**).

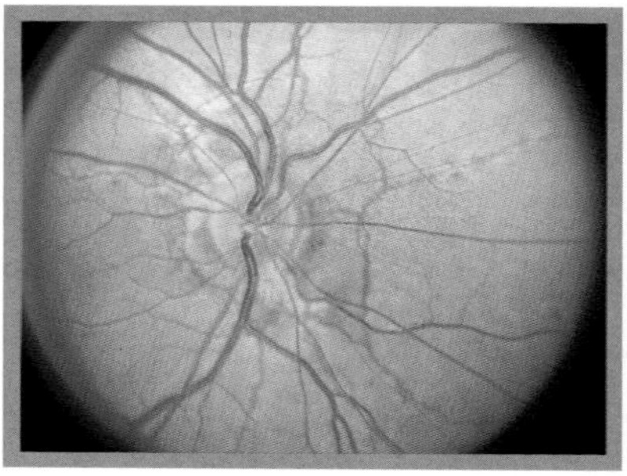

➔ Fig. 3.14
Pseudoxanthoma elasticum: ocular fundi. Angioid streaks in a patient with pseudoxanthoma elasticum. These pale areas in the retinal photograph surround the optic disc and extend along the retinal arteries and veins. They represent tears in Bruch's membranae of the retina (see Chapter 8).

Jaundice with Hepatitis and High Cardiac Output State

The cardiac output may be increased in several liver diseases, including cirrhosis and infectious hepatitis (**Fig. 3.15**). The patient pictured in Figure 3.15 is a young woman with jaundice caused by acute alcoholic hepatitis. She had tachycardia, a wide arterial pulse pressure, and other signs of a high cardiac output state. The mechanism of the increased output remains

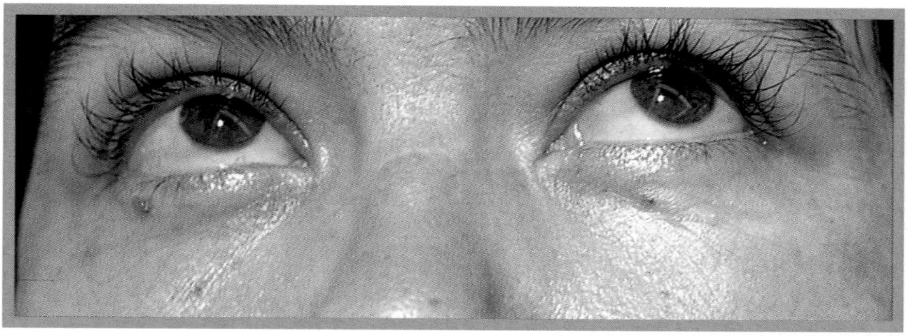

↑ Fig. 3.15
Hyperdynamic state. Jaundice in a young woman with alcoholic hepatitis and a high cardiac output state. Note arterial spiders on the cheeks. She had a wide arterial pulse pressure, tachycardia, and other signs of a high cardiac ouput state. (See Fig. 3.16 and Chapter 1.)

uncertain but has been attributed to increased blood volume, intrahepatic arteriovenous shunts, mesenteric arteriovenous shunts, and defects in inactivation of a circulating vasodilator (**Fig. 3.16**). Congestive heart failure may develop but the patient usually dies of liver disease first.

Hepatic disease: mechanisms of increased cardiac output
Increased blood volume
Failure of inactivation of vasodilator material
Intrahepatic arteriovenous shunts
Mesenteric arteriovenous shunts
Hypoxia caused by intrapulmonary and portopulmonary shunts

← Fig. 3.16
Hepatic disease: mechanisms of increased cardiac output.

Conjunctival Petechiae in Infective Endocarditis

Conjunctival petechiae (**Fig. 3.17**) are very suggestive of infective endocarditis. In patients with this disease, embolic phenomena may also involve the fingers or the toes, including their nail beds, the brain, the spleen, and the coronary arteries. However, these embolic manifestations may have other causes, and are not considered diagnostic.

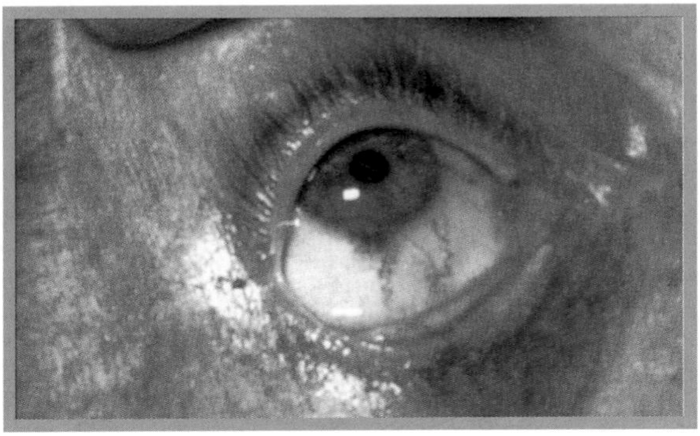

← Fig. 3.17
Infective endocarditis. Subacute bacterial endocarditis: conjunctival petechiae. (With permission from Hurst JW, ed. *The heart, arteries, and veins, 8th ed.* McGraw–Hill, 1994.)

The diagnosis of infective endocarditis usually depends upon three major findings: fever, a cardiac murmur, and a positive blood culture (**Fig. 3.18**). Durack *et al.* proposed new major and minor criteria for the diagnosis of infective endocarditis; a definitive diagnosis requires the presence of two major criteria, or one major and three minor criteria, or five minor criteria.

The two major criteria identified by Durack's group were a minimum of two positive blood cultures at least 12 hours apart, with organisms typical of the disease, and evidence of endocardial involvement. The latter could be provided either by echocardiogram or by the clinical finding of a new regurgitant murmur. Echocardiographic evidence could consist of an

→ Fig. 3.18 Infective endocarditis.

Infective endocarditis
Clinical Features
Fever (>38°C for 1 week or more), cardiac murmur, positive blood culture (95%) Murmur may be absent if acute and on a previously normal valve (especially tricuspid) Aortic and mitral valves most often involved; tricuspid and aortic valves in parenteral drug abusers Embolic phenomena: petechiae; coronary or cerebral embolism may occur Splenomegaly and clubbing may occur, especially in subacute forms Transthoracic echocardiogram shows vegetations in about 60% and transesophageal echocardiogram in about 90%
Most Common Organisms
Streptococci (30–65%) Enterococci (5–15%) *Staphylococcus aureus* (25–40%) Gram-negative bacteria (4–8%)
Indications for Surgical Replacement of Valve
Congestive failure caused by severe valvular regurgitation Systemic embolism Continued positive blood cultures Prosthetic valve involvement with instability

oscillating intracardiac mass (**Fig. 3.19**), a paravalvular abscess, or new partial dehiscence of a prosthetic valve. A new murmur of valvular regurgitation might arise from the aortic valve (**Fig. 3.20**), the mitral valve, or, especially in

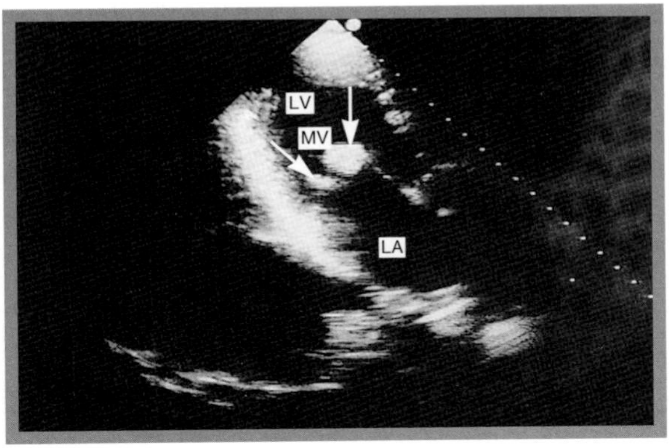

← Fig. 3.19 Infective endocarditis. Two-dimensional echocardiogram showing vegetation (arrows) on the mitral valve (MV). LA, left atrium; LV, left ventricle. (With permission from Fowler NO. *Diagnosis of heart disease*. Springer–Verlag, 1991.)

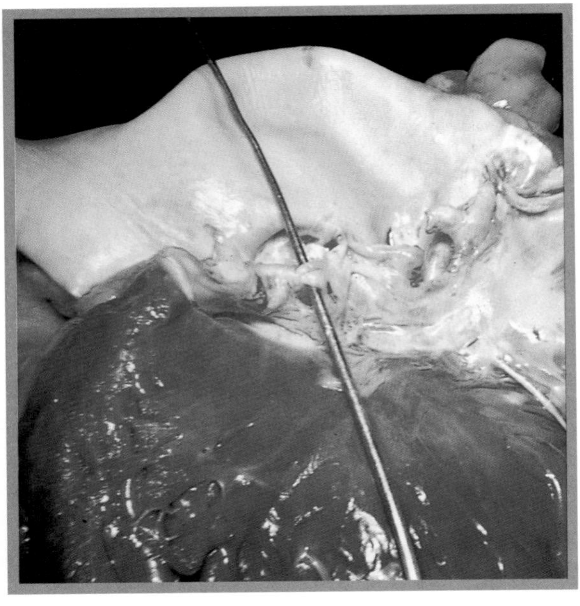

← Fig. 3.20 Infective endocarditis. This autopsy heart specimen shows a metal probe passing through a perforated aortic cusp resulting from acute infective endocarditis.

intravenous drug abusers, the tricuspid valve. Pulmonic valve involvement is rare.

Minor criteria proposed for the diagnosis were: a predisposing heart condition or drug use; fever >38.0°C; vascular phenomena; immunologic phenomena (glomerulonephritis, Osler's nodes, Roth spots in the retina, rheumatoid factor); an echocardiogram showing findings consistent with infective endocarditis but not meeting major criteria; blood cultures positive for atypical organisms. It should be noted that fever was absent in 13% of the definite cases in this study. Blood cultures were negative in 5% in the study by von Reyn *et al.*

References

Durack DT, Lukes AS, Bright DK. New criteria for diagnosis of infective endocarditis: utilization of specific echocardiographic findings. *Am J Med* 1994, **96**:200–209.

von Reyn CF, Levy BS, Arbeit RD, Friedland G, Crumpacker GS. Infective endocarditis: an analysis based on strict case definitions. *Ann Int Med* 1981, **94**:505–517.

4 Cervical Vessels

Congestive Heart Failure

Congestive heart failure is a clinical syndrome in which the cardiac output is inadequate for the metabolic needs of the body. The inadequate cardiac output leads to weakness and fatigue with effort (forward failure). Inadequate blood flow to the kidney causes sodium and water retention. In order to maintain a better cardiac output, the heart tends to dilate, thus increasing its ventricular filling pressure, causing systemic and pulmonary congestion (backward failure). The systemic and pulmonary congestion are due to increases in systemic venous pressure and pulmonary venous pressure, which are aggravated by neurohumoral mechanisms, including increased circulating catecholamines, angiotensin, vasopressin, and aldosterone.

Congestive heart failure is a common condition; it is estimated that there are at least 2,000,000 adults with congestive heart failure in the USA. The most common causes in adults are coronary artery disease and hypertension; valvular heart disease is perhaps the third most common cause. About 5–10% of cases are caused by cor pulmonale, and a similar percentage by cardiomyopathy. In adults, congenital heart disease is a relatively uncommon cause, but heart failure may be seen with atrial septal defect (ASD).

History

There is commonly a history of effort fatigue and dyspnea. The patient may complain of dependent edema, especially about the ankles and legs if ambulatory. Fluid accumulation leads to weight gain, which conceals the fact that there is a loss of lean body mass. Orthopnea and paroxysmal nocturnal dyspnea are common, and acute pulmonary edema may lead to increased dyspnea, orthopnea, wheezing, and pinkish sputum. Insomnia is a frequent complaint.

Physical findings

One of the most striking findings is that related to the increased systemic venous pressure of right ventricular failure. The systemic venous pressure increase is demonstrated by examination of the recumbent patient with the head, neck, and trunk elevated to 30° from the horizontal (**Fig. 4.1**). Other findings related to increased systemic venous pressure include hepatomegaly, dependent edema, and ascites. In milder cases, one may

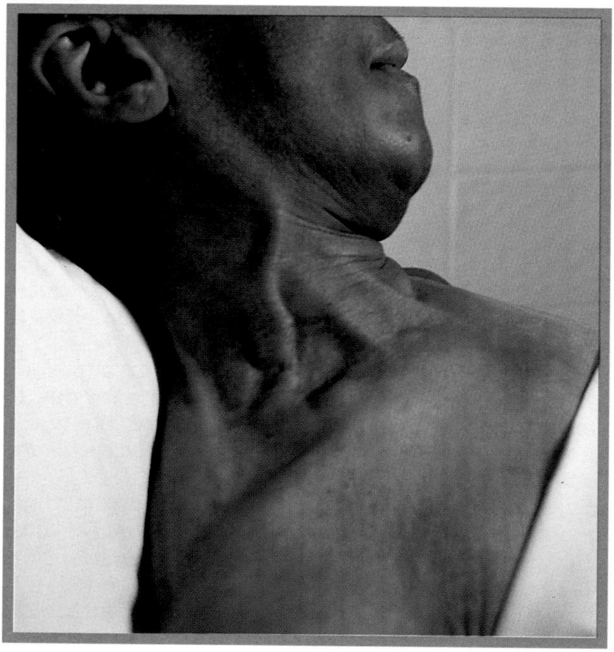

← Fig. 4.1 Congestive heart failure. Photograph of a patient with severe heart failure. The patient is lying with the head and trunk elevated at an angle of 30° from the horizontal. The external jugular vein is distended to the angle of the mandible. The systemic venous pressure was greater than 30cmH_2O.

demonstrate jugular venous distention in response to moderate abdominal pressure (hepatojugular reflux).

Other aspects of the physical examination relate to the pulmonary congestion of left ventricular failure. The patient may be orthopneic, and the ventilatory rate is often increased. Pulsus alternans is occasionally found in advanced cases (**Fig. 4.2**). Examination of the heart is important. Cardiac enlargement is usually present, and valvular heart disease may be found. An important finding is the S_3 gallop (**Fig.4.3**). In persons older than 30 years this finding at the cardiac apex usually, but not always, equates with an increased left ventricular end-diastolic pressure and left ventricular dysfunction. The pulmonary congestion of left ventricular failure may also be indicated by fine and medium basilar pulmonary rales. In more advanced heart failure, the rales are more generalized and perhaps accompanied by wheezing. The physical signs of pulmonary congestion may be confirmed by chest radiography (**Figs 4.4–4.6**). Pleural effusion is common when there is biventricular failure. Cheyne–Stokes respiration may be seen with left ventricular failure.

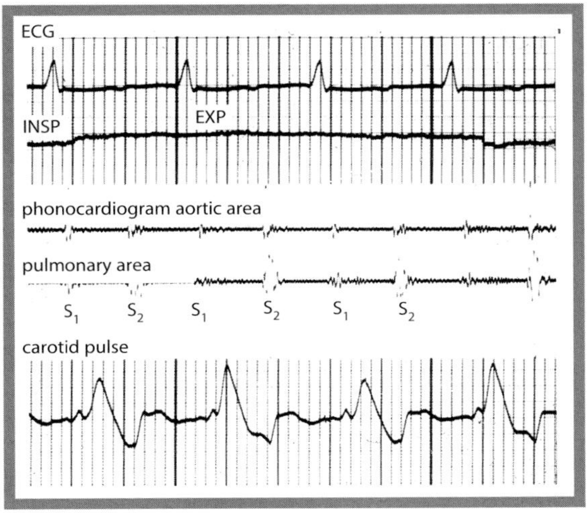

→ Fig. 4.2
Congestive heart failure. Pulsus alternans in the carotid pulse of a patient with congestive heart failure. This sign of left ventricular dysfunction can be brought out by having the patient sit or stand. It must be distinguished from an alternating pulse amplitude caused by premature systoles in a bigeminal pattern. S_1, first heart sound; S_2, second heart sound.

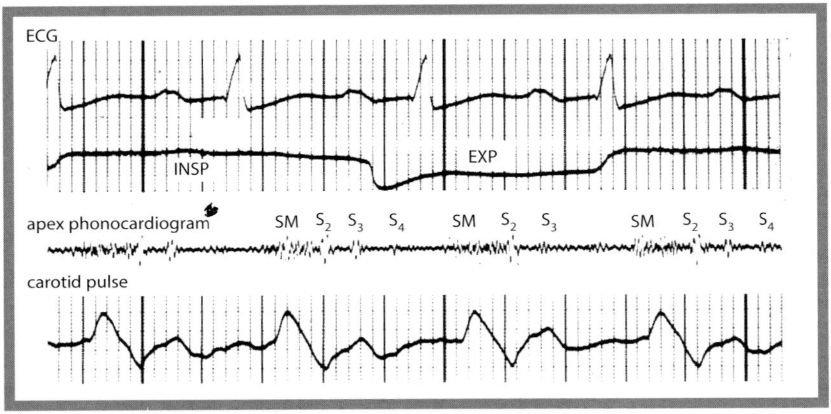

↑ Fig. 4.3
Congestive heart failure. S_3 (protodiastolic gallop) in a 20-year-old woman with cardiomyopathy. A presystolic gallop (S_4) is also recorded. An apical S_3 gallop usually means that the left ventricular diastolic pressure is increased, and is a confirmatory sign of congestive heart failure. However, an S_3 may be normal in patients younger than 30 years. S_1, first heart sound; S_2, second heart sound.

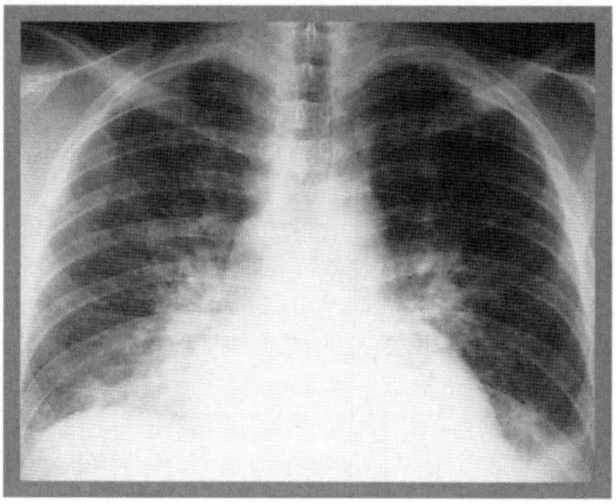

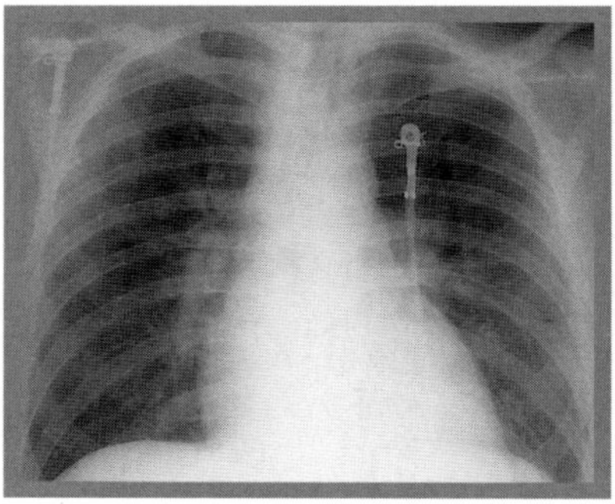

↑ Fig. 4.4a **↑ Fig. 4.4b**

Congestive heart failure. (**a**) Chest radiogram of a 33-year-old man with AIDS-related cardiomyopathy and congestive heart failure. Note cardiac enlargement, bilateral alveolar infiltrate, hilar engorgement, and left pleural effusion. (**b**) Chest radiogram of the same patient after 10 days of treatment for congestive heart failure. Note clearing of alveolar infiltrate and pleural effusion.

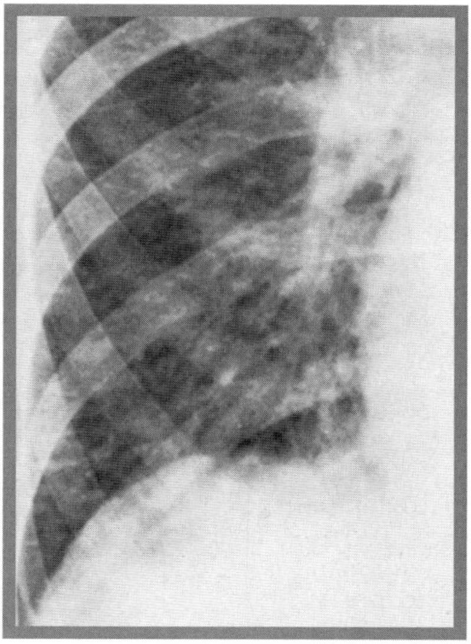

← Fig. 4.5

Congestive heart failure. Chest radiogram showing transverse basal septal lines, also known as Kerleys B lines, in the right costophrenic angle of a patient with congestive heart failure. This is a valuable sign of increased pulmonary capillary pressure as a result of left ventricular failure, but may also occur with lymphatic obstruction caused, for example, by lung cancer. (With permission from Fowler NO. *Diagnosis of heart disease*. Springer–Verlag, 1991.)

→ Fig. 4.6a
Congestive heart failure. Chest radiogram showing pseudotumor attributable to interlobar pleural effusion in a patient with congestive heart failure. Note cardiac enlargement.

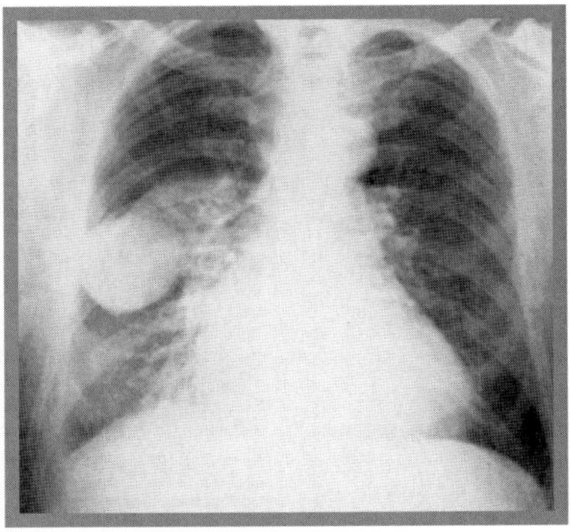

→ Fig. 4.6b
The same patient, 8 days later, after treatment for congestive heart failure. The pleural effusion has almost disappeared.

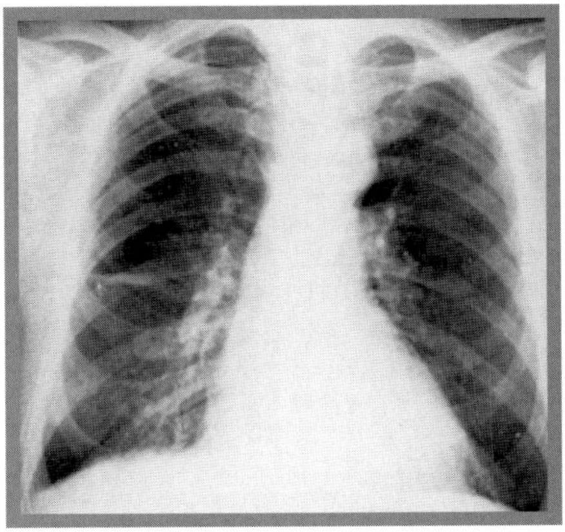

Echocardiograms are useful in the study of patients with congestive heart failure. Localized left ventricular contraction abnormalities suggest coronary disease as the etiology. Valvular or congenital heart disease may be recognized or quantitated, and chamber size and function can be measured. With left ventricular failure, the systolic ejection fraction is usually less than 50%. However, in as many as 40% of patients with left ventricular failure, the left ventricular ejection fraction is normal, especially in hypertensive patients. In these patients, the echocardiogram may demonstrate diastolic dysfunction (**Fig 4.7**). Maintenance of increased blood pressure during the Valsalva maneuver is a useful sign (**Fig. 4.8**).

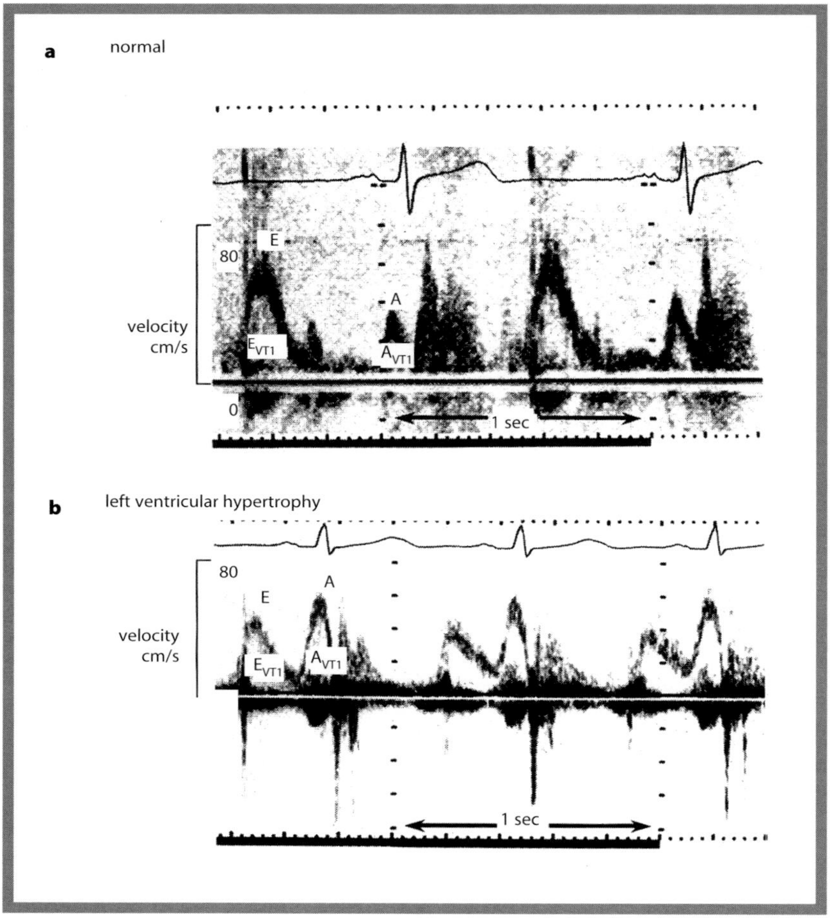

↑ Fig. 4.7
Congestive heart failure. Two-dimensional Doppler echocardiogram. In this patient with left ventricular hypertrophy, the A wave of mitral valve flow velocity is larger that the early diastolic E wave, indicating decreased left ventricular compliance, as may be seen in some patients with left ventricular failure and diastolic dysfunction.

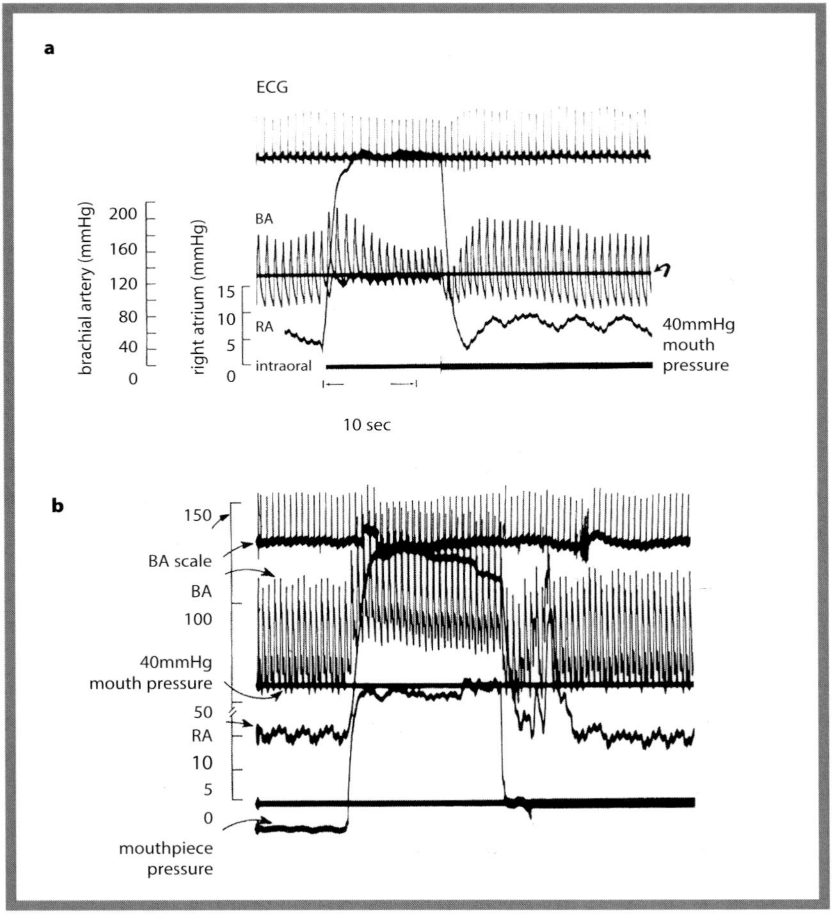

↑ Fig. 4.8

Congestive heart failure. 'Square-wave' response to Valsalva maneuver in a patient with congestive heart failure. (**a**) In the normal individual, the blood pressure declines during the latter part of the strain. (**b**) In the patient with heart failure, the blood pressure is maintained during the strain. BA, brachial arterial pressure; RA, right atrial pressure. (With permission from Fowler NO. *Diagnosis of heart disease*. Springer–Verlag, 1991.)

Diagnosis

An important aspect of the diagnosis is the determination of the underlying cause, and one should also investigate precipitating factors (**Fig. 4.9**). The diagnosis of congestive heart failure depends upon the clinical criteria enumerated in **Fig. 4.10.** Major and minor criteria for the diagnosis were given in the Framingham study paper by McKee *et al*. Major criteria included

Precipitating factors in congestive heart failure
Cardiac arrhythmias, especially atrial fibrillation; also atrial flutter, ventricular tachycardia, and other tachycardias
Excessive intake of sodium, either dietary or by intravenous route
Discontinuation of cardiac medication
Myocardial infarction
Pulmonary embolism
Pulmonary infections
Pregnancy
Hyperthroidism
Severe anemia
Physical or emotional stress
Infective endocarditis
Myocarditis
Sudden severe valvular dysfunction: rupture of mitral chordae tendineae, prosthetic valve dehiscence, fracture, or rupture; severe aortic valve prolapse or perforation from infective endocarditis; papillary muscle infarction
Inappropriate medication: androgens, estrogens, β-adrenergic blocking agents, sodium-retaining steroids, adriamycin, verapamil, non-steroidal agents
Renal failure
Aggravation of hypertension

↑ Fig. 4.9
Precipitating factors in congestive heart failure.

paroxysmal nocturnal dyspnea or orthopnea, increased systemic venous pressure, rales, cardiomegaly, acute pulmonary edema, S_3 gallop, prolonged circulation time, and hepatojugular reflux. Minor criteria were ankle edema, night cough, exertional dyspnea, hepatomegaly, pleural effusion, decreased vital capacity, tachycardia at 120 beats/min. Two major or one major and two minor criteria present concurrently sufficed for the diagnosis. If hemodynamic studies are undertaken, the pulmonary wedge and left ventricular diastolic pressures are increased above the normal range of 6–12mmHg in left ventricular failure, whereas the right atrial and right ventricular diastolic pressures are increased above the normal range of 0–7mmHg in right ventricular failure.

Diagnostic criteria for congestive heart failure

Increased jugular venous pressure or hepatojugular reflux

Cardiac enlargement or valvular disease

Dependent edema

Pulmonary crackling rales or alveolar infiltrate in absence of fever

S_3 apical gallop

Dyspnea, orthopnea, or tachypnea

Improvement in findings with ≥5pounds (≥2.27kg) weight loss after diuretics

Two criteria = Diagnosis of probable heart failure
Three criteria = Diagnosis of definite heart failure

← Fig. 4.10 Diagnostic criteria for congestive heart failure.

Reference

McKee PA, Castelli WP, McNamara PM, Kannel WB. The natural history of congestive heart failure: The Framingham Study. *N Engl J Med* 1971, **285**:1441–1446.

Further reading

Braunwald E. The pathogenesis of congestive heart failure: then and now. *Medicine* 1991, **70**:68–81.

Stevenson LW, Perloff JK. The limited reliability of physical signs for estimating hemodynamics in chronic heart failure. *JAMA* 1989, **261**:884–888.

Constrictive Pericarditis

Constrictive pericarditis has been defined as a chronic fibrous thickening of the pericardium, which is so contracted that normal diastolic filling of the heart is impaired. It is a relatively uncommon disease, and most large hospitals see no more than a few cases over a period of a year. Almost any cause of acute pericarditis may cause constrictive pericarditis, but in industrialized countries the great majority of patients present with no recognized antecedent of the condition (**Fig. 4.11**). In India, however, the majority of cases are related to tuberculosis.

History

The most common symptoms are slowly developing dyspnea with effort, along with dependent edema and abdominal swelling caused by ascites (**Figs 4.12** and **4.13**). Fatigue is relatively common. In contrast to the usual

Etiology of constrictive pericarditis in 231 patients	
Factor	**No.**
Unknown	169
Acute pericarditis	22
Tuberculosis	14
Radiation	11
Cardiac operation	4
Rheumatic	4
Amyloid	2
Others (Whipple's, Dressler's, hemorrhagic disorder, blunt trauma, rheumatoid arthritis)	5

↑ Fig. 4.11
Etiology of constrictive pericarditis. Data from a study of 231 patients. (From McCaughan BC, Schaff HV, Piehler JM, et al. *J Thorac Cardiovasc Surg* 1985, **89**:340.)

Clinical features of constrictive pericarditis
History
Exertional dyspnea and fatigue Abdominal swelling and discomfort Cough Orthopnea
Physical Findings
Jugular venous distention Hepatomegaly Dependent edema Ascites Kussmaul's sign Pericardial knock (minority) Pulsus paradoxus (minority) Absence of cardiac murmur

↑ Fig. 4.12
Clinical features of constrictive pericarditis.

complaints in congestive heart failure, orthopnea and paroxysmal nocturnal dyspnea are relatively less common. Some patients complain of abdominal pain, possibly caused by hepatic congestion.

Physical examination

In patients with constrictive pericarditis, the systemic venous pressure is invariably increased. This can usually be determined at the bedside by careful examination of the jugular veins (**Fig. 4.14**). Additional information may be obtained from

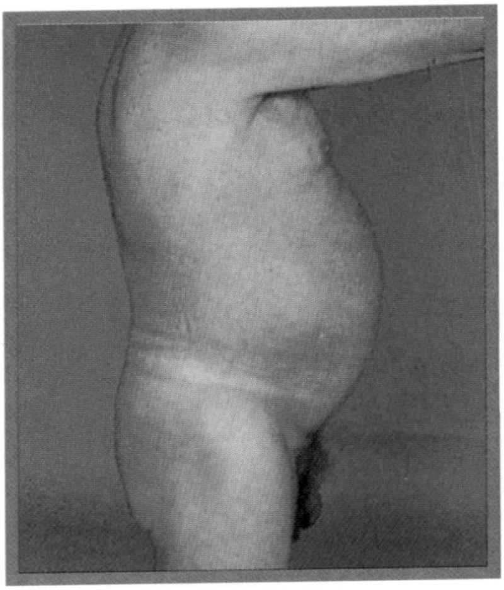

→ Fig. 4.13
Ascites in a patient with increased systemic venous pressure and salt and water retention. This may occur with either congestive heart failure or constrictive pericarditis. It is usually accompanied by hepatomegaly and edema of the lower extremities. Abnormal distention of the neck veins distinguishes this form of ascites from that associated with liver disease or abdominal malignant disease. (With permission from Timmis A, Brecker B. *Diagnosis in color: cardiology*. London, Mosby–Wolfe, 1997.)

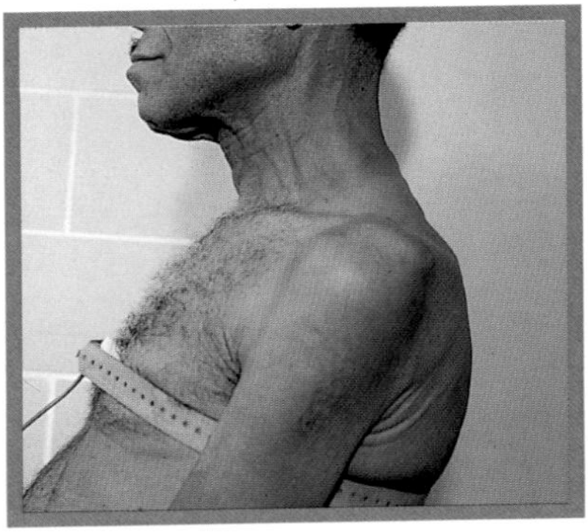

→ Fig. 4.14
Constrictive pericarditis. Distended external jugular veins in a seated patient with effusive-constrictive pericarditis. See Figs 4.21 and 4.22.

more detailed examination of the jugular veins: typically, there is a prominent diastolic Y descent (**Fig. 4.15**). Another characteristic finding is inspiratory swelling of the neck veins, known as Kussmaul's sign (**Fig. 4.16**), which, however, is not specific for constrictive pericarditis (**Fig. 4.17**). An early S_3, the pericardial knock, can be heard in a variable percentage of cases (**Fig. 4.18**): various reports have stated its prevalence to be from 5% to 58%. Pulsus paradoxus, an inspiratory decline of systolic blood pressure of more than 10mmHg, is found in a minority of patients (**Fig. 4.19**). Ascites is found in the majority of patients in most studies, and hepatomegaly and dependent edema are usually present.

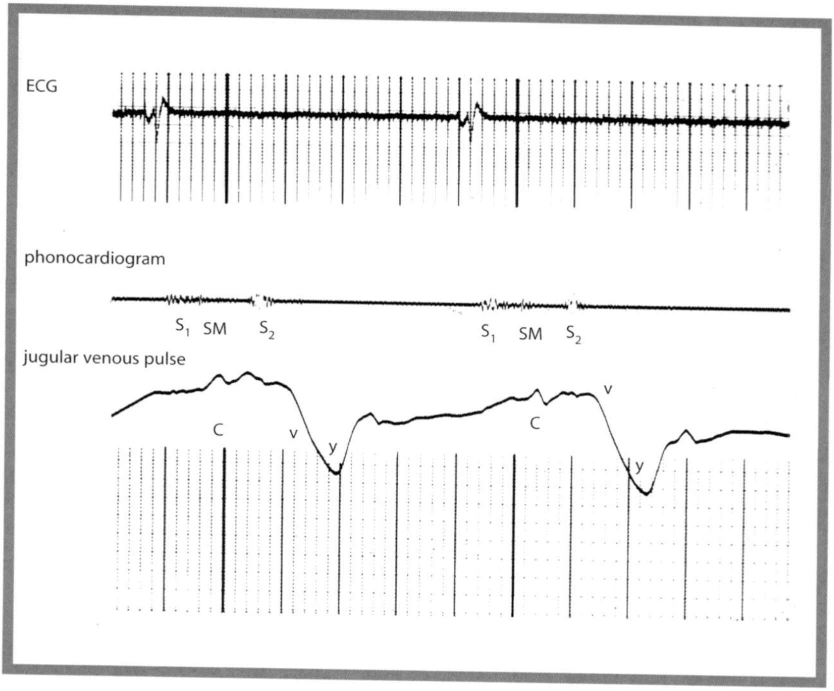

↑ Fig. 4.15
Constrictive pericarditis. Jugular venous pulse recording showing prominent Y descent. S_1, first heart sound; S_2, second heart sound; SM, systolic murmur.

Chest radiogram

Typically, the heart size appears normal on the chest radiogram (**Fig. 4.20**), although some cardiac enlargement is found in a minority of patients—especially those with effusive-constrictive pericarditis (**Figs 4.21** and **4.22**). The lungs are usually free of congestion or alveolar infiltrate, but pulmonary congestion is found in perhaps 5–10% of patients (**Fig. 4.23**). Pleural effusion is a common radiologic finding. Pericardial calcification was found in 40% of

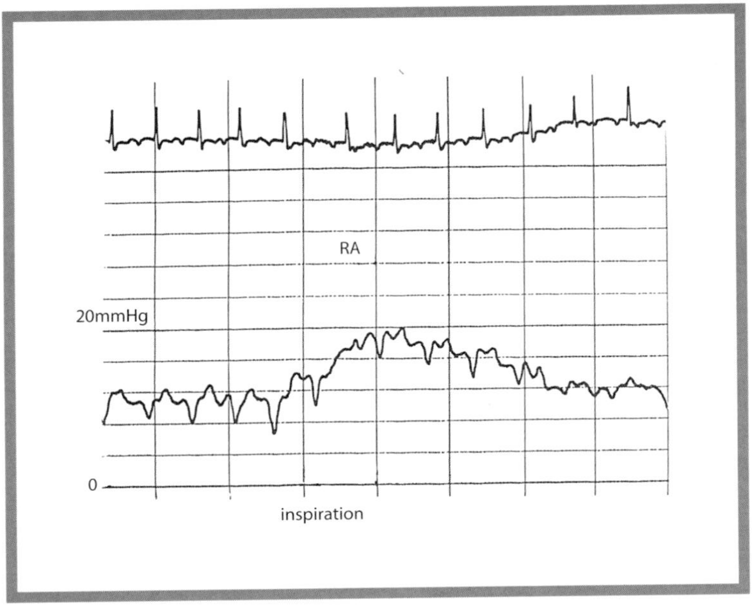

↑ Fig. 4.16
Constrictive pericarditis. Kussmaul's sign. Right atrial (RA) pressure record, showing increased mean pressure of 12mmHg (normal range 0–7mmHg). With inspiration, instead of the normal decline, the right atrial pressure increases. There is a prominent Y descent. The ECG shows that the rhythm is atrial flutter with varying A–V block. (With permission from Fowler NO. *Diagnosis of heart disease*. Springer–Verlag, 1991.)

Kussmaul's sign

Defined as inspiratory swelling of the neck veins

Found in 13% of 95 constrictive pericarditis cases (Stanford series)

Also occurs with tricuspid stenosis, right ventricular infarction, right ventricular failure, restrictive cardiomyopathy

Does not occur with cardiac tamponade

More commonly associated with failure of right heart pressures to decrease with inspiration than with inspiratory pressure increase*

Mechanism uncertain—attributed to traction on veins by Kussmaul

Lancet* 1989, **1:1337.

← Fig. 4.17
Constrictive pericarditis: Kussmaul's sign.

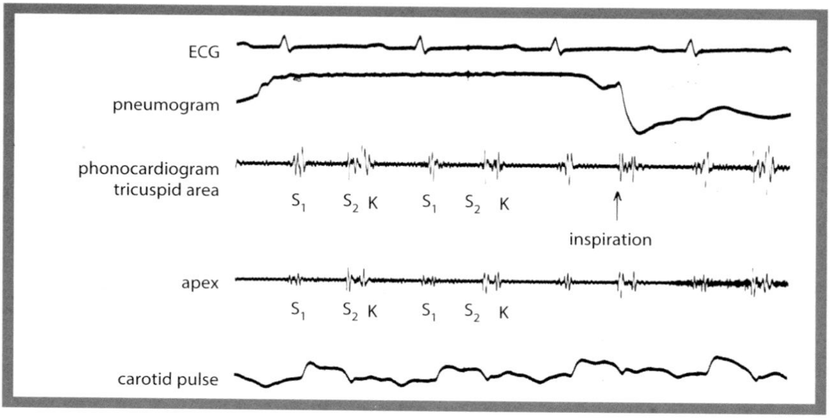

↑ Fig. 4.18
Constrictive pericarditis. Phonocardiogram, showing pericardial knock (K) in a patient with constrictive pericarditis. In this example, this early third sound follows the aortic component of the second sound by 0.06 seconds. The S_3 gallop of left ventricular dysfunction occurs later, 0.12–0.18 seconds after the aortic component of S_2.

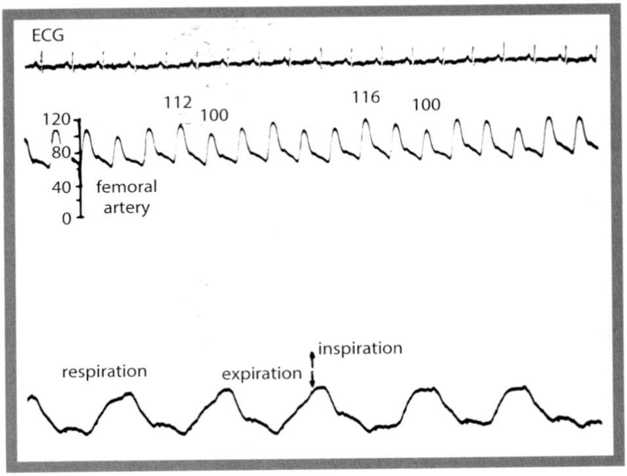

→ Fig. 4.19
Constrictive pericarditis. Pulsus paradoxus. Femoral arterial pressure record, showing an inspiratory decline in systolic pressure of up to 16mmHg. (With permission from Fowler NO. *Ann Int Med* 1953, **38**:478–511.)

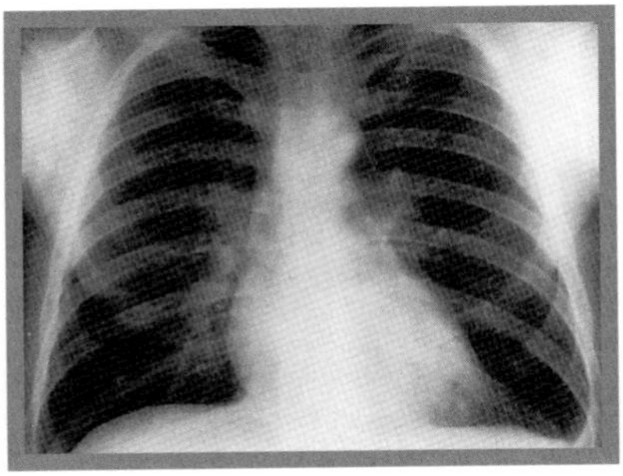

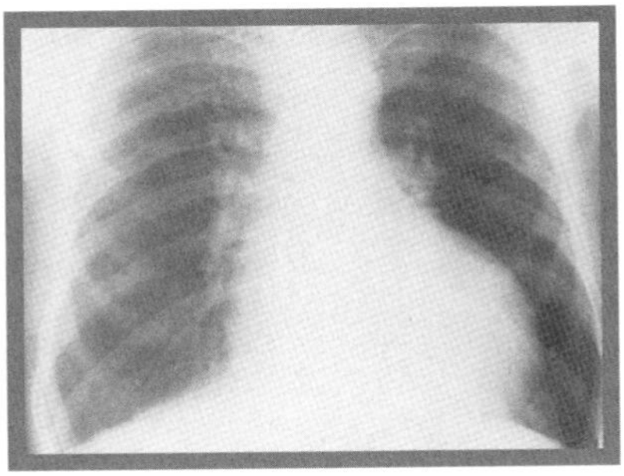

↑ Fig. 4.20
Constrictive pericarditis. The normal heart size and clear lung fields are characteristic of constrictive pericarditis, unlike the enlarged heart and alveolar infiltrate usually seen in congestive heart failure. (With permission from Fowler NO. *The pericardium in health and disease*. Futura Publishing Co., 1985.)

↑ Fig. 4.21
Constrictive pericarditis. The heart is moderately enlarged, and more characteristic of effusive-constrictive pericarditis than of pure constrictive pericarditis. The enlarged cardiopericardial silhouette is explained by the presence of about 300ml of pericardial fluid, in addition to thickened visceral and parietal pericardium in this patient.

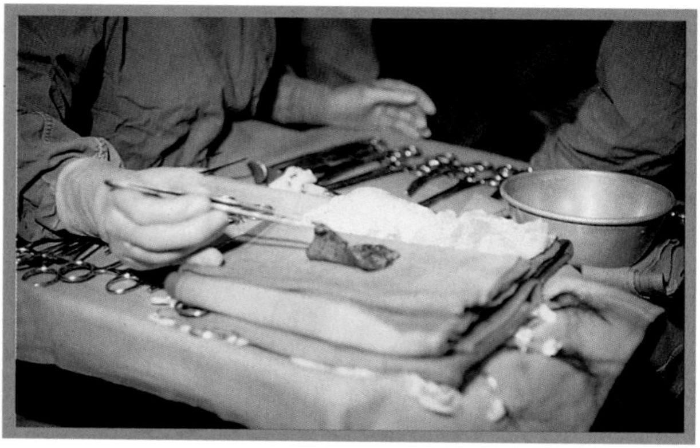

↑ Fig. 4.22
Constrictive pericarditis. Photograph of thickened parietal pericardium of the same patient as in Figures 4.14 and 4.21. There was 300ml of pericardial fluid between the visceral and parietal pericardium in this patient with effusive-constrictive pericarditis.

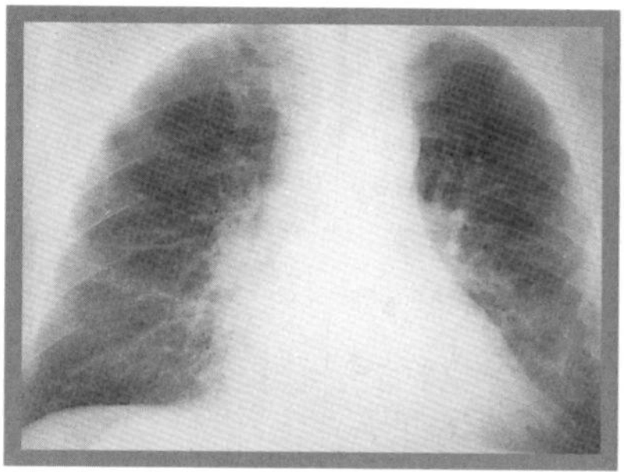

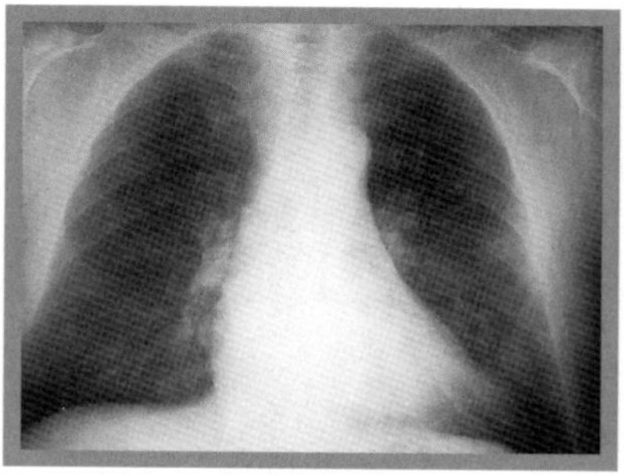

↑ Fig. 4.23a **↑ Fig. 4.23b**
Constrictive pericarditis. (**a**) Cardiac enlargement and pulmonary congestion. (**b**) Improvement after 6 days of diuretic therapy. This patient later underwent successful pericardiectomy. Pulmonary congestion is uncommon in constrictive pericarditis but may be seen in as many as 10% of patients. (With permission from Fowler NO. *The pericardium in health and disease*. Futura Publishing Co., 1985.)

patients in older series, but was found in only 5% in some recent studies (**Figs 4.24** and **4.25**). Rarely, the thickened parietal pericardium may be seen overlying the epicardial fat on plain chest radiogram (**Fig. 4.26**).

The ECG is not specific. Common findings are low-voltage QRS complexes and abnormal T waves (**Fig. 4.27**). The P waves often show evidence of left atrial enlargement, and atrial fibrillation is found in 20% of patients, or more; about 5% have atrial flutter. Patterns of bundle branch block or ventricular hypertrophy are uncommon.

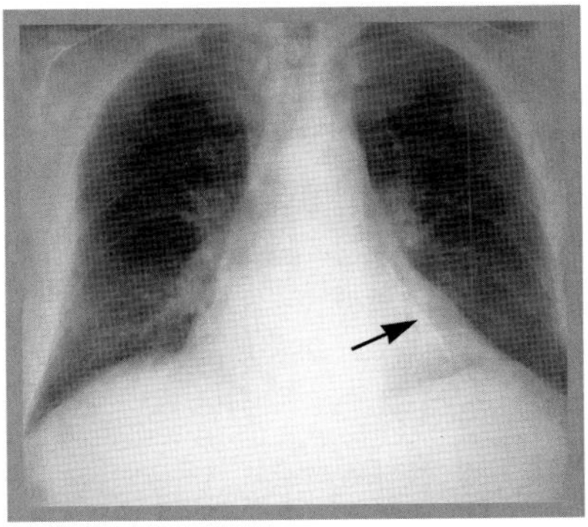

→ Fig. 4.24
Constrictive pericarditis. Chest radiogram showing pericardial calcification (arrow). This was formerly seen in up to 50% of patients with constrictive pericarditis. In recent series, radiologic evidence of pericardial calcification has been reported in only 5–21% of patients. Pericardial calcification alone is not diagnostic of constrictive pericarditis; the characteristic hemodynamic features must also be present.

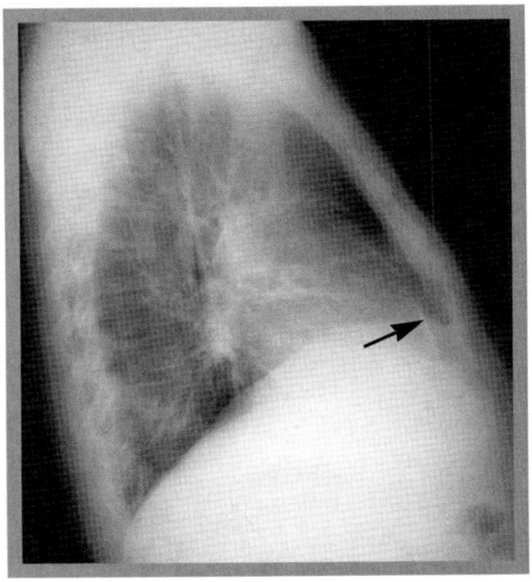

→ Fig. 4.25
Constrictive pericarditis. Chest radiogram, lateral view, showing pericardial calcification in the patient in Figure 4.24 (arrow).

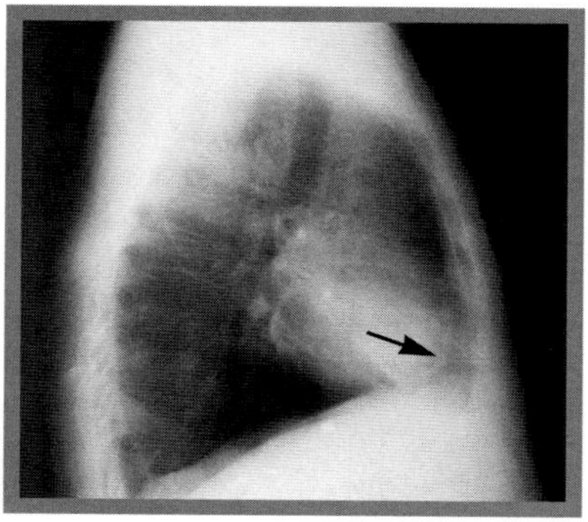

← Fig. 4.26
Constrictive pericarditis. Chest radiogram, lateral view. The thickened parietal pericardium can be visualized (arrow), even though it is not calcified. This is because there is an epicardial fat pad of low radiologic density underneath it.

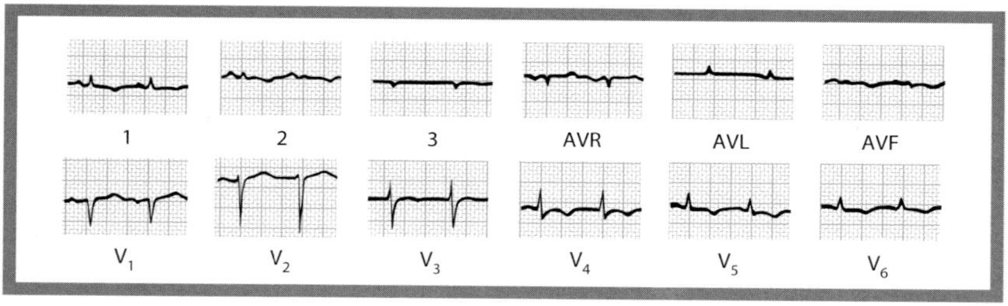

↑ Fig. 4.27
Constrictive pericarditis. Characteristic ECG, showing low voltage of QRS complexes and non-specific T wave abnormalities. (With permission from Fowler NO. *The pericardium in health and disease*. Futura Publishing Co., 1985.)

Hemodynamic study
The findings on right and left heart catheterization are characteristic. There is an equalization of right and left ventricular filling pressures; thus right atrial and right ventricular diastolic mean pressures are equal to or within 4mmHg of pulmonary wedge or left ventricular diastolic pressures. These filling pressures are usually between 12 and 30mmHg. In addition, both right and left ventricular pressure records show an early diastolic dip, followed by a plateau, the 'square-root' sign (**Fig. 4.28**). With effusive-constrictive pericarditis, the pressure tracings resemble those of cardiac tamponade. After pericardiocentesis, the pressure recordings change to resemble those of constrictive pericarditis (**Figs 4.29** and **4.30**).

Diagnosis

The diagnosis should be considered in patients who have increased jugular venous pressure and hepatomegaly in whom there is no or slight cardiac enlargement, and when there is no significant valvular, coronary, pulmonary,

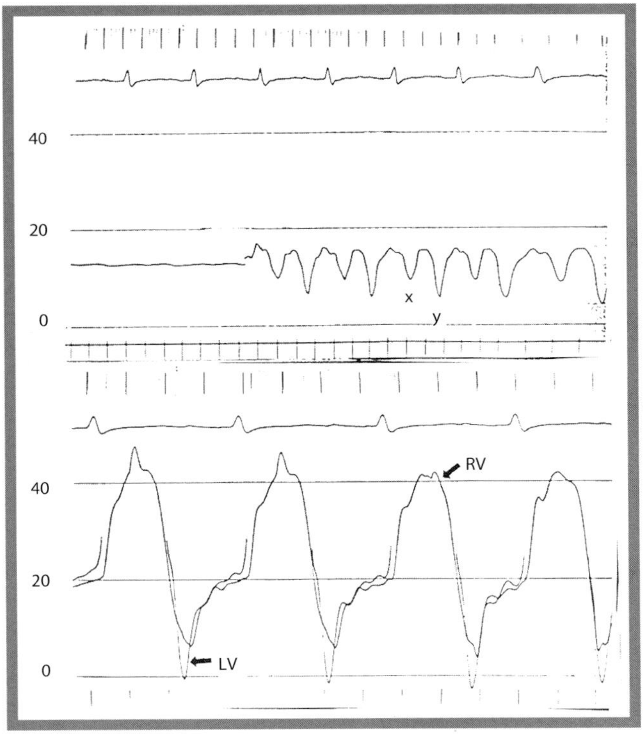

↑ Fig. 4.28

Constrictive pericarditis. Characteristic pressure recordings. The right atrial pressure, above, is increased, with prominent X and Y descents and little respiratory variation. Note that the paper speed is increased toward the end of the record. The right ventricular (RV) pressure shows a typical diastolic dip and plateau ('square-root sign'). The left ventricular (LV) and right ventricular diastolic pressures are equally increased to 20mmHg.

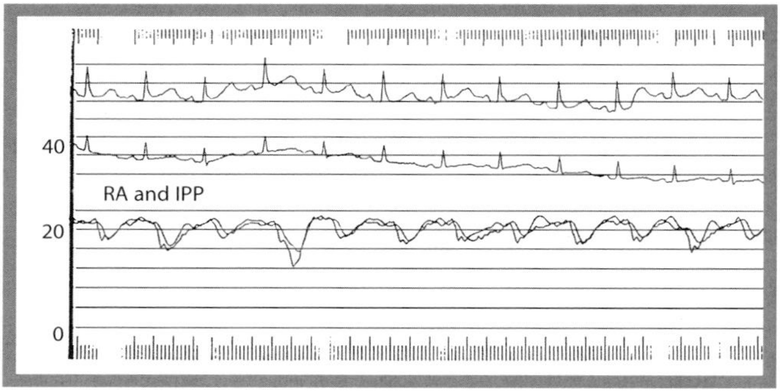

↑ Fig. 4.29
Constrictive pericarditis. Effusive-constrictive pericarditis. Right atrial (RA) and intrapericardial (IPP) pressures are equally increased, to 20mmHg, as one would expect with cardiac tamponade. The Y descent is not prominent. Compare with Figure 4.30.

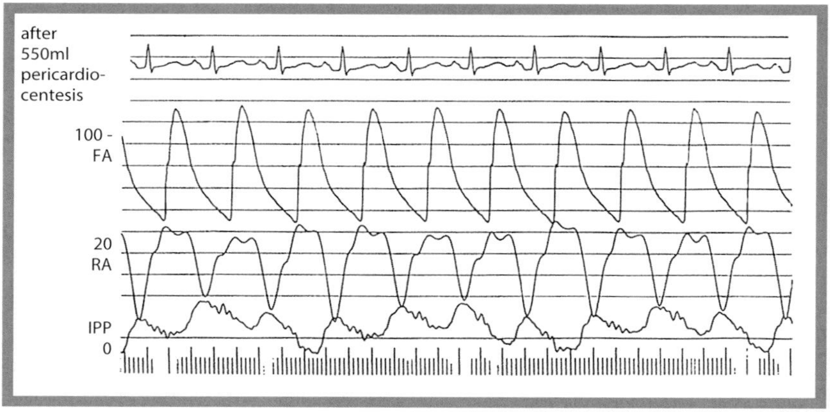

↑ Fig. 4.30
Constrictive pericarditis. Post-pericardiocentesis record of the same patient as in Figure 4.29, who had effusive-constrictive pericarditis. The intrapericardial pressure (IPP) has decreased to nearly zero, but the right atrial pressure remains increased and now shows the prominent Y descent characteristic of constrictive pericarditis. FA, femoral arterial pressure; RA, right atrial pressure.

or hypertensive disease. The diagnosis ultimately depends upon two things: the hemodynamic findings described above, and the demonstration of increased pericardial thickening by pericardial calcification, by magnetic resonance imaging or by computerized tomography (CT) pericardial scanning (**Figs 4.31** and **4.32**). Conventional echocardiography characteristically shows preserved ventricular function and biatrial enlargement but is not very useful in demonstrating increased pericardial thickness. However, study of ventilatory variation in mitral and tricuspid valve flow patterns is useful in distinguishing constrictive pericarditis from restrictive cardiomyopathy, which may have similar hemodynamic features (**Fig. 4.33**).

→ Fig. 4.31
Diagnosis of constrictive pericarditis.

Diagnosis of constrictive pericarditis
Depends upon hemodynamic pattern plus evidence of pericardial thickening or calcification
Pericardial calcification may occur without constriction
Pericardial calcification plus increased venous pressure nearly always implies constriction
Hemodynamic pattern alone may occur with restrictive cardiomyopathy

→ Fig. 4.32
Constrictive pericarditis. CT scan of the chest in a patient with constrictive pericarditis verified at thoracotomy. The thickened pericardium is seen as a rim surrounding the heart (arrow). (With permission from Fowler NO. *Diagnosis of heart disease*. Springer–Verlag, 1991.)

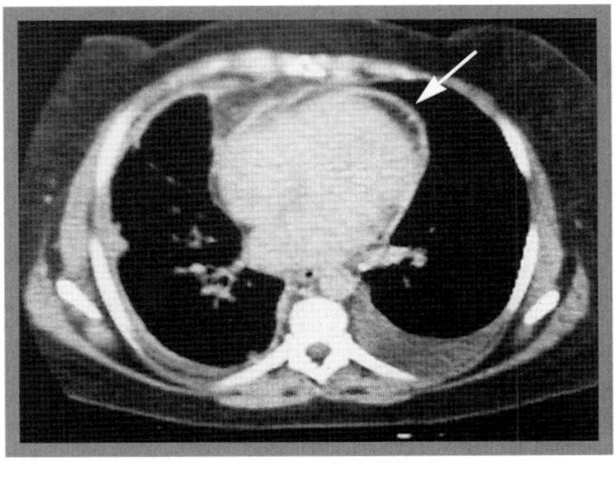

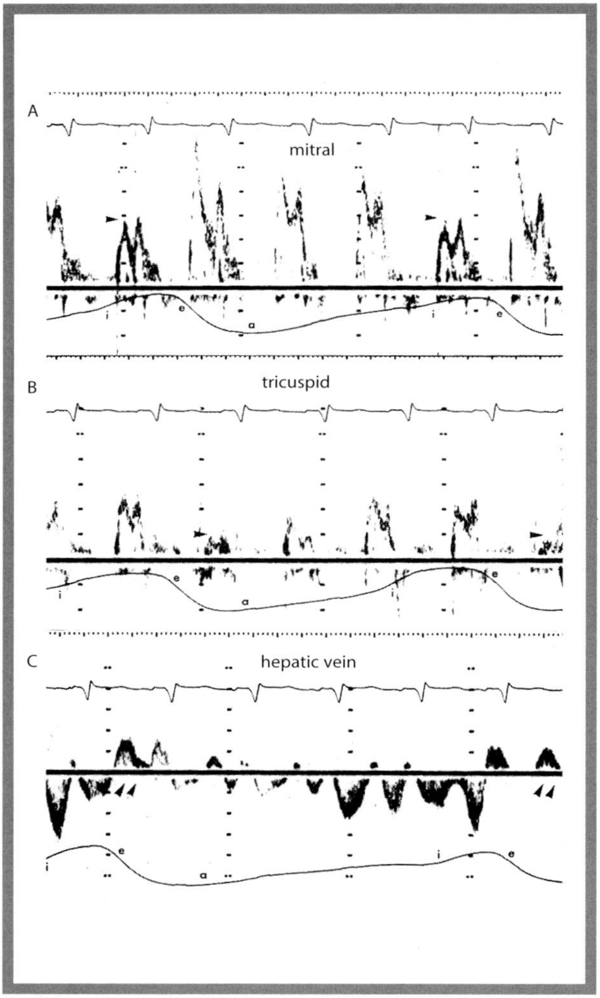

← Fig. 4.33 Constrictive pericarditis. Doppler echocardiogram of mitral and tricuspid flow velocity pattern, showing abnormal inspiratory increase in tricuspid flow velocity and abnormal inspiratory decrease in mitral flow velocity. Normally, the ventilatory variation should be less than 25%. This pattern is useful in distinguishing constrictive pericarditis from restrictive cardiomyopathy. However, a similar variation in A–V valve flow velocity may be seen with obstructive airway disease, right ventricular infarction, or cardiac tamponade.

Further reading

Fowler NO. Constrictive pericarditis: its history and current status. *Clin Cardiol* 1995, **18**:341–350.

Superior Vena Caval Syndrome

The superior vena caval syndrome is a clinical syndrome caused by narrowing or complete obstruction of the superior vena cava, causing an increase in pressure in the superior vena cava and its tributaries. A half-century ago, most cases were caused by syphilitic aortic aneurysm but today the great majority are caused by malignant neoplasms (**Fig. 4.34**). The clinical features of the syndrome largely involve the face, neck and chest (**Fig. 4.35**).

The diagnosis of the superior vena caval syndrome depends upon careful examination of the neck veins, which usually remain distended even when the patient is sitting up (**Figs 4.36** and **4.37**). Two features distinguish this syndrome from the cervical vein distention of congestive heart failure or pericardial disease: one is the absence of venous pulsations; the other is the presence of tortuous collateral veins over the chest (**Figs 4.37** and **4.38**). Swelling of the face and eyelids may also be a feature. In contrast, swelling of the face is rare in adults with congestive heart failure, but may be seen in infants and young children. Radiologic examination can provide evidence of superior mediastinal tumor causing the superior vena caval syndrome (**Fig. 4.39**).

Causes of superior vena caval syndrome
Bronchogenic carcinoma (85%)
Lymphoma (10%)
Mediastinal fibrosis (histoplasmosis, tuberculosis, hemorrhage, methysergide) (<3%)
Aortic aneurysm (dissection)
Miscellaneous (goiter, other metastatic carcinoma, spontaneous thrombosis)

↑ Fig. 4.34
Causes of superior vena caval syndrome.

Superior vena cava syndrome
Swelling of face, neck, chest
Dilated veins over face, neck, chest
Plethora and cyanosis of face
Proptosis and edema of eyelids
Headache

↑ Fig. 4.35
Clinical features of superior vena caval syndrome.

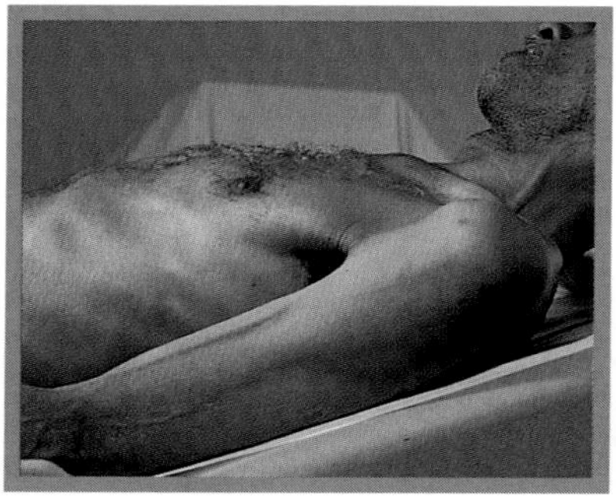

← Fig. 4.36
Superior vena caval syndrome. Distended left external jugular vein in a patient with mediastinal involvement by carcinoma.

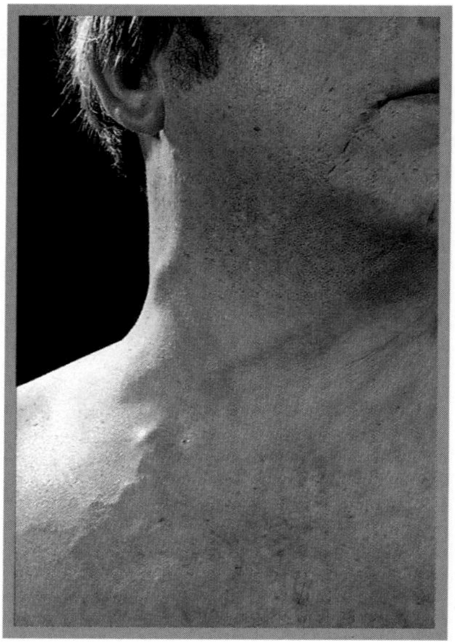

→ Fig. 4.37
Superior vena caval syndrome. Distended jugular veins in a patient with mediastinal fibrosis. Note the tortuous collateral veins on the chest wall. The same process also produced constrictive pericarditis in this patient.

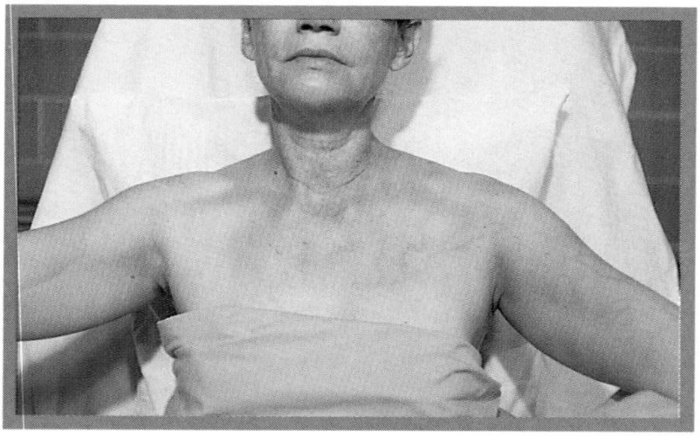

← Fig. 4.38
Superior vena caval syndrome. Note the collateral venous pattern on the chest wall.

→ Fig. 4.39
Superior vena caval syndrome. Chest radiogram of a patient showing a widened superior mediastinum and right pleural effusion as a result of metastatic carcinoma.

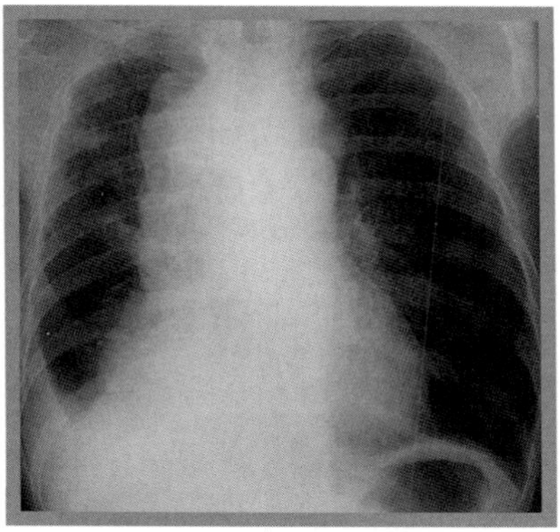

Kinked Left Innominate Vein

Distention of the left external jugular vein may result from pressure upon the left innominate vein (**Fig. 4.40)**, which can be demonstrated by venography (**Fig. 4.41**). The left innominate vein, being longer than the right, is more susceptible to pressure from mediastinal structures (**Fig. 4.42**). It is important to observe that the jugular vein distention is, in fact, unilateral, thereby effectively excluding bilateral cervical venous distention caused by congestive heart failure, pericardial disease, or superior vena caval obstruction. The most common cause of kinked left innominate vein, as in the patient in Figures 4.40 and 4.41, is an elongated atherosclerotic aorta. Aortic aneurysm, dissecting aortic aneurysm or mediastinal tumor may also be responsible. Less often, unilateral cervical venous distention may be caused, not by pressure upon the innominate vein, but by venous thrombosis.

Dissecting Aortic Aneurysm

This condition is also called aortic dissection or dissecting hematoma. It is relatively uncommon, and the diagnosis is often missed. The process usually begins with an intimal entry tear, either in the ascending aorta just above the aortic valve, or in the descending aorta just beyond the left subclavian artery. There are three types in the DeBakey classification: type I begins in the ascending aorta and propagates beyond the aortic arch; type II is confined to the ascending aorta; type III begins beyond the left subclavian artery and extends distally.

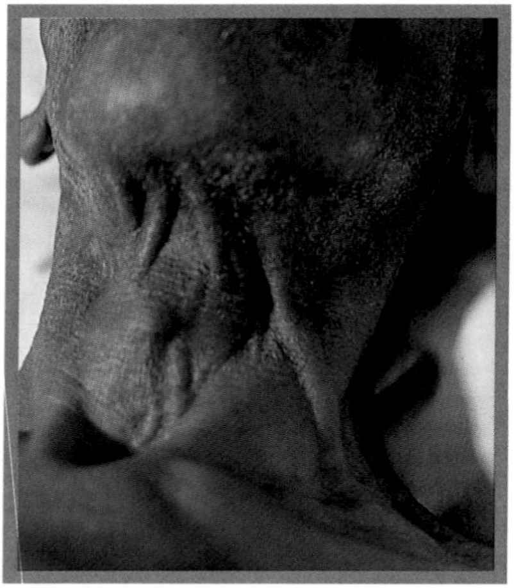

← Fig. 4.40
Kinked left innominate vein. The patient photographed shows distention of the left external jugular vein as a result of pressure of a tortuous aorta upon the left innominate vein. The anatomy is demonstrated in Figures 4.41 and 4.42. This benign condition must be distinguished from left innominate vein obstruction by neoplasm, aortic aneurysm, or thrombosis.

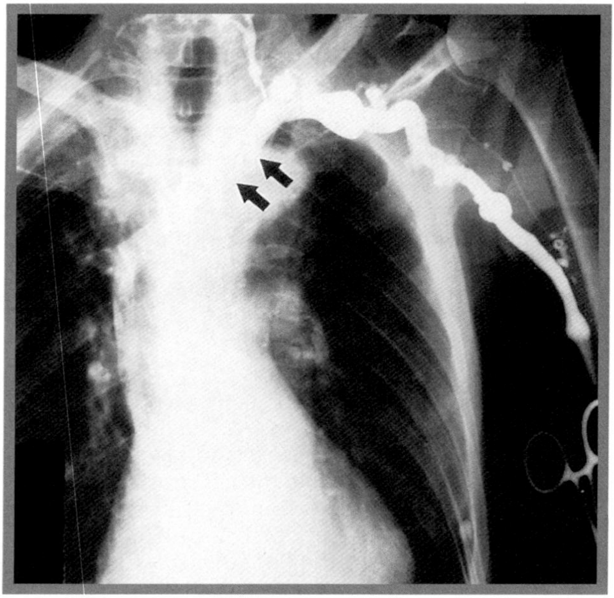

← Fig. 4.41
Kinked left innominate vein. Venogram demonstrating compression of the left innominate vein by a tortuous aorta (arrows). (With permission from Fowler NO. *Diagnosis of heart disease.* Springer–Verlag, 1991.)

There are a number of conditions that predispose to aortic dissection; by far the most common is hypertension (**Fig. 4.43**). Although aortic dissection may occur in persons of any age, it is most common in men in the sixth and seventh decades of life. Aortic dissection may be a catastrophic event in patients with Marfan syndrome, and is a particular risk in pregnant women with Marfan syndrome.

In addition to the many other presenting features of aortic dissection (**Fig. 4.44**), severe anterior chest pain is seen most commonly and is often described as tearing or ripping in quality; however, about 10% of patients have no history of chest pain. The pain may radiate to the back or to the abdomen. Such radiation suggests aortic dissection rather than myocardial infarction as the cause of severe chest pain but is not specific for that distinction.

Physical findings

The physical examination is helpful in making the diagnosis (**Fig. 4.45**). Hypertension is common, but may be absent because shock has intervened.

→ Fig. 4.42
Diagram showing the anatomy of superior vena cava and its tributaries. Note greater length of left innominate vein as compared to the right innominate vein. SUB, subclavian vein; EJ, external jugular vein; IJ, internal jugular vein; LIV, left innominate vein; RIV, right innominate vein; SVC, superior vena cava; IVC, inferior vena cava; RA, right atrium; RV, right ventricle.

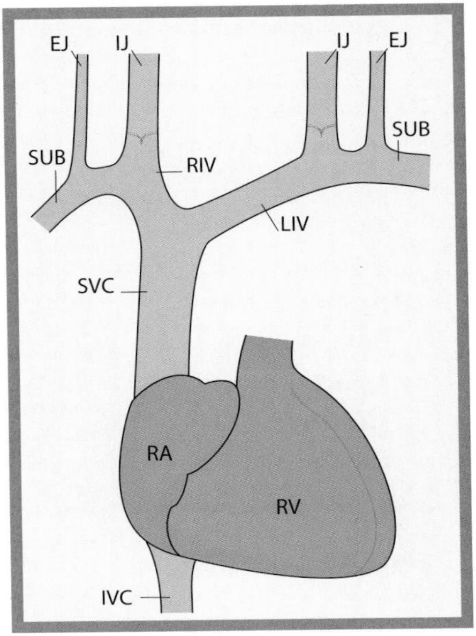

About 50% of patients with proximal dissection have aortic insufficiency (**Fig. 4.46**). A helpful finding in some patients is distention of the left jugular veins as a result of compression of the left innominate vein (**Figs 4.47–4.49**). In some patients with proximal dissection, there is rupture into the pericardial sac, with cardiac tamponade as the presenting feature.

Electrocardiogram

The ECG does not show specific changes but is useful in tending to exclude myocardial infarction as a cause of chest pain. It often shows evidence of left ventricular hypertrophy caused by antecedent hypertension. When the dissection has ruptured into the pericardial sac, one may see diffuse ST

Factors that predispose to acute aortic dissection
Hypertension
Marfan syndrome
Cystic medial necrosis
Aortic coarctation
Bicuspid aortic valve
Trauma, including surgical cannulation, aortic balloon pumping, insertion of prosthetic aortic valve
Relapsing polychondritis
Noonan's syndrome
Ehlers–Danlos syndrome
Turner's syndrome
Pregnancy
Aortic stenosis

↑ Fig. 4.43
Factors that predispose to acute aortic dissection.

Presenting features of dissecting aortic aneurysm
Pericarditis
Hypertensive crisis
Myocardial infarction
Aortic regurgitation
Cerebrovascular accident
Spinal cord ischemia
Mesenteric infarction
Mediastinal tumor
Superior vena caval syndrome
Acute pulmonary disorder
Cardiac tamponade
Paraplegia
Syncope
Aortic arch syndrome

↑ Fig. 4.44
Presenting features of dissecting aortic aneurysm.

segment elevation because of pericarditis. Uncommonly, in patients with dissection, one may see evidence of acute myocardial infarction when proximal dissection has encircled a coronary artery.

→ Fig. 4.45
Physical findings in dissecting aortic aneurysm.

Physical findings in dissecting aortic aneurysm

Predisposing: hypertension, Marfan's, pregnancy, and others

Unequal pulses (approx. 50%)

Aortic insufficiency in 25% (50% proximal)

Neurologic signs: hemiparesis, paraplegia

Pulsating sternoclavicular joint

Distention of left jugular veins

Left pleural effusion

Cardiac tamponade

→ Fig. 4.46
Dissecting aortic aneurysm. Phonocardiogram, showing aortic insufficiency murmur in a patient with acute aortic dissection. DM, diastolic murmur; ESM, ejection systolic murmur; RICS, right intercostal space; LICS, left intercostal space.

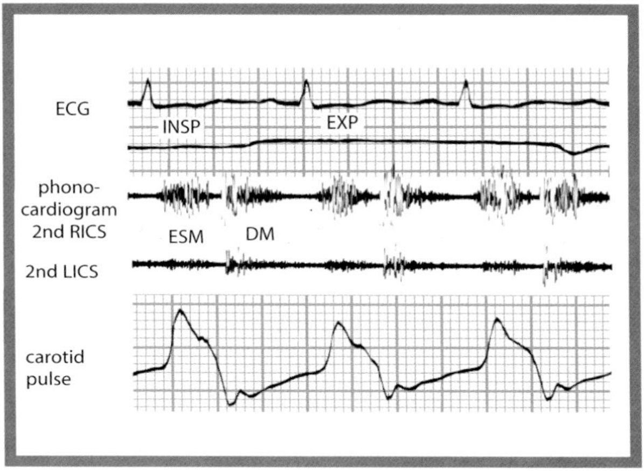

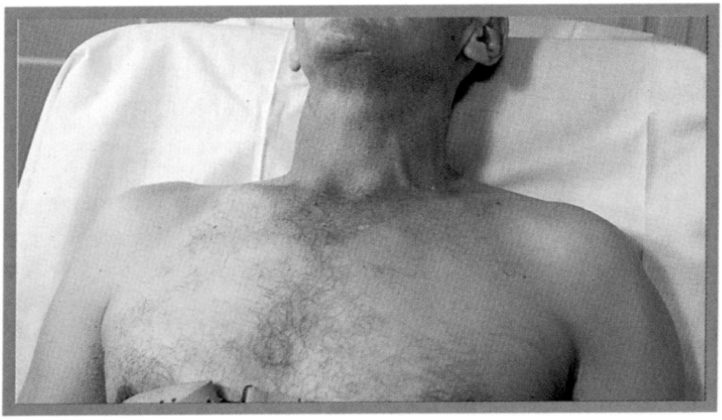

← Fig. 4.47 Dissecting aortic aneurysm. Distention of the left external jugular vein as a result of compression of the left innominate vein by a dissecting aneurysm. See Fig. 4.49.

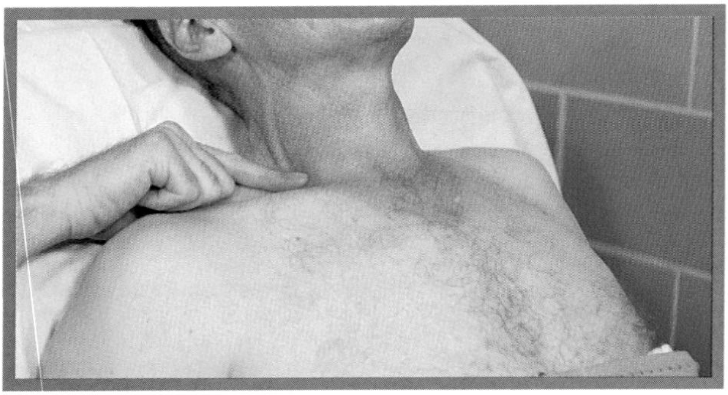

← Fig. 4.48 Dissecting aortic aneurysm. Digital compression of the lower right external jugular vein, showing that this vein is patent, although not distended by the dissecting aneurysm.

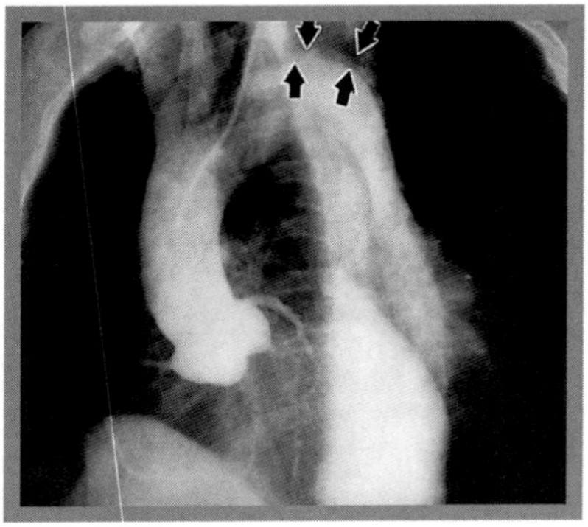

← Fig. 4.49 Dissecting aortic aneurysm. Aortogram of the patient in Figure 4.47. The arrows indicate the site of compression of the left innominate vein by the dissecting aneurysm. Distal to this point, the true aortic lumen is narrowed by the false channel.

Chest radiogram

The chest radiogram shows an increase in the width of the superior mediastinum in 80–90% of cases. When the aortic intima is calcified, increased width of the aortic wall can be seen (**Fig. 4.50**). There may be a leakage of blood into the left pleural space. However, a normal chest radiogram does not exclude the diagnosis.

Diagnosis

There are four widely used means of making the diagnosis, all of which are highly reliable. The 'gold standard' has been contrast aortography (**Fig. 4.51**; see also Fig. 4.49) but other techniques are becoming as reliable. Transesophageal echocardiography is becoming increasingly popular (**Figs 4.52** and **4.53**). Contrast-enhanced CT is also commonly used (**Fig. 4.54**); however, it often fails

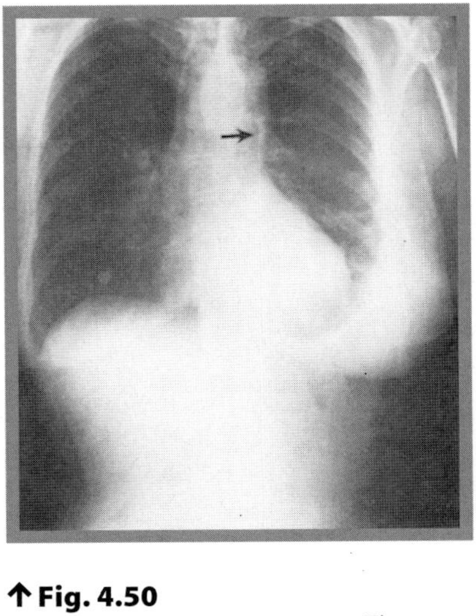

↑ **Fig. 4.50**
Dissecting aortic aneurysm. The chest radiogram shows thickening of the aortic wall, evident as an increased distance between the calcified intima and the outer aortic wall (arrow).

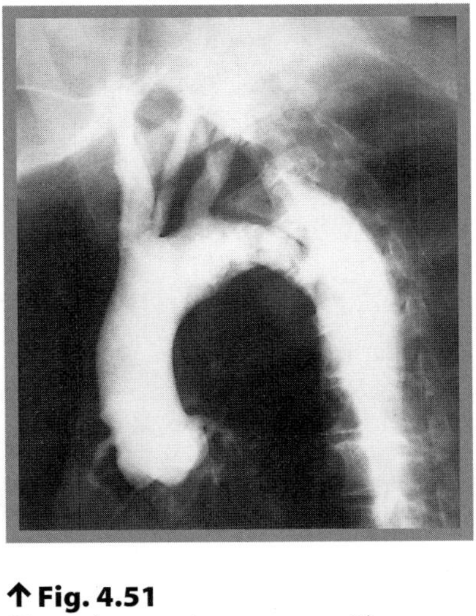

↑ **Fig. 4.51**
Dissecting aortic aneurysm. The aortogram demonstrates an intimal tear just beyond the left subclavian artery. Beyond this point, there is a large false channel that compresses the true lumen.

to show the entry tear. Magnetic resonance imaging is reliable, but less popular because of the time required and the isolation of the patient, who may need emergency care.

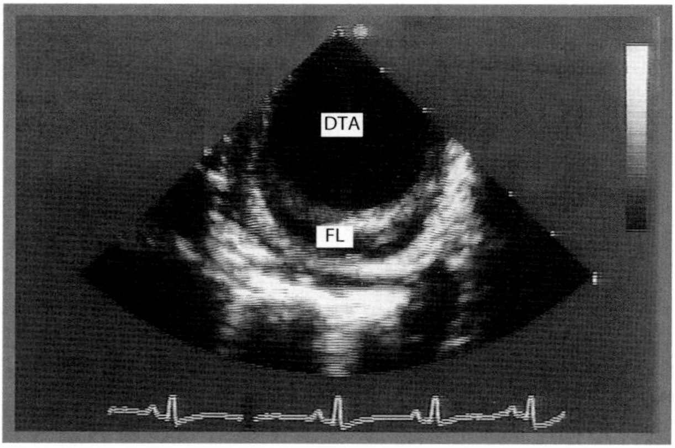

← Fig. 4.52 Dissecting aortic aneurysm. Two-dimensional echocardiogram, showing the true aortic lumen, above; it is separated from the false lumen below by an intimal flap. DTA, descending thoracic aorta; FL, false lumen.

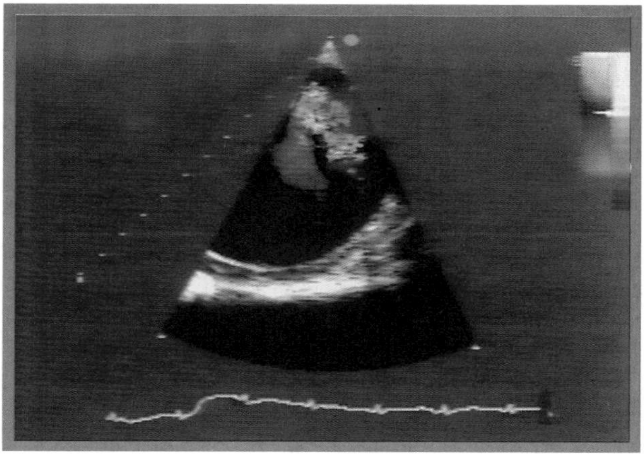

← Fig. 4.53 Dissecting aortic aneurysm. Doppler echocardiogram, showing blood flow from the large true lumen, below, to the false lumen, above. Turbulent flow is indicated by the polychromatic jet in the false lumen.

→ Fig. 4.54a
Dissecting aortic aneurysm. CT scan of the abdomen with contrast enhancement of an aortic dissection that began just beyond the left subclavian artery. See Fig. 4.54b for an explanatory diagram of this scan.

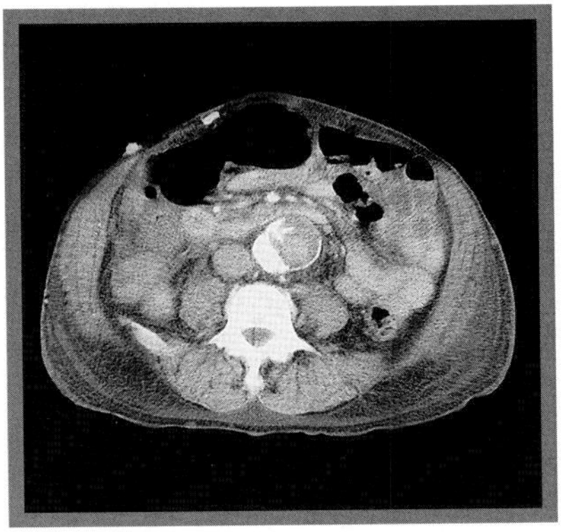

→ Fig. 4.54b
Dissecting aortic anneurysm.
TL indicates the true lumen and FC indicates the false channel produced by the dissection.

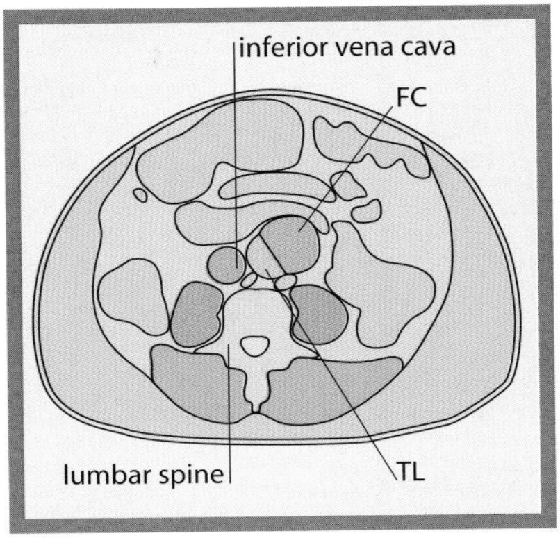

Further reading

DeSanctis RW, Doroghazi RM, Austen WG, Buckley MJ. Medical progress. Aortic dissection. *N Engl J Med* 1987, **317**:1060–1067.

Khanderia BK. Aortic dissection. The last frontier. *Circulation* 1993, **87**:1765–1768.

Kinked Carotid Artery

In a patient presenting with a pulsating mass just superior to the medial end of the right clavicle, arteriography may reveal the cause to be, not a carotid arterial aneurysm, but an elongated uncoiled carotid artery (**Fig. 4.55**). Arteriograms of a number of such patients have almost always shown a U-shaped or S-shaped, elongated common carotid artery, rather than a true aneurysm. The patient with this finding is usually a hypertensive woman of middle age. The kinked carotid artery is usually on the right side, but may be bilateral. It is seldom found on the left side alone.

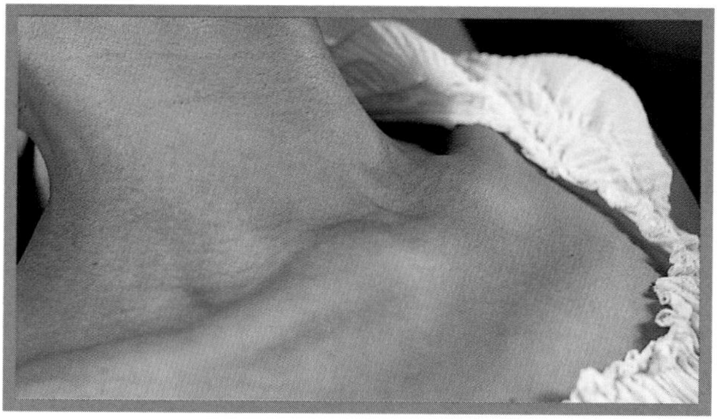

↑ Fig. 4.55
Kinked carotid artery. The swelling just superior to the right sternoclavicular joint is produced by an elongated, tortuous common carotid artery. This finding is most common in middle-aged, hypertensive women. It is more common on the right but may be bilateral. It is often mistaken for a carotid artery aneurysm.

5 Thorax

Syphilitic Aortic Aneurysm

In the 1940s, syphilitic aortitis was relatively common, accounting for 5–10% of cardiovascular deaths. Today, because of early recognition and treatment of syphilis, syphilitic aortitis has become a rarity. This manifestation of tertiary syphilis usually develops after a latent period of 10–25 years, and thus is uncommon in persons younger than 30 years. Syphilitic aortitis may remain asymptomatic; however, it may produce aortic aneurysm, aortic insufficiency, or coronary ostial stenosis with angina pectoris. It is estimated that about 50% of patients with syphilitic aortitis develop aortic aneurysm. The most common location for such aneurysms is the ascending aorta; the second most common site is the aortic arch, and about 15% are found in the descending thoracic aorta. In Heggtveit's study, 9% were found in the abdominal aorta.

Syphilitic aortic aneurysm may be asymptomatic, but symptoms are common. There may be a brassy cough and hoarseness as a result of recurrent laryngeal nerve paralysis. Angina pectoris may result from coronary ostial stenosis. There may be pain from sternal or rib erosion. Rupture into the trachea, bronchi or esophagus may be a terminal event. Rupture into the mediastinum and left pleural space may also occur.

Physical findings are variable. At times, there is a pulsating mass to the right of the sternum or beneath the left scapula (**Fig. 5.1**). A tracheal tug may be felt as a result of pulsatile pressure upon a main stem bronchus. Obstruction of the superior vena cava may produce the superior vena caval syndrome (see Chapter 4). Evidence of Horner's syndrome may be seen, because of compression of the left stellate ganglion. This produces left-sided ptosis and miosis, with decreased sweating of the left side of the face. About 33% or more of patients with syphilitic aortic aneurysm also have evidence of aortic valvular insufficiency on physical examination.

Diagnosis

When there is doubt concerning the nature of a mediastinal mass, computerized tomography (CT) scanning or magnetic resonance imaging will determine whether or not there is an aneurysmal mass or a neoplasm or cyst. Calcification within the wall of the ascending aorta is very suggestive of syphilitic aortitis (**Fig. 5.2**), although it may be seen in other varieties of aortitis.

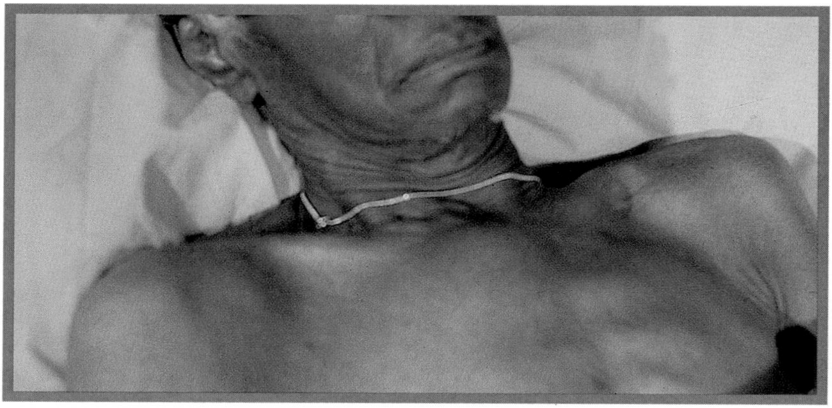

↑ Fig. 5.1
Syphilitic aortic aneurysm. The bulge beneath the right clavicle is caused by a syphilitic aortic aneurysm eroding through the chest wall. It is unusual for other varieties of ascending aortic aneurysm, such as aortic dissection, Marfan syndrome, or congenital aneurysm, to produce a visible erosion in this fashion.

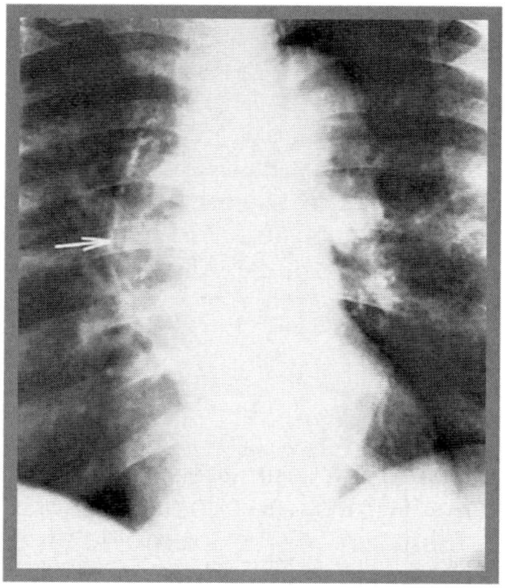

← Fig. 5.2
Syphilitic aortitis. The chest radiogram shows calcification of the ascending aorta. This finding is very suggestive of syphilitic aortitis, although it may be seen in other varieties of aortitis. With atherosclerosis, intimal calcification may be seen in the ascending aorta, but then is usually more extensive beyond the left subclavian artery. (With permission from Fowler NO. *Diagnosis of heart disease*. Springer–Verlag, 1991.)

Calcification as a result of atherosclerosis is usually more pronounced distal to the brachiocephalic arteries. Kahn, Wassermann and Venereal Disease Research Laboratory serologic tests are negative in 15–30% of instances, but the *Treponema pallidum* immobilization test is almost always positive.

Reference

Heggtveit HA. Syphilitic aortitis. A clinicopathologic autopsy study of 100 cases, 1950 to 1960. Circulation 1964, 29:346–355.

Further reading

Boyd LJ. A study of four thousand reported cases of aneurysm of the thoracic aorta. Am J Med Sci 1924, 168:654–668.

Cor Pulmonale Caused by Poliomyelitis

The World Health Organization defined chronic cor pulmonale as hypertrophy of the right ventricle resulting from diseases affecting the function or the structure of the lung, except when these pulmonary alterations result from diseases that primarily affect the left side of the heart or from congenital heart disease.

Cor pulmonale usually results from one or more of four factors that tend to produce pulmonary hypertension: anatomic decrease in the pulmonary vascular bed; hypoxia and acidosis causing vasoconstriction of pulmonary resistance vessels; increased pulmonary blood flow; increased blood viscosity as a result of secondary polycythemia. In advanced cases, left ventricular failure may further increase the pulmonary arterial pressure. By far the most common cause of chronic cor pulmonale is chronic obstructive airway disease resulting from either chronic bronchitis or pulmonary emphysema. Chronic cor pulmonale may also be caused by interstitial lung disease; that caused by pulmonary vascular disease (for example primary pulmonary hypertension) was discussed in Chapter 2. Hypoventilation states caused by respiratory center insensitivity to carbon dioxide, obesity, or disease of the chest wall also may be the cause.

In this chapter, we present two examples of disease of the chest wall producing hypoventilation and pulmonary hypertension, which in turn caused cor pulmonale. Atrophy of the chest wall muscles subsequent to poliomyelitis is one example of such a cause (**Figs 5.3** and **5.4**). The patient illustrated had severe hypoxia and hypercapnia. To avoid coma caused by hypercapnia, he required a permanent tracheostomy, and assisted ventilation with an external chest ventilator (cuirass) at night. His ECG (**Figs 5.5** and **5.6**) showed right axis deviation in the limb leads and evidence of right atrial hypertrophy and right ventricular hypertrophy in lead V_1. T wave inversions in the right precordial leads probably reflected right ventricular strain. Patients with long-standing poliomyelitis are known to develop a syndrome consistent with pulmonary vasoconstriction, cor pulmonale, and congestive heart failure. Both the phrenic and the intercostal nerves may be involved in producing the hypoventilation in these patients.

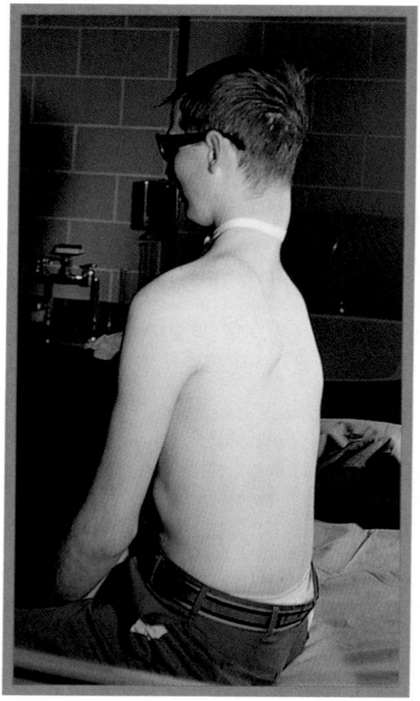

↑ Fig. 5.3
Cor pulmonale caused by poliomyelitis. The photograph shows atrophy of the muscles of the chest wall secondary to lower motor neuron disease in this patient with cor pulmonale. There was also involvement of intercostal muscles and the diaphragm, leading to hypoxia and hypercapnia.

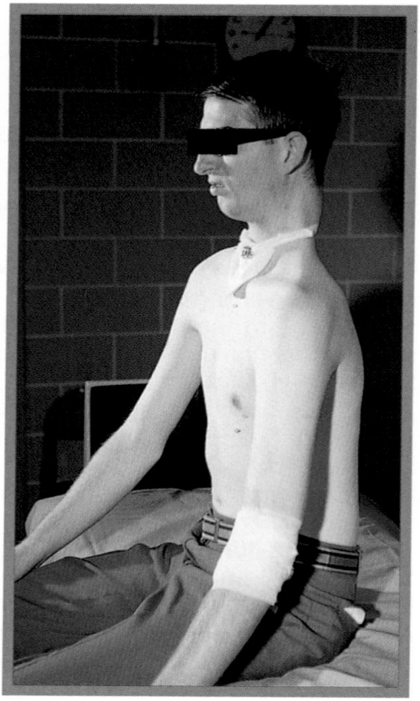

↑ Fig. 5.4
Cor pulmonale caused by poliomyelitis. Atrophy of the thoracic muscles is shown. Because of hypoventilation, the patient required a permanent tracheostomy.

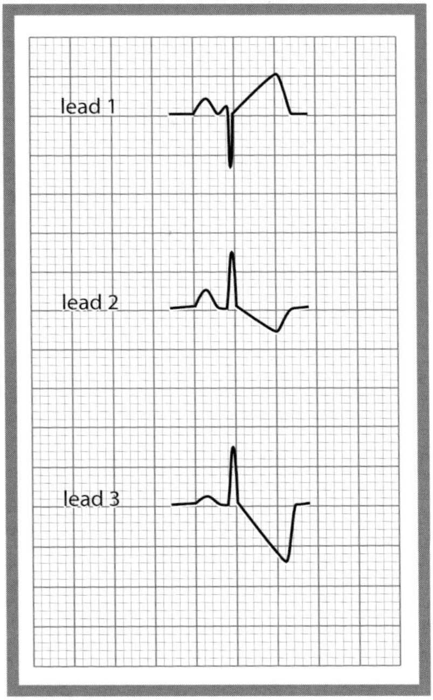

↑ Fig. 5.5
Cor pulmonale caused by poliomyelitis. ECG of the patient shown in Figures 5.3 and 5.4. There is right axis deviation of the QRS complex with inferior T wave changes attributable to right ventricular hypertrophy.

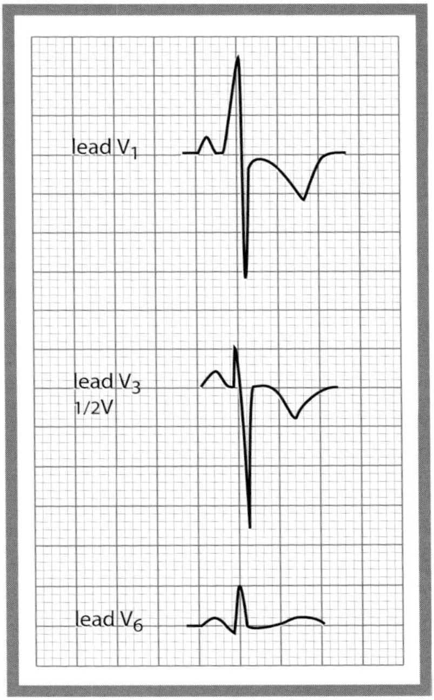

↑ Fig. 5.6
Cor pulmonale caused by poliomyelitis. ECG of the patient shown in Figures 5.3 and 5.4. The prominent R wave in lead V_1 and negative T waves in the right precordial leads are due to right ventricular hypertrophy and strain. The P wave in lead V_1 exceeds 1.5 mm in height, and is consistent with right atrial enlargement.

Further reading

Bergofsky EH. Respiratory failure in disorders of the thoracic cage. Am Rev Respir Dis 1979, 119:643–669.

Kyphoscoliotic Heart Disease

Severe kyphoscoliosis may also lead to hypoventilation with pulmonary hypertension and cor pulmonale, also known as 'heart failure of the hunchback' (**Figs 5.7** and **5.8**). Kyphoscoliosis may result from empyema, tuberculosis, trauma, rickets, Duchenne muscular dystrophy, or poliomyelitis, but most often it is idiopathic. Some patients have scoliosis alone; others have both kyphosis and scoliosis. Patients with this disorder may have cyanosis and digital clubbing. The total lung capacity is reduced and the vital capacity may be as little as 25% of normal. Hanley *et al.* studied nine patients with kyphoscoliosis and heart

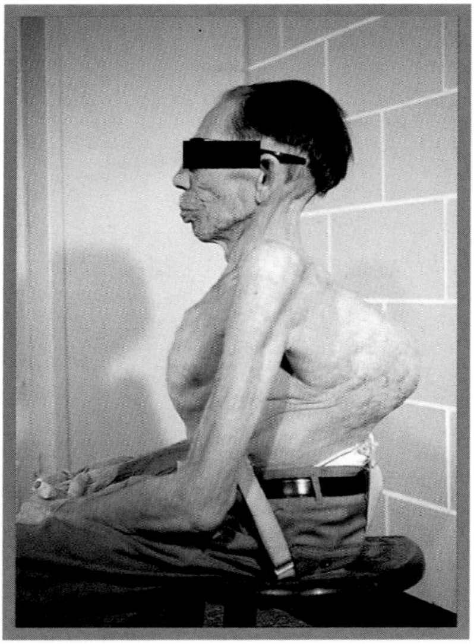

↑ Fig. 5.7
Heart failure of patient with severe kyphoscoliosis. This patient's condition caused hypoventilation and pulmonary hypertension, with resultant cor pulmonale. (With permission from Fowler NO. *Diagnosis of heart disease*. Springer–Verlag, 1991.)

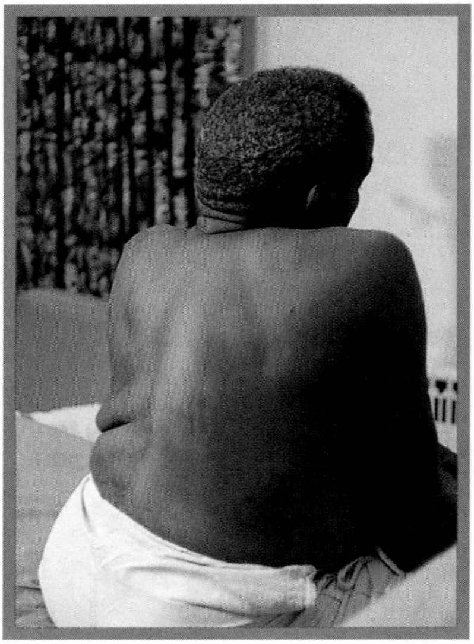

↑ Fig. 5.8
Heart failure of the hunchback. Severe kyphoscoliosis caused cor pulmonale in this patient.

failure and found that eight of them had severe arterial hypoxia and increased arterial P_{CO_2}, but such abnormalities were found in only two of 14 patients with kyphoscoliosis without heart failure. Pulmonary hypertension in kyphoscoliosis has been attributed to a combination of pulmonary vasoconstriction and pulmonary vascular alteration.

Reference

Hanley T, Platts MM, Clifton M, Morris TL. Heart failure of the hunchback. Q J Med 1958, 27:155–171.

Pectus Excavatum

Pectus excavatum (**Fig. 5.9**) is also known as funnel breast or *Schusterbrust*. It may be an isolated disorder, or may be associated with Marfan syndrome, homocystinuria, Hunter–Hurler syndrome, Ehlers–Danlos syndrome, or mitral valve prolapse. The condition, although unsightly, seldom causes a significant cardiac or pulmonary abnormality. However, because of cardiac displacement or compression, it may falsely suggest organic heart disease. Thus it is a cause of 'pseudo-heart disease'. It is considered severe when the distance between the posterior sternum and the vertebral column is less than 5cm, and moderate when the distance is 5–7cm (the normal average is 10.5cm for men and 9cm for women).

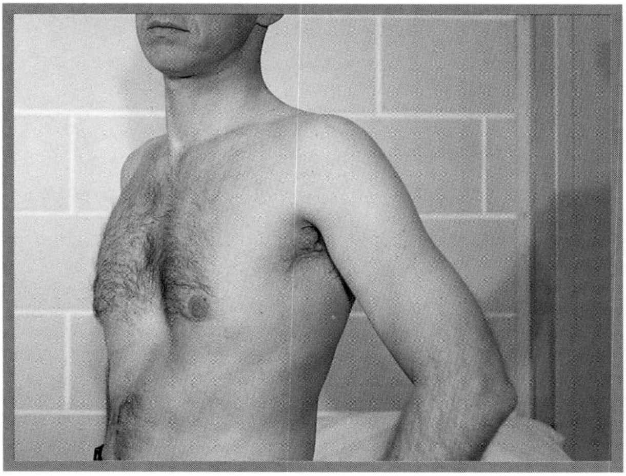

→ Fig. 5.9 Pectus excavatum. Severe funnel breast produced 'pancake heart', a variety of pseudo-heart disease, in this patient (see Fig. 5.10). (With permission from Fowler NO. *Diagnosis of heart disease.* Springer–Verlag, 1991.)

The physical examination often reveals an ejection pulmonic systolic murmur. Expiratory splitting of S_2 and a systolic ejection sound have been described. The intensity of the murmur may be increased by pressure over the sternum. The heart may be displaced to the left, and the location of the apical impulse may incorrectly suggest cardiac enlargement. The heart may be flattened anteroposteriorly and thus appear enlarged on chest radiogram; this is known as 'pancake heart' (**Fig. 5.10**).

The ECG may show a QR or RSR' pattern in lead V_1, with negative T waves in the right precordial leads. QRS voltage may be decreased in the right precordial leads, and increased in lead V_6. Because of displacement of the heart to the left, a sharply negative P wave is often seen in lead V_1. Cardiac catheterization findings are usually normal, but occasional increase in right atrial pressure has been reported. The vital capacity is often normal, but on average is slightly reduced.

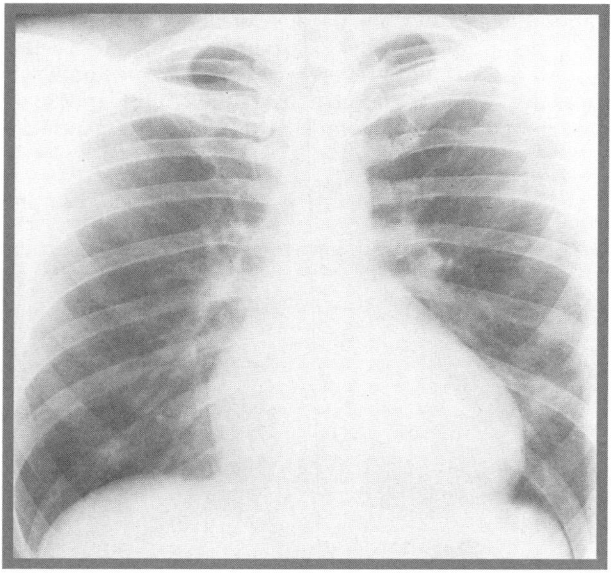

← Fig. 5.10 Pectus excavatum. Chest radiogram of the patient pictured in Figure 5.9. The heart is compressed by severe pectus excavatum, leading to 'pancake heart' and apparent cardiac enlargement. (With permission from Fowler NO. *Diagnosis of heart disease.* Springer–Verlag, 1991.)

Further reading

Evans W. The heart in sternal depression. Br Heart J 1946, 8:162–170.

Fink A, Rivin A, Murray JP. Pectus excavatum. An analysis of 27 cases. Arch Int Med 1961, **108**:427–437.

Straight Back Syndrome

'Straight back syndrome' is found in patients lacking the normal degree of thoracic kyphosis (**Figs 5.11** and **5.12**). This condition is another cause of pseudo-heart disease. Patients with this syndrome may have expiratory splitting of S_2, a midsystolic murmur, and apparent enlargement of the pulmonary artery on the chest radiogram. Thus, atrial septal defect (ASD) may be suggested. An association with mitral valve prolapse has been described.

Ansari studied 50 patients with cardiac murmurs and straight upper dorsal spines. Only two had expiratory splitting of S_2. None had diastolic murmurs. Twenty-nine patients had mitral valve prolapse and three had a bicuspid aortic valve on echocardiography. Cardiomegaly on chest radiogram was present in

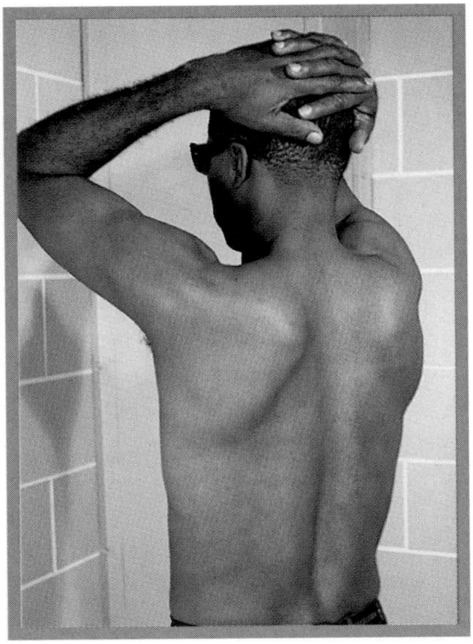

↑ **Fig. 5.11**
Straight back syndrome. Loss of normal upper dorsal spine kyphosis is shown in this patient. This can be a cause of pseudo-heart disease.

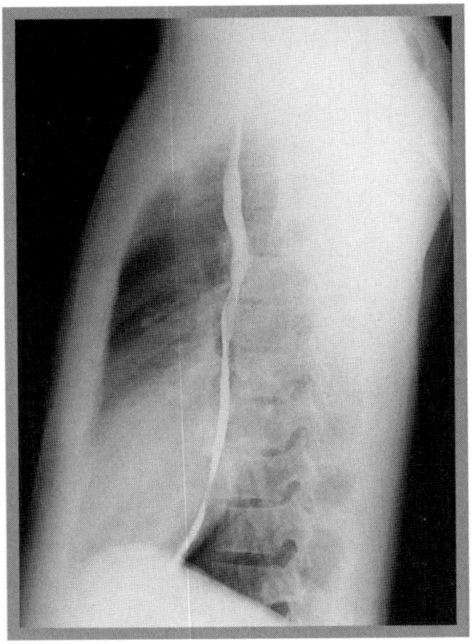

↑ **Fig. 5.12**
Straight back syndrome. Chest radiogram of the patient in Figure 5.11, showing loss of normal upper dorsal kyphosis.

five, and apparent enlargement of the pulmonary artery in two. Only seven were believed to have pseudo-heart disease.

Reference

Ansari A. The 'straight back' syndrome. Clin Cardiol 1985, **8**:290–305.

Further reading

Abrams J. Essentials of cardiac physical diagnosis. Philadelphia: Lea and Febiger, 1987.

Atrial Septal Defect

Atrial septal defect is the most common major congenital heart disease of adults. Because of the associated right ventricular enlargement in childhood, uncommonly one may see a bulge in the left parasternal region produced by deformity of the ribs overlying the dilated right ventricle (**Fig. 5.13**). The physical signs are subtle but, with careful auscultation, are usually diagnostic. Except

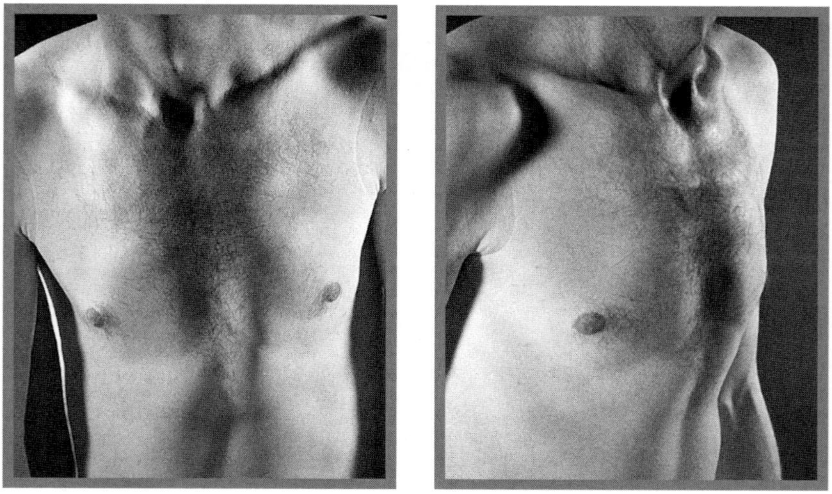

↑ Fig. 5.13a **↑ Fig. 5.13b**
Atrial septal defect. Left precordial bulge in a patient with congenital atrial septal defect. The bulge is produced by right ventricular enlargement occurring during the growth period.

with advanced pulmonary hypertension, the shunt through the defect is from left to right atrium, and the patient is acyanotic. There is nearly always an ejection pulmonic systolic murmur, maximal in the second left intercostal space adjacent to the sternum. This is produced by the increased pulmonary blood flow and is seldom more than grade 3 (of 6) intensity. There is usually no thrill. The most specific auscultatory finding is failure of S_2 to become single during expiration. The interval between the earlier aortic component (A_2) and the later pulmonic component (P_2) is usually constant throughout the respiratory cycle (**Figs 5.14** and **5.15**). The delay in P_2 is caused by a combination of decreased elasticity of the pulmonary artery and a prolonged right ventricular ejection time. With very large ASDs, there may be a low-pitched, delayed-onset diastolic murmur near the cardiac apex. This is produced by increased flow across the tricuspid valve and should not be confused with the murmur of mitral stenosis. When there is an ostium primum ASD, there is usually also an apical pansystolic murmur of mitral incompetence (see Chapter 1).

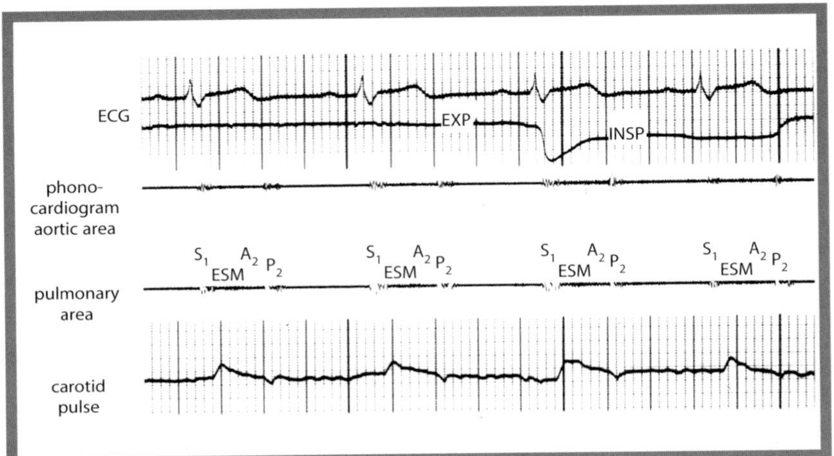

↑ Fig. 5.14
Atrial septal defect. Phonocardiogram showing an ejection systolic murmur (ESM) in the second left intercostal space adjacent to the sternum. There is fixed splitting of S_2, with a constant interval between the earlier aortic closure sound (A_2) and the later pulmonic closure sound (P_2). S_1, first heart sound. (With permission from Fowler NO. *Diagnosis of heart disease*. Springer–Verlag, 1991.)

The chest radiogram (**Figs 5.16** and **5.17**) demonstrates a small aortic knob and enlarged right ventricle and pulmonary artery, with enlarged hilar and peripheral pulmonary arterial branches. These findings may be absent or inconspicuous when the left-to-right shunt is small and the pulmonary blood flow is less than twice the systemic flow.

The ECG characteristically shows a pattern of incomplete right bundle branch block (**Fig. 5.18**). This pattern is seen in about 60–90% of adults with

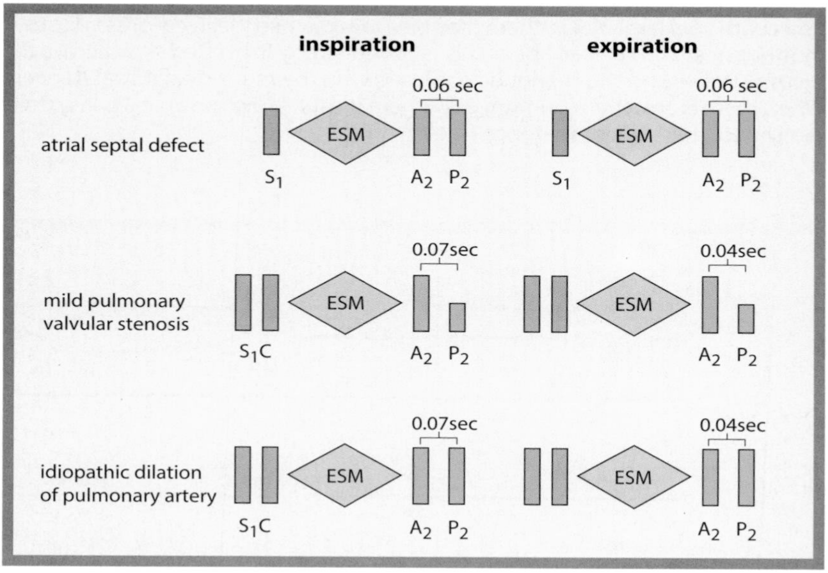

↑ Fig. 5.15
Atrial septal defect. Diagram of auscultatory findings in three varieties of congenital heart disease that produce an ejection systolic murmur in the pulmonary auscultatory area in the second left intercostal space adjacent to the sternum. In ASD there is fixed splitting of S_2, with no ventilatory variation of the interval between A_2 and P_2. With mild pulmonary valvular stenosis, there is an ejection sound (C), P_2 is diminished to absent, and the interval between A_2 and P_2 increases with inspiration. The ejection sound becomes faint during inspiration. With idiopathic dilatation of the pulmonary artery, there is an ejection sound, but P_2 is preserved.

ASD. The rhythm is usually normal sinus rhythm, but after the age of 40 years, as many as 10–20% of the patients have atrial fibrillation or, less commonly, atrial flutter. With ostium primum defect, the characteristic pattern is that of incomplete right bundle branch block and left axis deviation (**Fig. 5.19**).

The defect in the atrial septum can be demonstrated by two-dimensional echocardiography (**Fig. 5.20**) and the shunt can be seen by means of color Doppler echocardiography (**Fig. 5.21**).

→ Fig. 5.16
Atrial septal defect. Chest radiogram of a woman in the seventh decade of life. She had atrial fibrillation, which occurs in 10–20% of patients after the age of 40 years. There is a large pulmonary artery segment with a small aortic knob. The pulmonary vessels show evidence of increased blood flow, being enlarged peripherally.

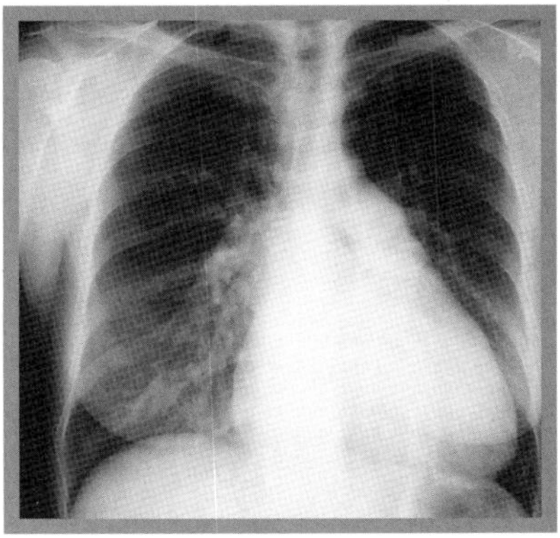

→ Fig. 5.17
Atrial septal defect. Chest radiogram of a 25-year-old woman, showing a large pulmonary artery segment and a small aortic knob. The peripheral pulmonary vessels are enlarged as a result of increased pulmonary blood flow.

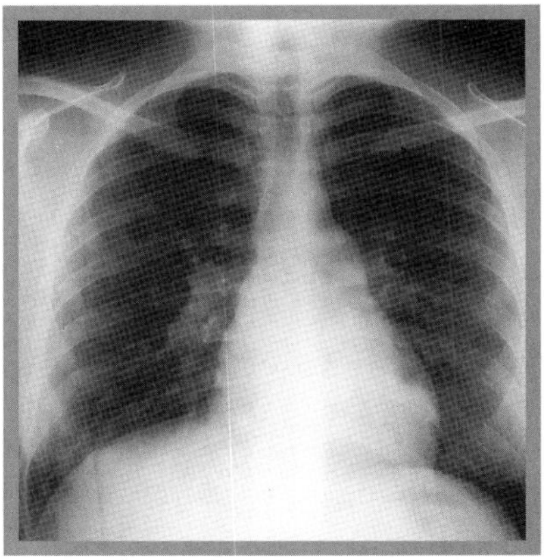

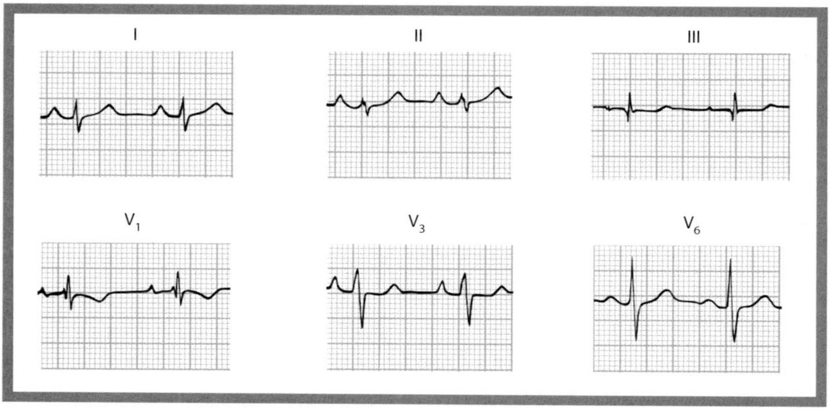

↑ Fig. 5.18
Atrial septal defect. Ostium secundum defect. ECG of a 31-year-old woman, showing the typical pattern of incomplete right bundle branch block in lead V_1. This pattern is seen in 60–90% of adults with ASD, and is probably caused by right ventricular outflow tract hypertrophy.

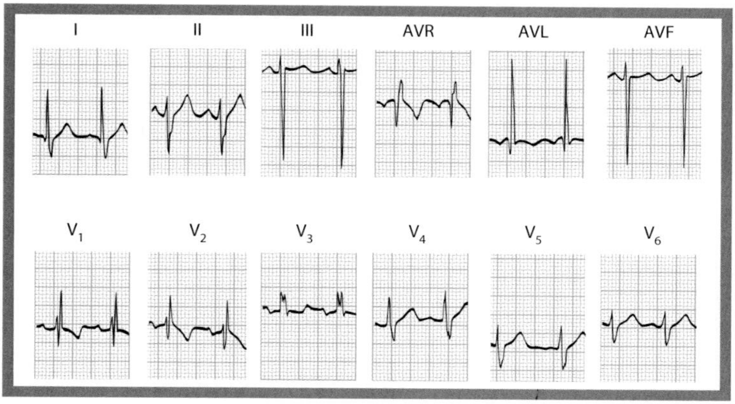

↑ Fig. 5.19
Atrial septal defect. Ostium primum defect. The ECG shows the typical pattern of abnormal left axis deviation of the QRS and incomplete right bundle branch block.

→ Fig. 5.20
Atrial septal defect. Two-dimensional echocardiogram, modified apical four-chamber view, showing ASD. AO, aorta; LA, left atrium; RA, right atrium; RV, right ventricle; TV, tricuspid valve. (With permission from Fowler NO. *Diagnosis of heart disease*. Springer–Verlag, 1991.)

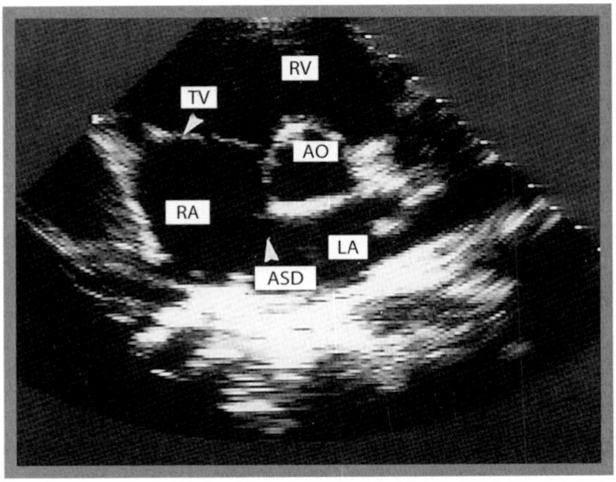

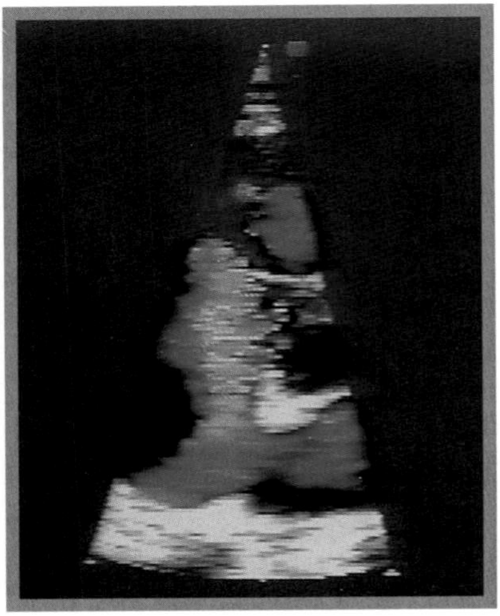

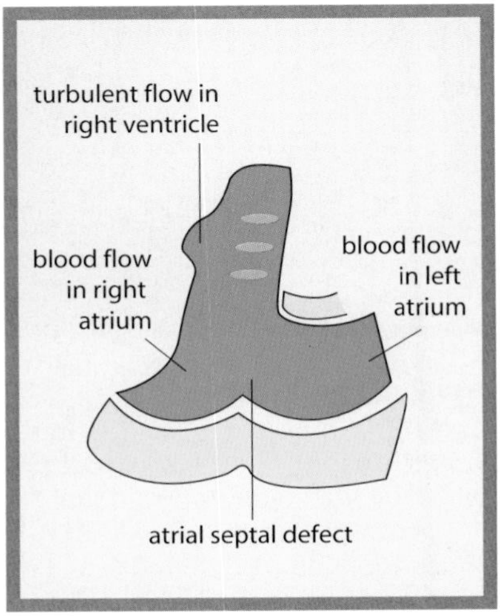

↑ Fig. 5.21a **↑ Fig. 5.21b**
Atrial septal defect. Two-dimensional echocardiogram with color-flow Doppler technique. The flow from left atrium to right atrium through the ASD is shown.

The left-to-right shunt can be demonstrated also by right heart catheterization, which shows a step-up or increase in blood oxygen saturation in the right atrium to a value 10% or more greater than that in the superior vena cava. The shunt can also be shown by injection of radio-opaque contrast medium into the left atrium (**Fig. 5.22**).

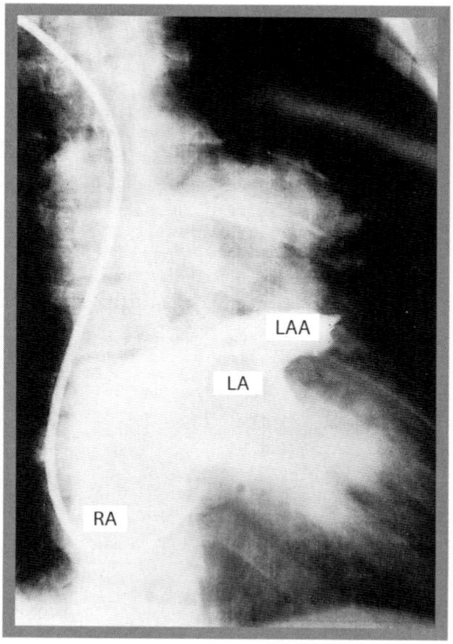

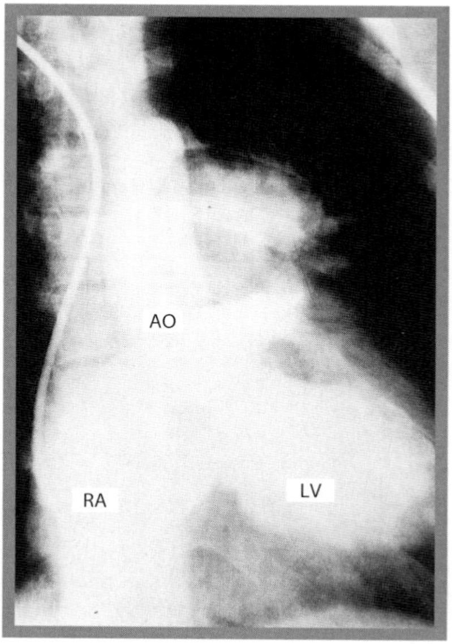

↑ Fig. 5.22a **↑ Fig. 5.22b**

Atrial septal defect. Cardiac catheterization with angiocardiogram. The cardiac catheter tip has been advanced through the ASD into the left atrium and injection of radio-opaque contrast demonstrates passage of contrast from left atrium to right atrium. AO, aorta; LA, left atrium; LAA, left atrial appendage; LV, left ventricle; RA, right atrium.

6 Hands

Jaccoud's Arthritis

Typically, in Jaccoud's post-rheumatic-fever arthritis (**Figs 6.1–6.3**) there is ulnar deviation of the fingers. However, unlike rheumatoid arthritis, there is no true synovitis; rather, there is subluxation of the joints and, as shown here, the ulnar deviation is reversible. The great majority of patients with this disorder have rheumatic aortic or mitral valve disease, or both (**Fig. 6.4**). Reversible ulnar deviation of the fingers may also be seen with systemic lupus erythematosus (SLE) and Ehlers–Danlos syndrome.

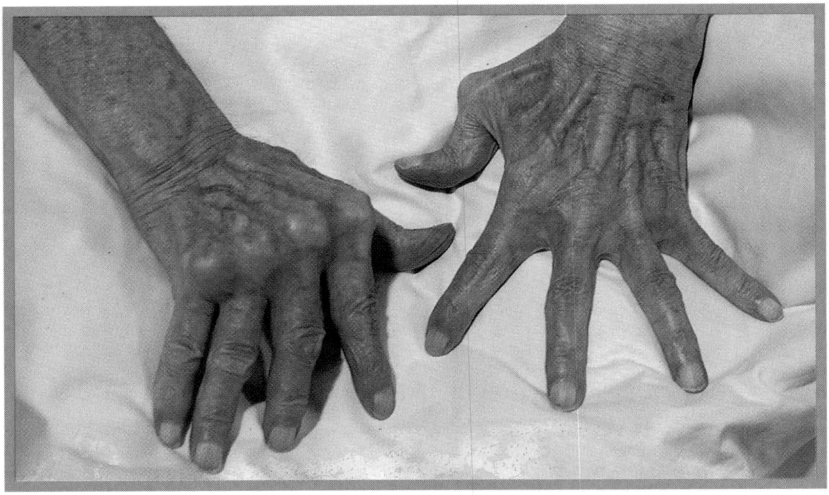

↑ Fig. 6.1
Jaccoud's arthritis. Characteristic subluxation of the metacarpophalangeal joints is seen in the patient's right hand (viewer's left). The fingers of the left hand were easily moved into the correct position.

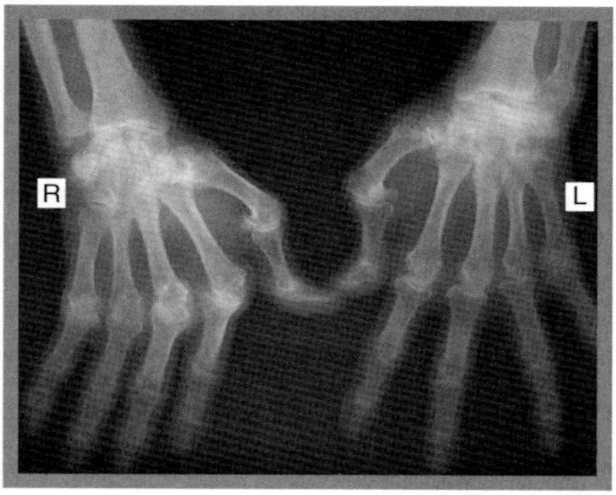

← Fig. 6.2
Jaccoud's arthritis. Radiogram of hands of the patient seen in Figure 6.1. Ulnar deviation of the fingers of the right hand is seen (R). The metacarpophalangeal joints show subluxation, but no true arthritis.

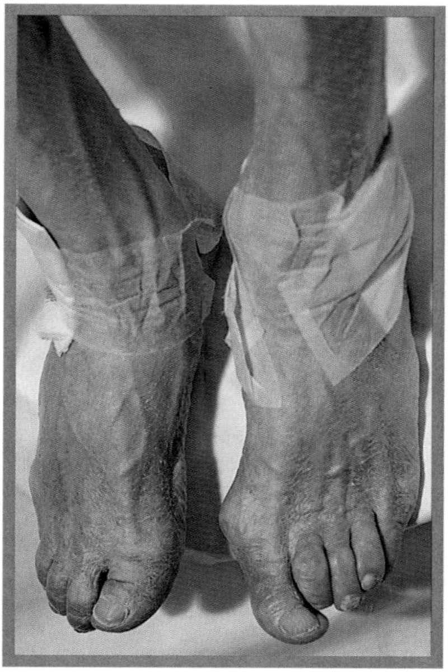

↑ Fig. 6.3
Jaccoud's arthritis. Involvement of the toes in the patient shown in Figures 6.1 and 6.2.

Jaccoud's arthritis
Described by Jaccoud in 1869.
Metacarpophalangeal subluxation without erosion, narrowing, or fusion of joints.
Of 29 cases, 27 had aortic regurgitation or mitral regurgitation (mitral regurgitation, 21; aortic regurgitation, 17; mitral stenosis, 5; aortic stenosis, 6).
Rheumatoid factor and ANA are negative.
Lax ligaments may cause reversible ulnar deviation in SLE and Ehlers–Danlos syndrome (hypereosinophilia syndrome).

↑ Fig. 6.4
Jaccoud's arthritis. (Modified from *Am heart J* 1983, **105**:515–517.)

Scleroderma

Scleroderma, also known as progressive systemic sclerosis, is a systemic disease of unknown cause. It is characterized by generalized spasm of arteries 150–500μm in diameter, followed by inflammation and fibrosis of these vessels. The areas most affected include the skin, kidneys, lungs, heart, skeletal muscles, and gastrointestinal tract (**Fig. 6.5**). There are numerous effects upon the cardiovascular system (**Fig. 6.6**). Cardiomyopathy (scleroderma heart disease) may occur with or without fibrosis of the small intramural coronary arteries (**Fig. 6.7**). Epicardial coronary disease is rare, and major valvular involvement is unusual. Ventricular arrhythmias are common. Pericarditis is common, and may occur with or without renal failure (**Figs 6.8** and **6.9**). Renal involvement may cause hypertension or rapidly developing renal failure. Cor pulmonale may result from pulmonary fibrosis or involvement of pulmonary resistance vessels.

Patients with scleroderma often develop one or more components of the CREST syndrome (calcinosis, Raynaud's syndrome, esophageal dysfunction, sclerodactyly, telangiectasia). Raynaud's syndrome develops in most patients. It is characterized by painful spasm of the digital arteries of the

→ Fig. 6.5
Scleroderma.

Scleroderma

Profuse spasm of arteries 150–500μm in diameter, followed by low grade inflammation, fibrosis, and obliteration. (Increased activity of endothelial cells, mast cells, fibroblasts)

Peripheral exposure to cold reduces blood flow to heart

Decreased vascularization of skin, skeletal muscles, lung, heart, gastrointestinal tract, followed by fibrosis

Obliteration of interlobular arteries of the kidney may cause rapid renal failure, often with severe hypertension

Hereditary aspects uncertain

Cardiovascular features of scleroderma

Raynaud's syndrome common; also CREST syndrome (calcinosis, Raynaud's syndrome, esophageal dysfunction, sclerodactyly, telangiectasia)

Cardiomyopathy, with or without intimal sclerosis of small coronary arteries. Atrioventricular block (Stokes–Adams), arrhythmias (ventricular tachycardia), heart failure occur

Pulmonary hypertension (cor pulmonale) with or without pulmonary fibrosis

Systemic hypertension (renal disease)

Pericardial disease is common (20% or more; 67% caused by renal failure); usually asymptomatic

Epicardial coronary disease and valvular disease are rare

← Fig. 6.6 Cardiovascular features of scleroderma.

Summary of autopsy data from 34 patients with scleroderma

Physical Finding	% of patients
Pericardial disease	62*
Myocardial disease	
fibrosis, diffuse	12
total with fibrosis	30
left ventricular hypertrophy	47
right ventricular hypertrophy	28
biventricular hypertrophy	25
Lung fibrosis	65

*Three had clinical evidence of tamponade

← Fig. 6.7 Summary of autopsy data from 34 patients with scleroderma. (Ages 39–76 years; 7 male, 27 female.) (Modified from McWhorter JE IV, LeRoy EC. *Am J Med* 1974, **57**: 566–575.)

Clinical cardiac features of scleroderma

Congestive heart failure
- cardiomyopathy
- cor pulmonale
- systemic hypertension (renal disease)
- mitral valve disease

Cardiac arrhythmias
- atrioventricular block Stokes–Adams syncope)
- ventricular tachycardia
- atrial fibrillation, atrial flutter, atrial tachycardia

Pericarditis (uremia)
- acute pericarditis
- asymptomatic effusion
- constrictive pericarditis (rare)

Raynaud's syndrome

← Fig. 6.8
Clinical cardiac features of scleroderma.

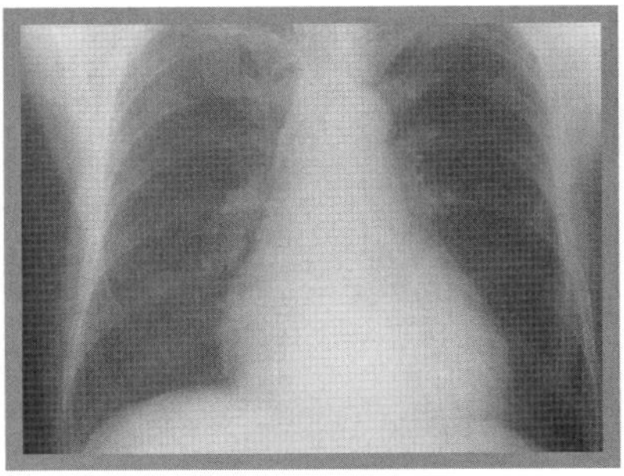

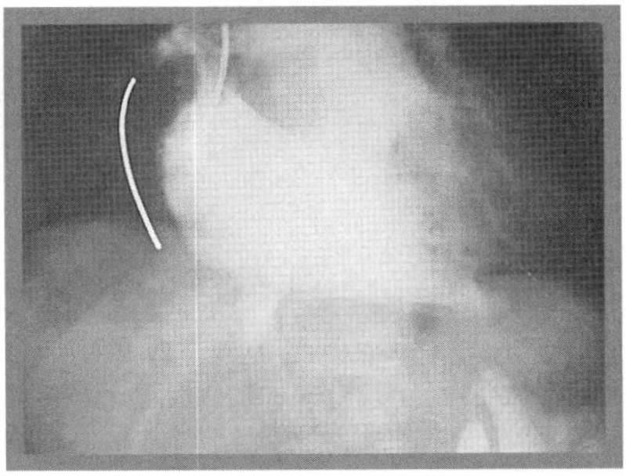

↑ Fig. 6.9a **↑ Fig. 6.9b**
Scleroderma. Chest radiogram and angiocardiogram of a patient with scleroderma and pericardial effusion. (**a**) The characteristic enlargement of the cardiopericardial silhouette, with clear lung fields. (**b**) The angiocardiogram shows a space between the outside border of the contrast medium in the right atrium and the curved bright line that shows the location of the parietal pericardium.

fingers and toes upon exposure to cold or with emotional stress. The digits at first turn white, and then become cyanotic (**Figs 6.10–6.13**). This vasospastic period usually lasts for 3–10 minutes, and is followed by a period of hyperemia. Continued involvement may lead to obliteration of digital arteries, with necrosis of the terminal phalanges (acromicria) (**Fig. 6.14**). Raynaud's syndrome is not specific for scleroderma, but also occurs with other connective tissue diseases, microemboli, cryoglobulinemia, macroglobulinemia, thromboangiitis obliterans, repeated trauma, and as a primary disease.

Another feature of scleroderma that may first suggest the disease is involvement of the skin. There may be a loss of normal wrinkling, and difficulty in frowning or opening the mouth widely. The skin of the fingers becomes shiny and bound down (sclerodactyly) (**Figs 6.15–6.18**). Limited joint movement may lead to a mistaken diagnosis of rheumatoid arthritis.

The disease tends to be progressive. Renal failure is the most common cause of death, and cardiac disease the next most common cause. Once heart failure develops, the prognosis is poor, and patients nearly always die within 7 years.

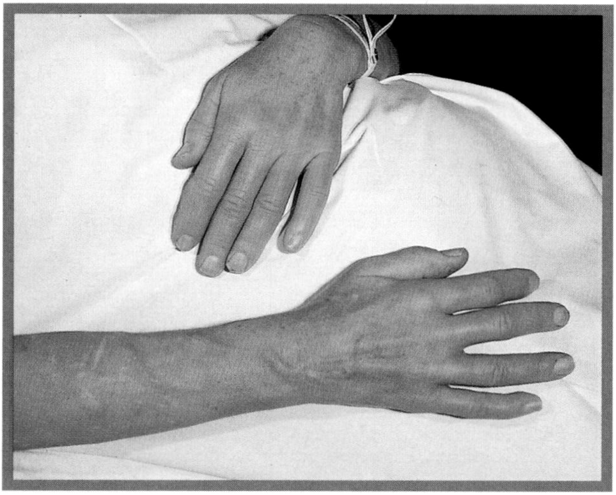

← Fig. 6.10 Scleroderma. Hands of a patient with scleroderma before exposure to cold.

→ Fig. 6.11
Scleroderma. Pallor of the fingers of the right hand after exposure to cold involving the right hand only.

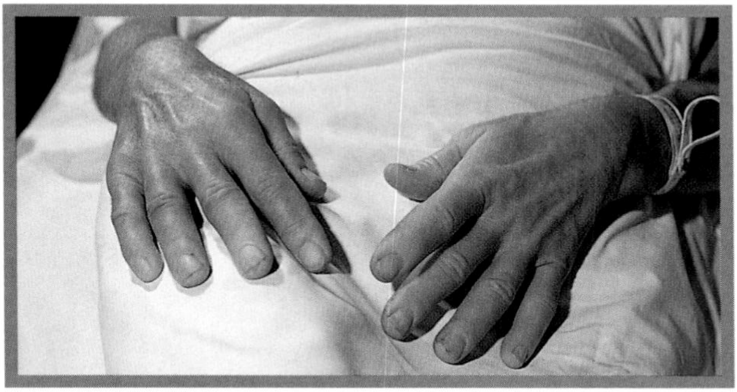

→ Fig. 6.12
Scleroderma. Raynaud's phenomenon, showing digital pallor caused by arterial spasm.

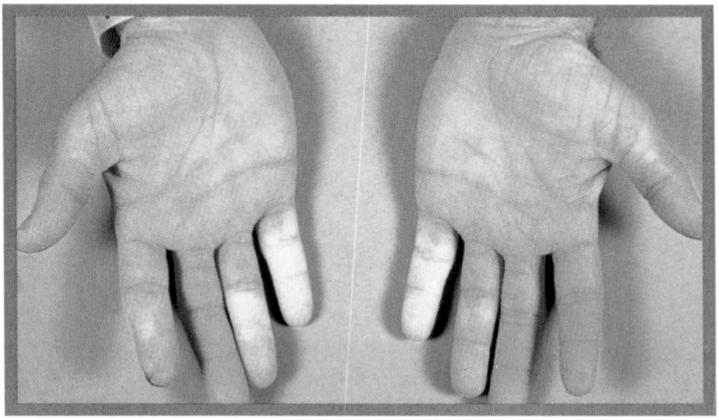

→ Fig. 6.13
Scleroderma. A later stage of Raynaud's phenomenon, showing cyanosis of the involved digits.

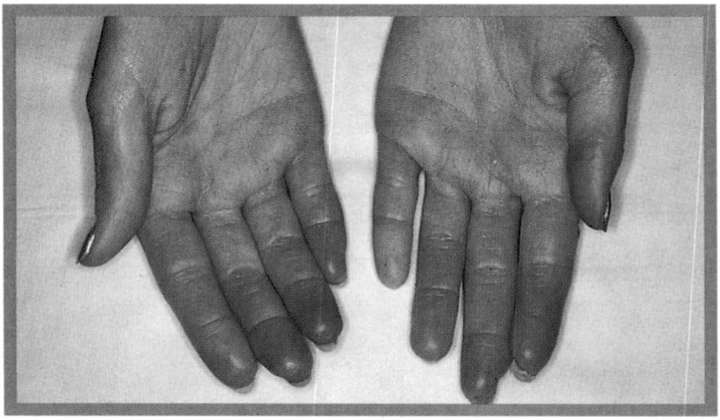

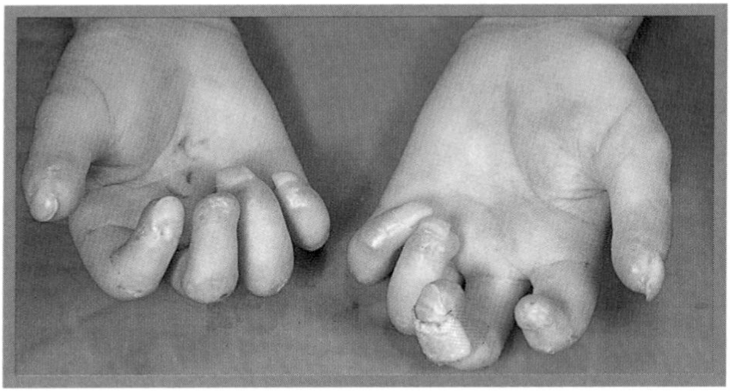

← Fig. 6.14
Scleroderma. Sclerodactyly with partial necrosis and scarring of the terminal digits. (With permission from Fowler NO. *Diagnosis of heart disease*. Springer–Verlag, 1991.)

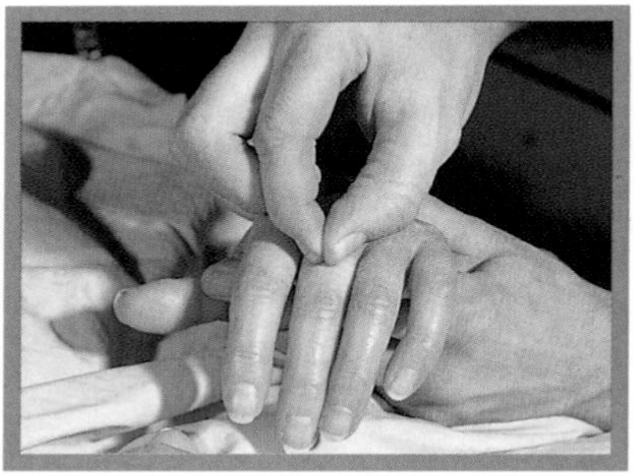

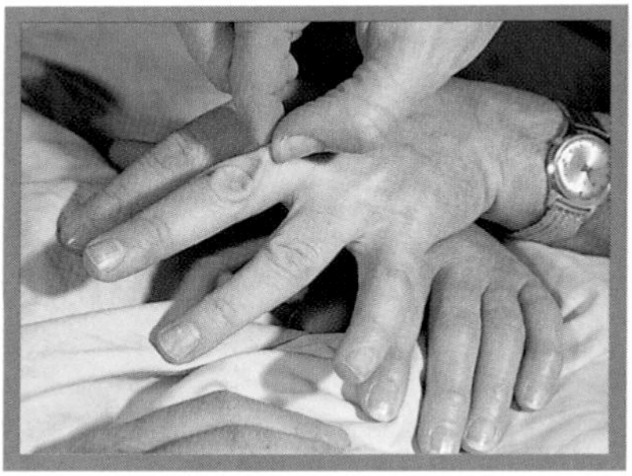

↑ Fig. 6.15a

↑ Fig. 6.15b

Scleroderma. (**a**) Shiny, inelastic skin of the fingers. (**b**) Normal elasticity.

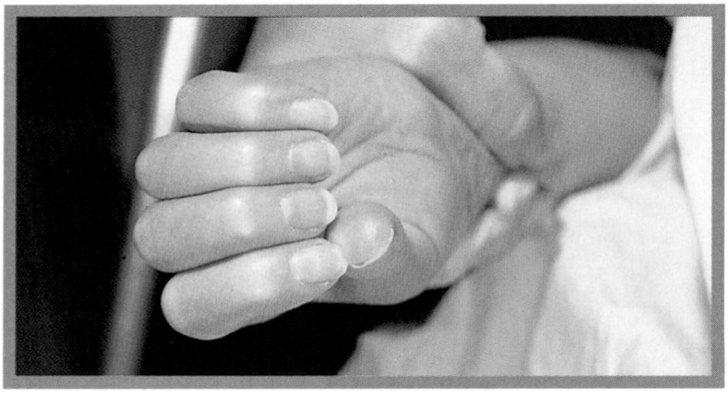

← Fig. 6.16
Scleroderma.
Note limited flexion of fingers and shiny skin.

→ Fig. 6.17
Scleroderma. Shiny skin of the fingers, with deformity of the proximal and distal interphalangeal joints. This may be mistaken for rheumatoid arthritis.

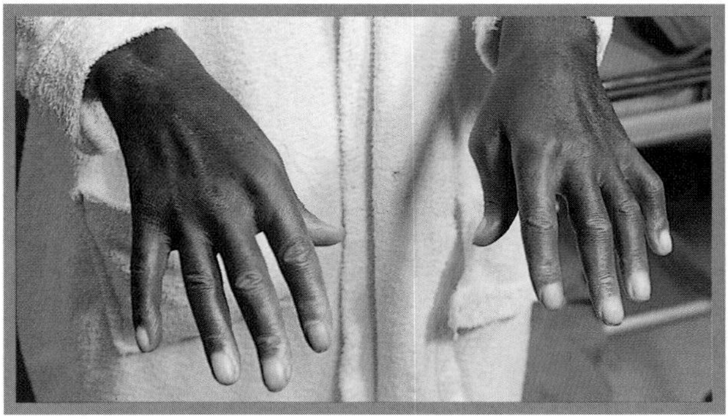

→ Fig. 6.18
Scleroderma. The fingers are puffy, with loss of hair.

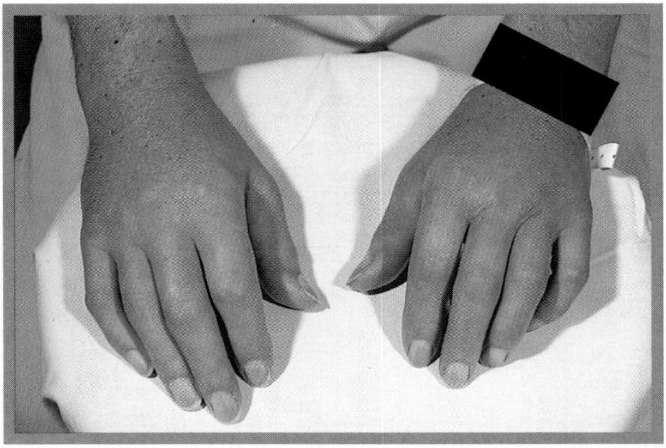

Further reading

Botstein JR, LeRoy EC. Primary heart disease in systemic sclerosis (scleroderma): advances in clinical and pathologic features, pathogenesis, and new therapeutic approaches. *Am Heart J* 1981, **102**:913–919.

LeRoy EC. The heart in systemic sclerosis. *N Engl J Med* 1984, **310**:188–190.

Patent Ductus Arteriosus

Patent ductus arteriosus is one of the more common congenital cardiac defects. In the absence of severe pulmonary hypertension, the condition is readily diagnosed from the typical continuous 'machinery' murmur (**Fig. 6.19**).

The fact that the maximal intensity of the murmur is in the second left intercostal space adjacent to the sternum serves to distinguish patent ductus arteriosus from other left-to-right shunts with continuous murmurs, such as

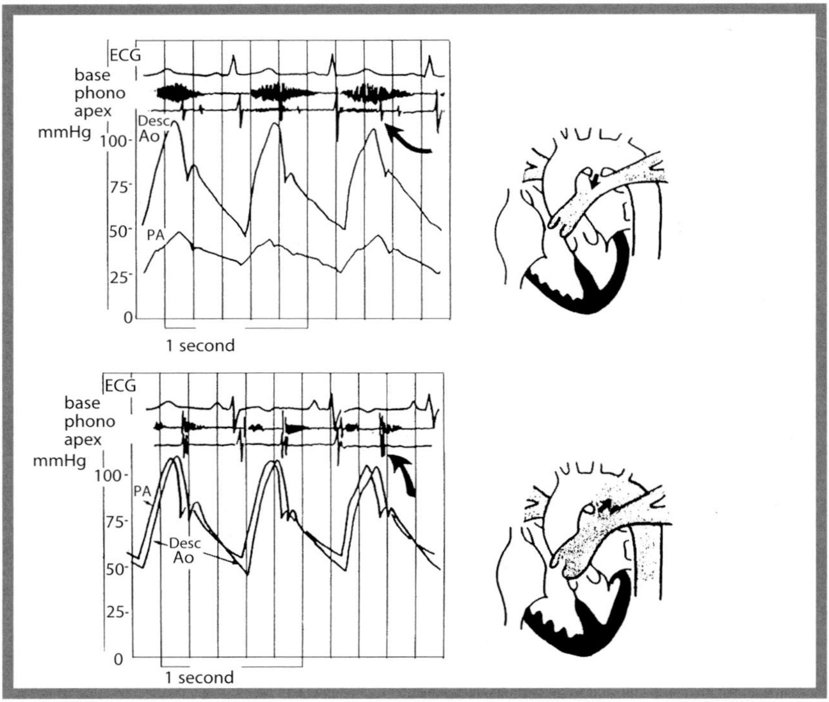

↑ Fig. 6.19
Patent ductus arteriosus. Upper panel: Left-to-right shunting ductus arteriosus (straight arrow) and continuous murmur at base. The curved arrow indicates S_2. Descending aortic (Desc Ao) pressure exceeds pulmonary arterial (PA) pressure throughout the cardiac cycle.
Lower panel: pulmonary hypertensive ductus with right-to-left shunting (straight arrow) and desaturation of differential cyanosis of blood in the descending aorta (shading). The curved arrow indicates the diastolic murmur of pulmonary regurgitation. There is no continuous murmur. (With permission from *Mod Concepts Cardiovasc Dis* 1990, **59**:19.)

coronary arteriovenous fistula and rupture of an aortic sinus of Valsalva aneurysm into the right heart. In patients with patent ductus arteriosus, usually the aortic pressure exceeds the pulmonary arterial pressure throughout the cardiac cycle; thus there is a shunt from aorta to pulmonary artery that continues from systole into diastole, producing the characteristic murmur (**Fig. 6.20**; see also Fig. 6.19). The shunt is from left to right and the patient is acyanotic. When the characteristic continuous murmur is present in the typical location in the second left intercostal space, the diagnosis can nearly always be made at the bedside. The diagnosis may be confirmed by cardiac catheterization or by two-dimensional echocardiography (**Fig. 6.21**).

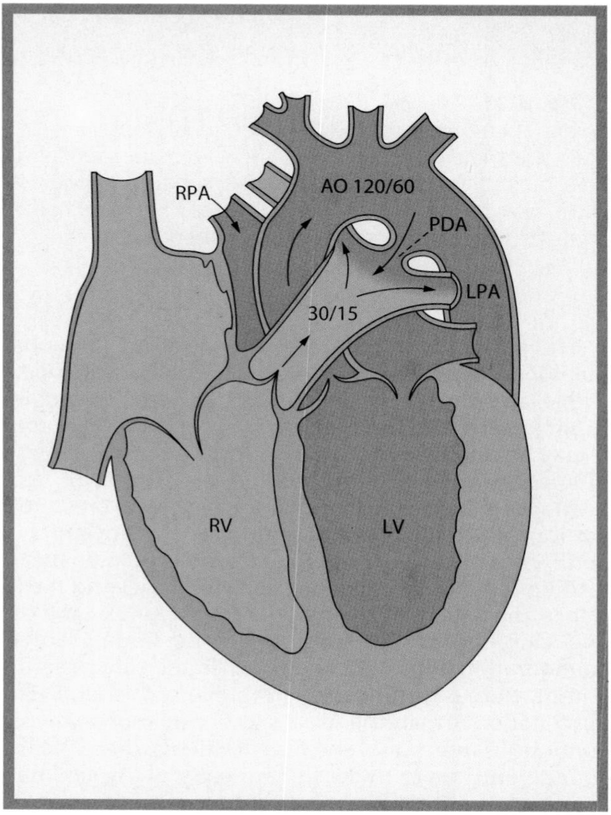

→ Fig. 6.20 Patent ductus arteriosus. The drawing shows the shunt of oxygenated blood from the aorta (AO) through the patent ductus arteriosus (PDA) into the pulmonary artery. The normal aortic pressure (120/60mmHg) exceeds the normal pulmonary arterial pressure (30/15mmHg) through the cardiac cycle; thus the shunt and the murmur are continuous. LPA, left pulmonary artery; LV, left ventricle; RPA, right pulmonary artery; RV, right ventricle.

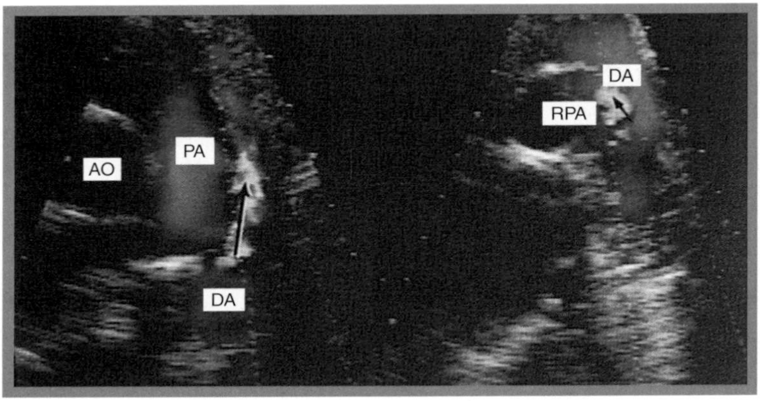

↑ Fig. 6.21
Patent ductus arteriosus. Two-dimensional Doppler echocardiogram of a patient with normal pulmonary arterial pressure and left-to-right shunt: parasternal short-axis view on the left; suprasternal view is on the right. In the latter view, the aorta is just superior to the right pulmonary artery (RPA). AO, aorta; DA, ductus arteriosus; PA, pulmonary artery.

The patient with patent ductus arteriosus may have, or may develop, pulmonary hypertension. This usually occurs in early life, and is more common with a large ductus. As pulmonary hypertension progresses, the left-to-right shunt lessens, and the characteristic continuous murmur is no longer heard. It may be replaced by an early blowing diastolic murmur that results from pulmonary valvular regurgitation (see Fig. 6.19). As pulmonary vascular resistance increases further, pulmonary arterial pressure approximately equals aortic pressure, and there is some reversal of flow through the ductus into the aorta. Thus mixed venous blood from the pulmonary artery enters the aorta, leading the arterial oxygen unsaturation beyond the left subclavian artery. Hence, the patient develops differential cyanosis and clubbing, with cyanosis and clubbing of the toes, while the fingers are pink and of normal configuration (**Figs 6.22** and **6.23**). In the clinical setting and physiology of patent ductus arteriosus with reversed shunt (**Fig. 6.24**), precordial auscultation reveals the usual signs of pulmonary hypertension. There is no continuous murmur of the patent ductus, there is a loud pulmonic closure sound, and there may be an early diastolic murmur of pulmonary regurgitation. The ECG shows right ventricular hypertrophy in approximately

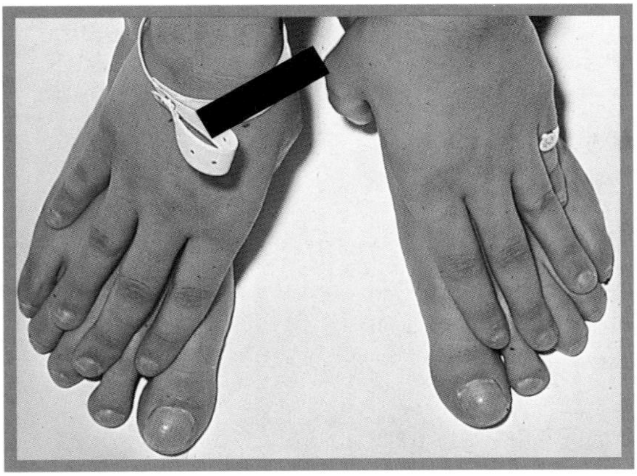

← Fig. 6.22
Patent ductus arteriosus. The photograph shows cyanosis and clubbing of the toes, with normal fingers, in a patient with pulmonary hypertension and reversed shunt through the ductus. See also Figures 6.19 and 6.23. (With permission from Fowler, NO. *Diagnosis of heart disease*. Springer–Verlag, 1991.)

→ Fig. 6.23
Patent ductus arteriosus. The diagram shows the flow pattern in a patient with patent ductus arteriosus and severe pulmonary hypertension and reversed shunt. Pressure in the pulmonary artery equals that in the aorta (AO), at 110/70mmHg. Because of the greater vascular resistance in the pulmonary circulation, desaturated blood flows through the ductus (PDA) into the aorta. See also Figures 6.19 and 6.22. LA, left atrium; LV, left ventricle; LPA, left pulmonary artery; LPV, left pulmonary vein; PT, pulmonary arterial trunk; RA, right atrium; RPA, right pulmonary artery; RV, right ventricle.

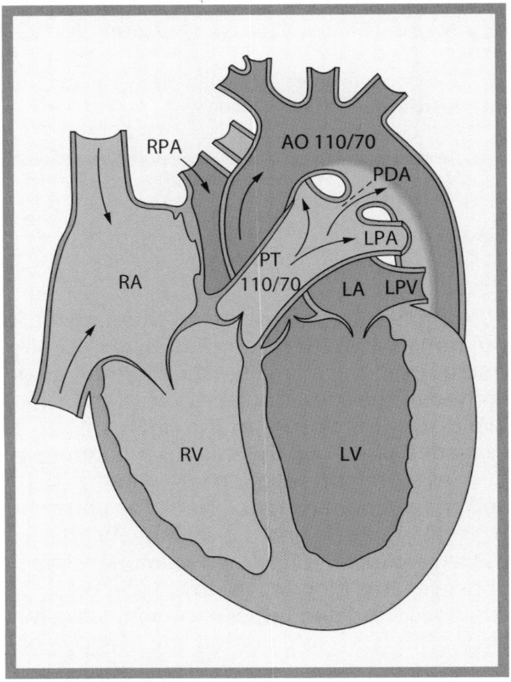

Patent ductus arteriosus with reversed shunt	% of patients
Onset in infancy	83
Eventually develop differential cyanosis and clubbing	50
A continuous murmur is not heard	100
Right ventricular hypertrophy on ECG	50
Dilated pulmonary trunk and right and left branches	90
Peripheral pulmonary oligemia on chest radiogram	>50
Bidirectional shunting	42
Average pulmonary vascular resistance	22 units
Develop prominent pulmonary artery impulse, systolic ejection sound, loud P_2	

← Fig. 6.24 Patent ductus arteriosus with reversed shunt.

50% of patients with reversed shunt, and the chest radiogram is typical of pulmonary hypertension (**Fig. 6.25**). As one cannot diagnose the patent ductus from the characteristic murmur, a finding of cyanosis and clubbing limited to the toes is both valuable and specific (see Fig. 6.22). One should avoid surgical closure of the ductus if the pulmonary vascular resistance exceeds 8 units, or if the shunt is predominantly right to left.

A less common situation is that in which there is transposition of the aorta and the pulmonary artery. Here, the aorta carries mixed venous blood from the right ventricle and the pulmonary artery carries oxygenated blood from the left ventricle. Thus, when pulmonary hypertension develops, there is flow of oxygenated blood to the lower part of the body through the patent ductus, while the head and upper extremities receive mixed venous blood from the aorta. This leads to clubbing and cyanosis of the fingers, while the toes are pink and without clubbing (**Figs 6.26** and **6.27**).

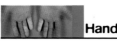

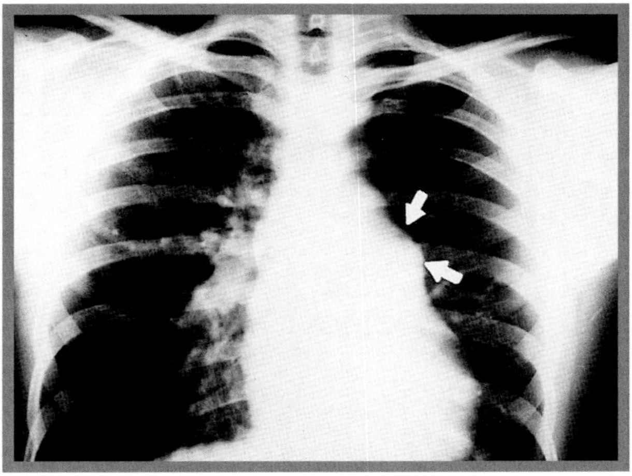

→ Fig. 6.25
Patent ductus arteriosus. Chest radiogram of a patient with patent ductus arteriosus, severe pulmonary hypertension, and reversed shunt. The arrows indicate the enlarged pulmonary artery segment.

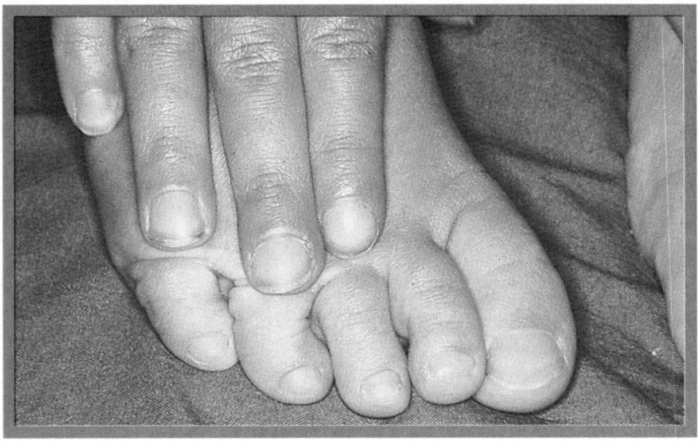

↑ Fig. 6.26
Patent ductus arteriosus. Photograph of hands and feet of a patient with patent ductus arteriosus, pulmonary hypertension, and transposition of the great arteries. There is cyanosis with clubbing of the fingers, and the toes are normal. Because of the transposition, the upper extremities and trunk receive desaturated aortic blood. Oxygenated blood is shunted through the ductus to mix with the bluish unsaturated blood in the descending aorta. See Figure 6.27.

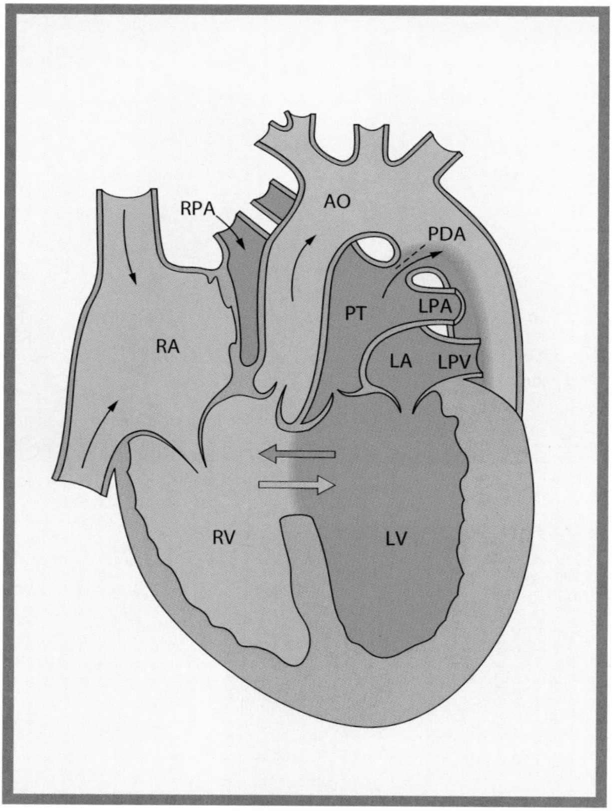

↑ Fig. 6.27
Patent ductus arteriosus. Drawing of a patient's circulation in the presence of patent ductus arteriosus, pulmonary hypertension, and transposition of the great arteries. The aorta (AO) arises from the right ventricle (RV), and carries desaturated blood. The pulmonary arterial trunk (PT) arises from the left ventricle (LV), and carries saturated blood. Because of pulmonary hypertension, oxygenated blood is shunted from the pulmonary artery through the ductus (PDA) into the aorta, giving rise to pink toes, while the fingers are clubbed and cyanotic. The paired arrows indicate a bidirectional shunt through a ventricular septal defect (VSD). See also Figure 6.26. LA, left atrium; LPA, left pulmonary artery; LPV, left pulmonary vein; RA, right atrium; RPA, right pulmonary artery.

Further reading

McManus BM, Hahn PF, Smith JA, Roberts WC, Jackson JH. Eisenmenger ductus arteriosus with prolonged survival. *Am J Cardiol* 1984, **54**:462–464.

Wood P. The Eisenmenger syndrome. *BMJ* 1958, **2**:701–709 and 755–762.

Absent Aortic Arch

Clubbing of the fingers, of the left hand only (**Fig. 6.28**), and cyanosis and clubbing of the toes (as was also present in the child pictured), occurs in patients with absence of the aortic arch. In this rare condition, the ascending aorta arises normally from the left ventricle and supplies normally oxygenated blood to the right upper extremity. The aortic arch is absent, and the descending aorta is supplied with unsaturated arterial blood from the pulmonary artery through a patent ductus arteriosus (**Fig. 6.29**). Pulmonary hypertension is present, as

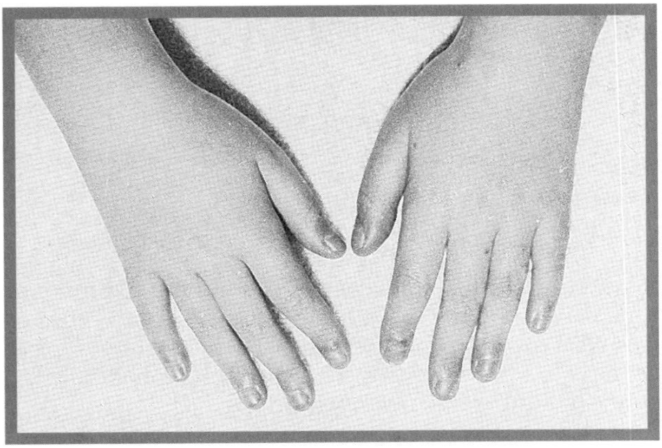

↑ Fig. 6.28
Absent aortic arch. The child in this photograph had clubbing of the fingers of the left hand and not of the right. This unusual finding occurs when the aortic arch is interrupted. The right hand receives oxygenated blood from the ascending aorta (see Fig. 6.29). The blood to the descending aorta and left arm is desaturated blood arising from the pulmonary artery and flowing through a patent ductus arteriosus to the left arm and lower body. Pulmonary hypertension is present. (Reprinted by permission of the publisher from Dorney E, *et al* Unilateral clubbing of the fingers due to absence of the aortic arch. *Am J Med* 1955, **18**:151. Copyright 1955 by Excerpta Medica, Inc.)

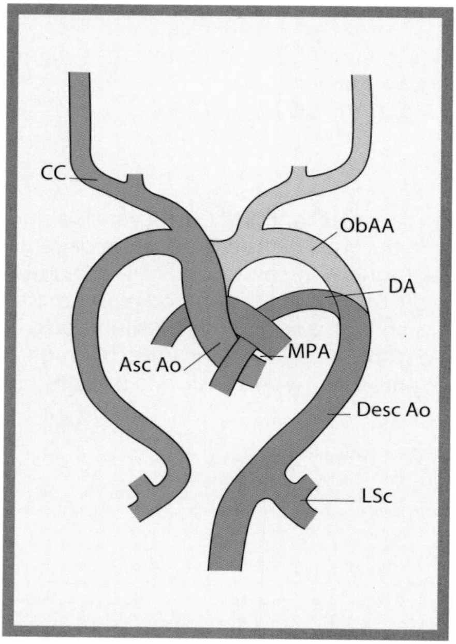

← Fig. 6.29
Absent aortic arch. Diagram of circulation. The clear area indicates the obliterated aortic arch. The black shading indicates oxygenated blood in the ascending aorta and its branches. The cross-hatched area indicates desaturated blood entering the descending aorta from the pulmonary artery through the ductus arteriosus. Asc Ao, ascending aorta; CC, common carotid artery; DA, ductus arteriosus; Desc Ao, descending aorta; LSc, left subclavian artery; MPA, main pulmonary artery; ObAA, obliterated aortic arch.

pulmonary arterial pressure must equal or exceed systemic arterial pressure. Patients with this condition have cardiac physical findings similar to those of patent ductus arteriosus with reversed shunt—that is, absence of the typical continuous ductus murmur, a loud P_2, a diastolic murmur of pulmonary valvular insufficiency, and evidence of right ventricular hypertrophy.

Reference

Dorney ER, Fowler NO, Mannix EP. Unilateral clubbing of the fingers due to absence of the aortic arch. *Am J Med* 1955, **18**:150–154.

Thyrotoxicosis (Onycholysis)

Onycholysis (separation of the nail from the nail bed) (**Fig. 6.30**; the same young woman as pictured in Figs 1.33 and 1.34), along with exophthalmos, stare, lid lag, fine tremor of the tongue and fingers, and warm moist pinkish skin, is one of the physical signs suggesting thyrotoxicosis. Common circulatory signs are wide arterial pulse pressure, sinus tachycardia or atrial fibrillation, a 'bruit de

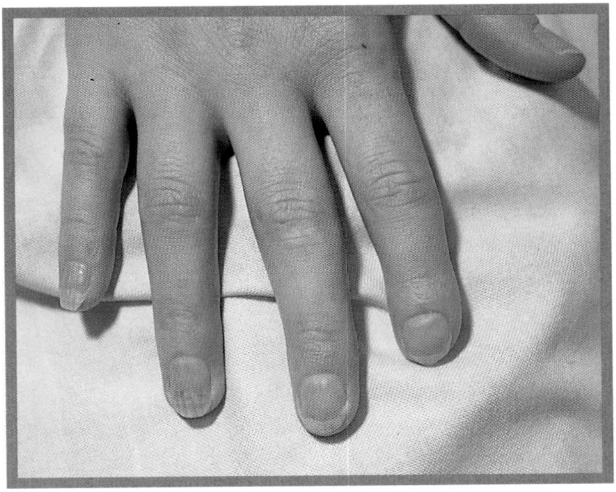

→ Fig. 6.30 Onycholysis. Separation of the nail plate from its bed in a 28-year-old woman with hyperthyroidism (see Figs 1.33 and 1.34).

diable' heard over the thyroid gland, a cervical venous hum, a loud S_1, and the presence of S_3 and S_4. Most of these circulatory signs are due to the high cardiac output state that usually accompanies this condition.

Holt–Oram Syndrome

The Holt–Oram syndrome has also been called the heart–hand syndrome, atriodigital dysplasia, and upper limb cardiovascular syndrome. It is an autosomal dominant condition characterized by dysplasia of the upper extremities. The genetic defect is believed to be present on the long arm of chromosome 12 (12q2). Expression within a pedigree is variable. The usual deformity involves the thumb, which is typically digitalized; that is, it is triphalangeal and lies in the same plane as the fingers (**Fig. 6.31**). In some cases, the thumb is missing entirely; in others, the thenar eminence is hypoplastic. Syndactyly and clinodactyly may occur. In other instances, the radius is missing or deformed (**Fig. 6.32**). There may be phocomelia; there may be hypoplasia of the clavicles. Carpal deformities also occur, and the ulna may be misshapen. The upper extremity anomalies are usually bilateral, but not necessarily symmetrical.

Approximately 50% of patients have congenital cardiac defects. The most common lesion is an atrial septal defect (ASD) of the ostium secundum variety. Ventricular septal defect (VSD) may also occur. Less common lesions are pulmonary valve stenosis, anomalous pulmonary venous return, transposition

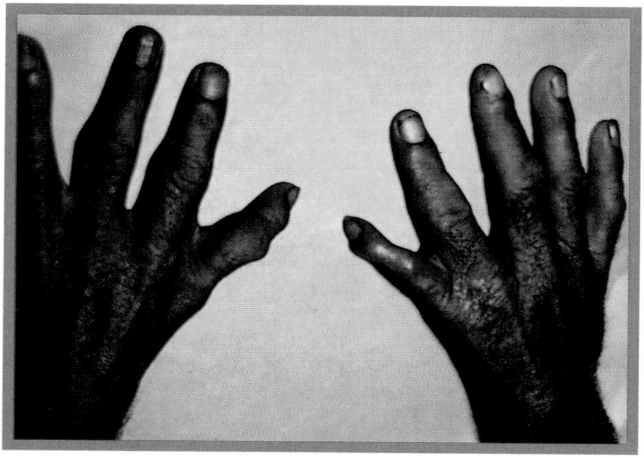

← Fig. 6.31
Holt–Oram syndrome. Note the triphalangeal thumb. (With permission from Schlant RC, Alexander RW, eds. *Hurst's the heart, arteries, and veins, 8th ed.* New York: McGraw–Hill, NY; 1994.)

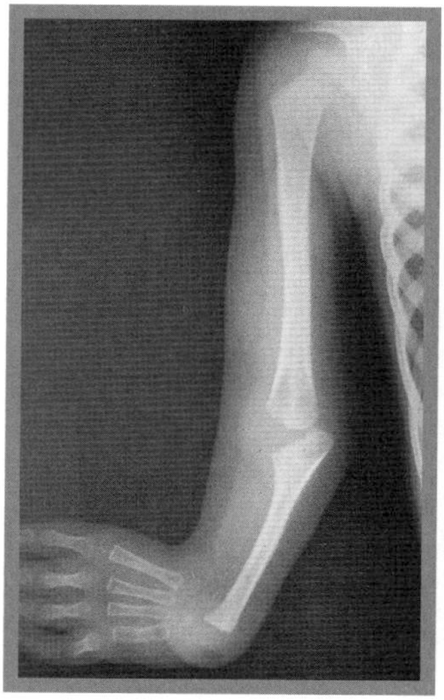

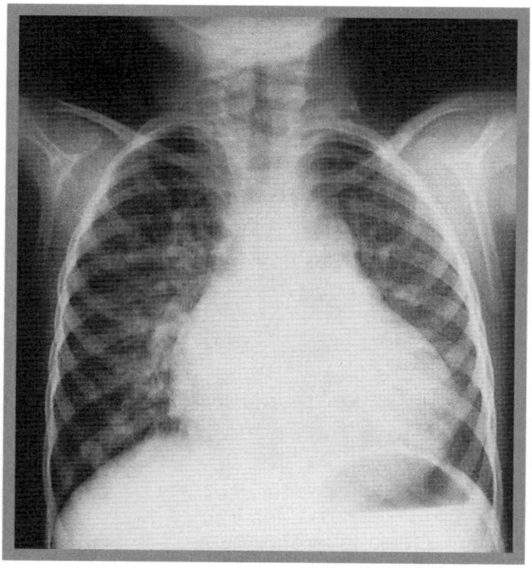

↑ Fig. 6.32a **↑ Fig. 6.32b**
Holt–Oram syndrome. (**a**) Radiogram showing absence of thumb and radius in a 3-year-old boy with a single ventricle. (**b**) The chest radiogram shows an enlarged heart and pulmonary over-circulation associated with a single ventricle.

of the great arteries, coarctation of the aorta, and hypoplastic left heart syndrome (**Fig. 6.33**). An association with mitral valve prolapse has been described. Atrioventricular conduction disturbances may be found, and sinus bradycardia has also been described. Zhang *et al.* described tetralogy of Fallot in this condition. Pectus excavatum and hypoplastic peripheral arteries also have been reported.

Three diagnostic criteria for Holt–Oram syndrome have been proposed: autosomal dominant transmission; ASD in at least one family member; skeletal anomalies in the upper extremity involving the thumb, metacarpus, wrist, and radius.

→ Fig. 6.33 Holt–Oram syndrome. (From Smith AT, Sack GHJr and Taylor GJ. *J Pediatr* 1979, **95**:538–543.)

Holt–Oram syndrome

Upper limb dysplasia: absent or triphalangeal thumb, radial aplasia, phocomelia

Heart disease (present in 50%): ASD; VSD; atrioventricular conduction disturbances; mitral prolapse; (also transposition, coarctation, pulmonary stenosis)

Variability within families; autosomal dominant

Possible relation to locus on chromosome 20g13

Reference

Zhang KZ, Sun QB, Cheng TO. Holt–Oram syndrome in China; a collective review of 18 cases. *Am Heart J* 1986, **111**:572–577.

Further reading

Basson CT, Cowley GS, Solomon SD, *et al.* The clinical and genetic spectrum of the Holt–Oram syndrome (heart–hand syndrome). *N Engl J Med* 1994, **330**:885–891.

Muller LM, DeJong G, Van Heerden KMM. The antenatal ultrasonographic detection of the Holt–Oram syndrome. *S Afr Med J* 1985, **68**:313–315.

Digital Clubbing

Digital clubbing may be an important physical sign in various kinds of cardiopulmonary disease; alternatively, it may be an incidental finding of no clinical significance. Early clubbing may be signaled by softening and fluctuation of the nail bed and loss of the angle between the nail bed and the skin at the base of the nail. Later, there is actual enlargement of the terminal digit. This enlargement has been attributed to increased vascularity, fibrous hyperplasia, and edema. Digital clubbing is usually painless, but in chronic suppurative pulmonary disease or lung cancer there may be pain over the tibia, radius, and ulna, associated with hypertrophy of the bony cortex (pulmonary hypertrophic osteoarthropathy or pulmonary acropachy).

Digital clubbing may or may not be accompanied by cyanosis (**Fig. 6.34**). Acyanotic clubbing may be caused by chronic pulmonary suppurative

Digital clubbing
Clubbing Without Cyanosis
Carcinoma of the lung
Chronic suppurative pulmonary infection: bronchiectasis, lung abscess, empyema
Subacute bacterial endocarditis
Pulmonary fibrosis, mesothelioma
Gastrointestinal disorders: biliary cirrhosis; regional enteritis
Familial
Clubbing With Cyanosis
Eisenmenger's syndrome
Tetralogy of Fallot
Ebstein's anomaly
Tricuspid atresia
Pulmonary arteriovenous fistula
Transposition of the great arteries
Differential cyanosis and clubbing: patent ductus arteriosus with pulmonary hypertension

← Fig. 6.34 Digital clubbing.

disease, lung cancer, or subacute infective endocarditis. It may be a benign familial condition. As it usually requires a few months to develop, digital clubbing is not usually seen with acute forms of infective endocarditis. Tetralogy of Fallot is a particularly unusual cause of acyanotic digital clubbing (**Fig. 6.35**). Several weeks before the Figure 6.35 photograph was taken, the patient had cyanotic digital clubbing caused by a right-to-left shunt at the ventricular level, associated with Fallot's tetralogy. At the time of the photograph, he had undergone surgical correction of the tetralogy. Thus he was no longer cyanotic, but the clubbing had not yet disappeared. Six months after surgical correction of his tetralogy of Fallot, he no longer had digital clubbing (**Fig. 6.36**).

Differential cyanosis and clubbing associated with patent ductus arteriosus and pulmonary hypertension have been discussed above, in the sections on patent ductus arteriosus and absent aortic arch.

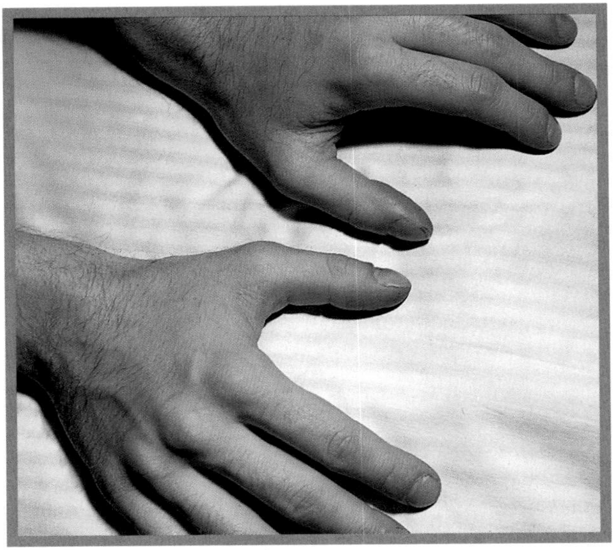

→ Fig. 6.35
Digital clubbing. This photograph shows digital clubbing without cyanosis in a 20-year-old man recently operated upon for surgical correction of tetralogy of Fallot. See also Figure 6.36.

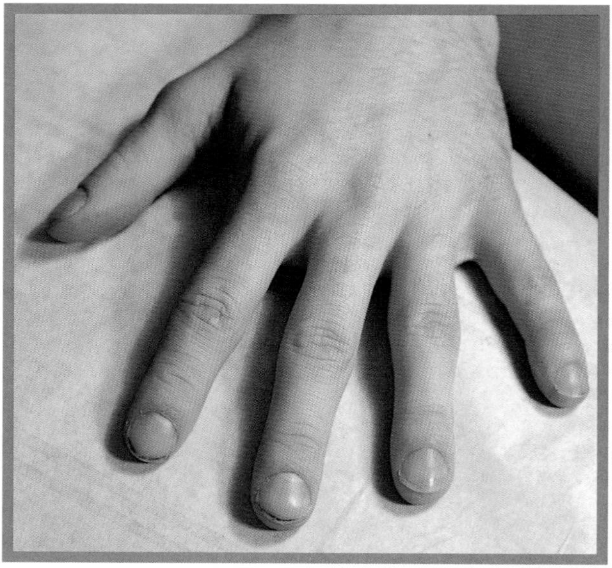

← Fig. 6.36 Digital clubbing. Photograph of the hands of the patient in Figure 6.35. Six months after surgical correction of tetralogy of Fallot, the digital clubbing has disappeared.

Further reading

Editorial. Finger clubbing. *Lancet* 1975, **1**:1285.

Fishman AP. *Pulmonary diseases & disorders, 2nd ed.* New York: McGraw-Hill Book Company; 1988:318.

Digital Petechiae and Hemorrhages

Digital petechiae and hemorrhages may be found in a patient with acute infective endocarditis (**Fig. 6.37**), when they may be due to either vasculitis or embolism. These findings are not specific for infective endocarditis, although they may suggest the condition. The diagnosis of infective endocarditis as their cause must depend upon the cardinal features of the disease: fever, cardiac valvular vegetations demonstrated by echocardiography, cardiac valvular insufficiency, and above all, a positive blood culture. Rather than infective endocarditis, various hematologic disorders may be responsible for digital petechiae and hemorrhages. Scurvy or atheroemboli may also be to blame. Splinter hemorrhages alone are most often due to trauma, and are less suggestive of infective endocarditis.

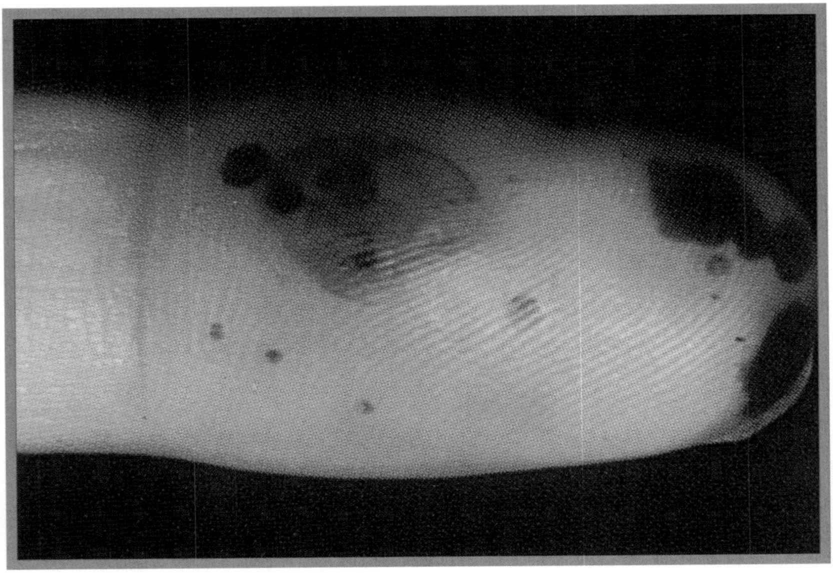

↑ Fig. 6.37
Digital petechiae and hemorrhages in a patient with acute infective endocarditis. Although splinter hemorrhages in the nail bed may be seen in infective endocarditis, they are most often caused by trauma. Other causes include hematologic disorders, vasculitis, scurvy, or atheroemboli. (With permission from Schlant RC, Alexander RW, eds. *Hurst's the heart, arteries, and veins, 8th ed.* New York: McGraw–Hill, NY; 1994.)

Shoulder–Hand Syndrome

The shoulder–hand syndrome has been called a reflex sympathetic dystrophy syndrome. It may be precipitated by myocardial infarction, cervical osteoarthritis, trauma, or other factors. The features of the syndrome include pain and swelling in an extremity, trophic skin changes, pain or limited motion of the ipsilateral shoulder, and a precipitating event.

This syndrome is an uncommon complication of coronary artery disease. It may occur in patients with stable angina pectoris or unstable angina pectoris, or may follow acute myocardial infarction. When it complicates myocardial infarction, its onset is usually delayed for a period ranging between 1 week and 7 months. In the 1950s, Russek observed this complication only once in 50 patients with acute myocardial infarction. It is probably even less common today, possibly because patients with acute myocardial infarction are no longer kept in bed for a period of up to 6 weeks, as was the practice in the past.

The shoulder–hand syndrome is characterized by pain and swelling in the hand of the affected upper extremity (**Figs 6.38** and **6.39**). More commonly, the left upper extremity and hand are involved, possibly because the pain of ischemic heart disease is more common on that side. Pain and limited motion of the shoulder usually precede discomfort in the hand and forearm. As the initial swelling subsides, there is a tendency for skin atrophy and osteoporosis to develop. Eventually, there may be a frozen shoulder. The fingers of the affected hand may be covered with shiny atrophic skin, resembling sclerodactyly. Flexion contraction of the tendons may follow.

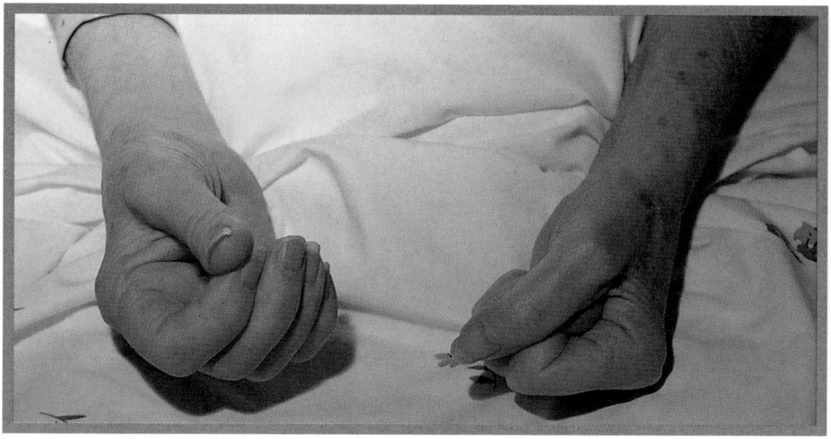

↑ Fig. 6.38
Shoulder–hand syndrome. The patient whose hands are pictured here had coronary artery disease with angina pectoris and myocardial infarction. She developed swelling of the right hand, with difficulty in making a fist, after a myocardial infarction. This syndrome is also called sympathetic osteodystrophy and is often accompanied by pain and limited motion of the painful upper extremity. Radiograms may show osteoporosis of the affected extremity. It is seldom seen today, possibly because the activity of such patients is less restricted than in the past.

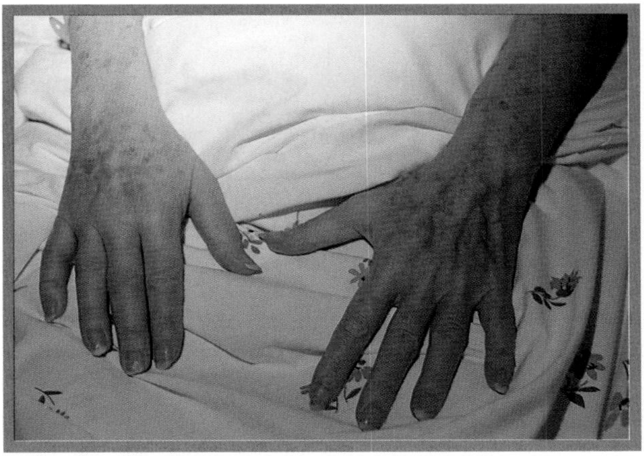

→ Fig. 6.39 Shoulder–hand syndrome. Further features of the patient in Figure 6.38.

Reference

Russek HI. Shoulder–hand syndrome following myocardial infarction. *Med Clin North Am* 1958, **42**:1555–1556.

Further reading

Kozin F, McCarty DJ, Sims J, Genant H. The reflex sympathetic dystrophy syndrome. *Am J Med* 1976, **60**:321–331.

Thromboangiitis Obliterans

Thromboangiitis obliterans, also known as Buerger's disease, is an uncommon disease. It is most commonly seen in males who smoke tobacco, but may occur in persons of either sex aged between 15 and 50 years. There is no racial bias. It is a panvasculitis involving both arteries and veins that usually begins distally in digital vessels, and tends to progress proximally. Symptoms are more common in the lower extremities, where calf vessels and the profunda femoris may be involved, with associated symptoms of calf claudication. Superficial thrombophlebitis is common. Later on, iliac, cerebral, and coronary arteries may be attacked. In a few patients, epicardial coronary artery involvement may lead to coronary thrombosis.

Involvement of the arteries of the upper extremities is not rare: in the angiographic study by Hirai & Shionoya, arterial obstruction in at least one upper limb was found in 31 of 34 patients, all of whom were male smokers. The radial or ulnar pulse may be absent. Involvement of arteries of the upper extremities suggests Buerger's disease rather than arteriosclerosis as the cause of arterial disease in the lower extremities. Involvement of the digital arteries may be signaled by Raynaud's syndrome; at times, Raynaud's syndrome, usually bilateral, is the presenting feature of thromboangiitis obliterans. The disease tends to progress slowly, and thrombotic occlusion of vessels may lead to ischemic necrosis (**Fig. 6.40**).

The diagnosis may be made by angiography or biopsy. The progress of the disease is usually halted by cessation of smoking, but in some instances amputation of an affected part is necessary. At times, autoamputation of terminal digits occurs.

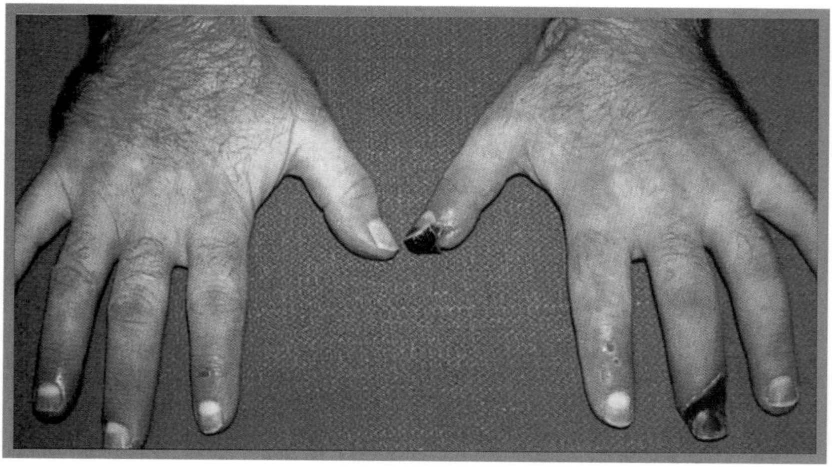

↑ Fig. 6.40
Thromboangiitis obliterans. Photograph of the hands of a 35-year-old man who had smoked approximately 40 cigarets daily for 20 years. The thumb and middle finger of the left hand demonstrate necrosis involving the terminal phalanges. Radial pulses were markedly diminished. (With permission from Rosencrance G, Thistlewaite T. *N Engl J Med* 1996, **334**:891.)

Reference

Hirai M, Shionoya S. Arterial obstruction of the upper limb in Buerger's disease; its incidence and primary lesion. *Br J Surg* 1979, **66**:124–128.

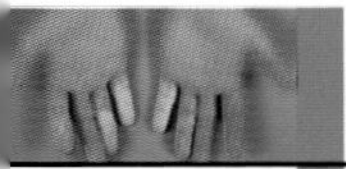

7 Extremities

Xanthoma in Hypercholesterolemia

Xanthomas represent an important clue to hyperlipoproteinemias and the possibility of coronary artery disease. They are, essentially, cholesterol-filled nodules that occur subcutaneously or overlying tendons (xanthoma tendinosum), and are of several varieties (**Fig. 7.1**). Xanthelasma, tendinous xanthoma, and corneal arcus have been considered to be a triad associated with hypercholesterolemia.

Xanthoma tendinosum occurs as nodular swellings over the Achilles tendons, elbows, and extensor surfaces of the hands (**Figs 7.2–7.4**). These are usually associated with type II hyperlipoproteinemia, a familial hyperlipoproteinemia in which serum cholesterol is increased and serum triglyceride values are normal. When the patient has the homozygous form of this disorder, xanthoma tendinosum may appear before puberty. This kind of xanthoma is unusual in type III hyperlipoproteinemia, in which both cholesterol and serum triglycerides tend to be equally increased. Xanthelasma, involving the eyelids, may also occur in type II hyperlipidemia, but is less specific (see Fig. 2.48).

Palmar xanthomas (also called xanthoma striata palmaris) and tuberoeruptive xanthomas occur in type III hyperlipoproteinemia. These patients may have xanthoma tuberosum, which may be soft, hard, eruptive, or pedunculated, and may be found over the tibial tubercles and the elbows. Although tendinous xanthomas are said to be rare in type III hyperlipoproteinemia, they were found in 25% of the patients studied by Morganroth *et al.* Eruptive xanthomas, 1–2mm in diameter, may occur anywhere on the body, and are associated with types I and V hyperlipoproteinemia.

Xanthelasma and corneal arcus are rare in type III hyperlipoproteinemia. Corneal arcus (annulus senilis) is not necessarily correlated with hypercholesterolemia or coronary artery disease, but when it is found in the young (arcus juvenalis), a correlation may exist (see Fig. 3.1). Pe'er *et al.* found a correlation between the width of the corneal arcus and serum cholesterol concentration in men averaging 61.9 years and women averaging 59 years of age.

Xanthomas and xanthelasma may also appear in patients with biliary cirrhosis (**Figs 7.5** and **7.6**).

Familial hyperlipidemia	
Type II	
50% reduction (heterozygote) or absence (homozygote) of hepatic low-density lipoprotein receptor	
Tendinous xanthomas	
Arcus juvenilis and xanthelasma	
Type III	
Increased serum cholesterol and triglycerides	
81% had xanthomas in one study:	
xanthoma striata palmaris	64%
xanthoma tuberosum (elbows, buttocks, knees)	50%
tendinous xanthomas (Achilles tendon, extensor tendons)	25%
May have corneal arcus and xanthelasma	
Types I and V	
May have eruptive xanthomas 1–4 cm in diameter all over the body	
Type IV	
Elevated triglycerides and very low density lipoproteins	
Xanthomas not commonly described	

← Fig. 7.1 Familial hyperlipidemia.

→ Fig. 7.2
Xanthoma in hypercholesterolemia. Xanthoma of the Achilles tendon in a young woman with familial hypercholesterolemia and coronary artery disease. This patient is also pictured in Figs 7.3 and 7.4.

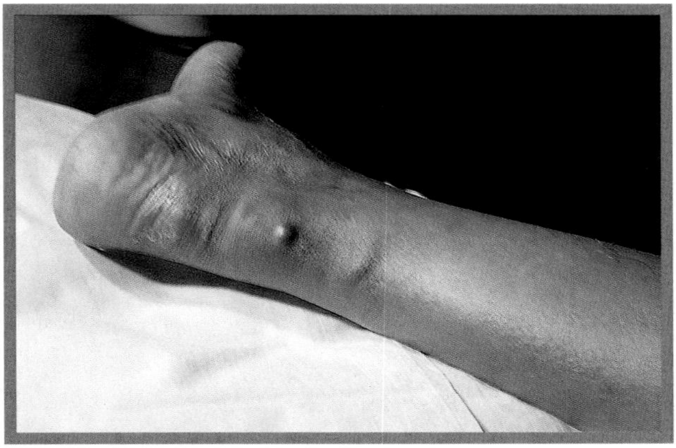

→ Fig. 7.3
Xanthoma in hypercholesterolemia. Tendinous xanthomas.

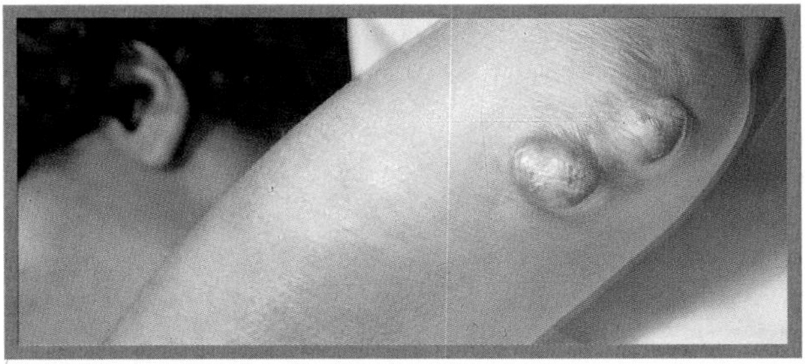

→ Fig. 7.4
Xanthoma in hypercholesterolemia. Tendinous xanthomas of the finger. (With permission from Fowler NO. *Diagnosis of heart disease*. Springer–Verlag, 1991.)

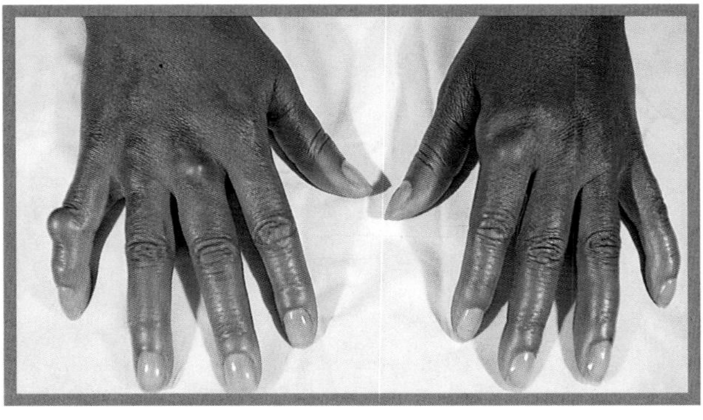

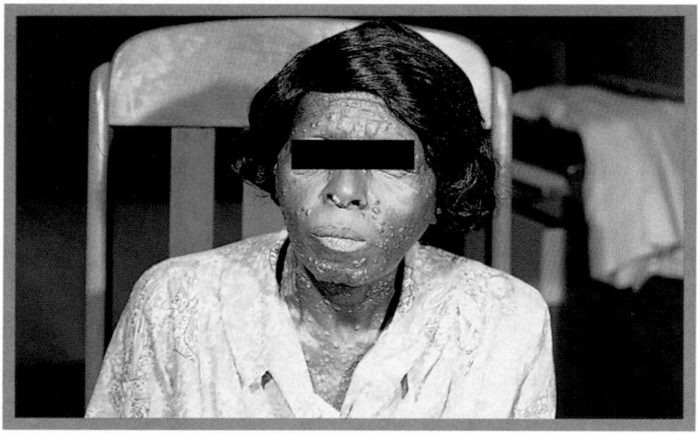

← Fig. 7.5 Facial xanthomas in a patient with biliary cirrhosis.

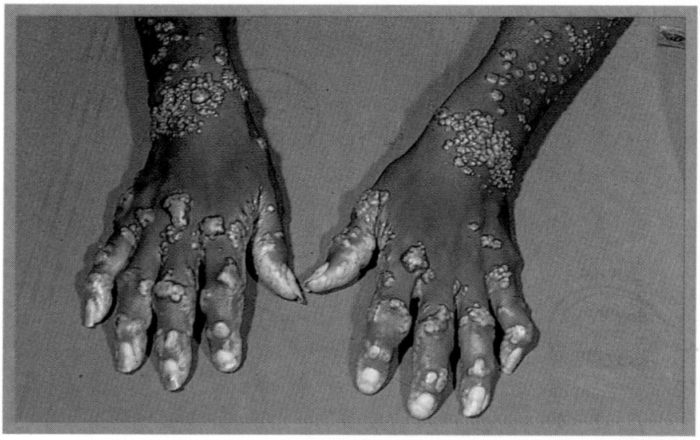

← Fig. 7.6 Xanthomas of the fingers in a patient with biliary cirrhosis.

References

Morganroth J, Levy RJ, Fredrickson DS. The biochemical, clinical, and genetic features of Type III hyperlipoproteinemia. *Ann Int Med* 1975, **82**:158–174.

Pe'er J, Vidaurri J, Halfon S-T, Eisenberg S, Zauberman H. Association between corneal arcus and some of the risk factors for coronary artery disease. *Br J Ophthalmol* 1983, **67**:795–798.

Further Reading

Winder AF. Relationship between corneal arcus and hyperlipidemia is clarified by studies in familial hypercholesterolemia. *Br J Ophthalmol* 1983, **67**:789–794.

Lymphedema

Lymphedema may be responsible for unilateral swelling of one lower extremity (**Fig. 7.7**), and may be primary or secondary. Primary lymphedema is caused by a primary abnormality or disease of the lymph-conducting elements of the lymph vessels of lymph nodes. It is more common in women and usually appears before the age of 40 years. The edema of primary lymphedema may be either unilateral or bilateral. Congenital lymphedema is a form of primary lymphedema that is present at birth and is associated with absent, malformed, or damaged lymphatic vessels. It may be found in Turner's syndrome (see Fig. 1.32), and in Noonan's syndrome. Simple congenital lymphedema is non-familial; one congenital familial form, called Milroy's disease, is an autosomal dominant.

Secondary lymphedema is caused by blockage of lymphatic vessels by infection, parasitism (filariasis), or neoplasm involving inguinal lymph nodes, or may be caused by surgical or traumatic damage to lymphatics. Radiation therapy directed at the lymph nodes for treatment of cancer may be responsible for lymphedema, especially when used after surgical excision of regional lymph nodes. This is commonly seen in an upper extremity after such treatment for breast cancer.

Lymphedema must be distinguished from venous disease as a cause of unilateral lower extremity edema; venous disease is by far the most common cause of such edema. Insufficiency of the valves in the communicating veins between superficial saphenous veins and deep femoral veins is a common explanation, and iliofemoral thrombophlebitis also may cause unilateral edema; a very common cause is surgical removal of saphenous veins for use in coronary artery bypass grafts. Venous disease as a cause of unilateral edema is suggested when superficial veins are prominent and tortuous, and when there are varicosities with hemosiderin-related skin pigmentation, varicose eczema, or ulcers. At lymphangiography, venous disease is associated with rapid uptake of the isotope, whereas the uptake is slow in lymphedema and the lymphatics are decreased or blocked. Venous disease as a cause of unilateral edema may be confirmed by the use of venography.

Unilateral edema may be seen with arthritis or fractures, or cellulitis, but then does not involve the entire extremity and is usually associated with pain, warmth, and tenderness. An arteriovenous fistula may cause edema of one lower extremity. An immobilized patient who is seated all day with one leg elevated may develop edema of the dependent leg. Congestive heart failure does not usually cause unilateral leg edema, unless a bed-ridden patient lies constantly on one side. The same may be said for other causes of more generalized edema, such as renal disease, hypoproteinemia, anemia, or medication.

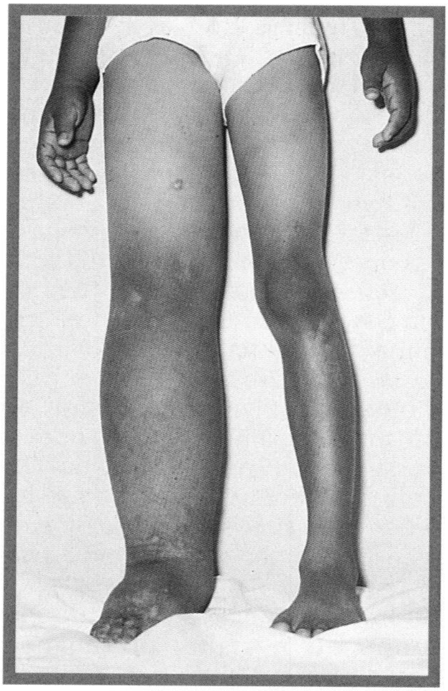

← Fig. 7.7
Lymphedema. Massive edema of the right lower extremity, caused by congenital lymphedema.

Further Reading

Browse NL. The diagnosis and management of primary lymphedema. *J Vasc Surg* 1986, **3**:181–184.

Browse NL, Stewart G. Lymphedema: pathophysiology and classification. *J Cardiovasc Surg* 1985, **26**:91–106.

Duchenne Muscular Dystrophy

Duchenne muscular dystrophy is an X-linked recessive disorder. It involves skeletal and cardiac muscle, smooth muscle of blood vessels, and the central nervous system. In this disease, dystrophin, produced by a defective gene at the xp21 locus of the short arm of the X chromosome, is absent from myogenic cells, or nearly so.

The typical physical findings are those of hypertrophy and pseudohypertrophy of skeletal muscle groups. Pseudohypertrophy is due to infiltration or replacement of skeletal muscle fibers by fat and connective tissue. The earliest expression clinically usually involves enlargement of the calves, but the deltoid and pectoralis major muscles are also commonly involved (**Fig. 7.8**). As a rule, there is difficulty in walking and in rising from a

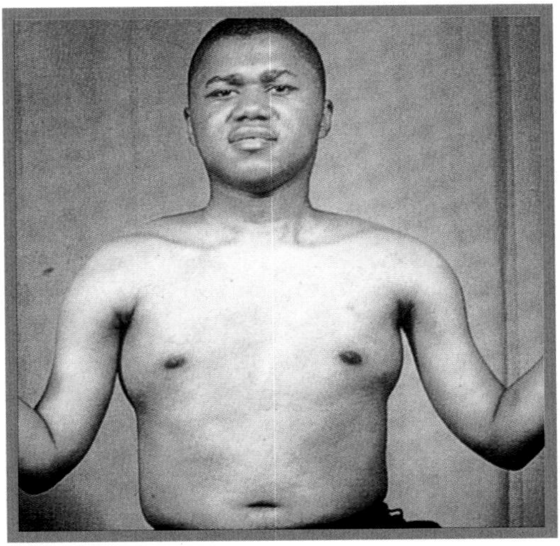

→ Fig. 7.8a
Duchenne muscular dystrophy. A 17-year-old boy with striking enlargement (hypertrophy–pseudohypertrophy) of the deltoid and pectoralis major muscles.

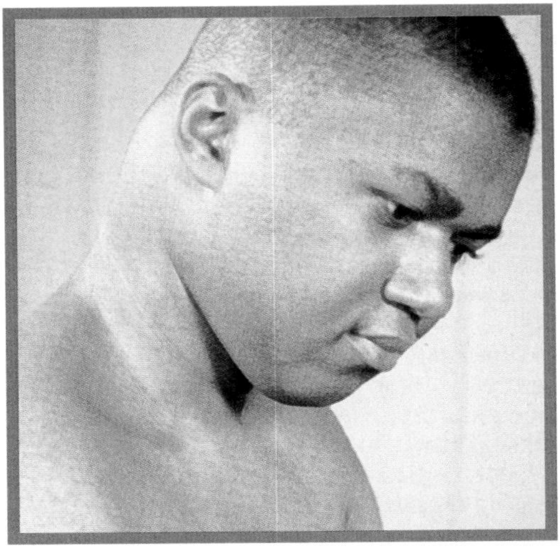

→ Fig. 7.8b
Duchenne muscular dystrophy. Enlargement of the trapezius. (With permission from Perloff JK: Cardiac manifestations of neuromuscular disease. In *Atlas of Heart Diseases, Vol 2: Cardiomyopathies, Myocarditis, and Pericardial Disease*, ed. Abelmann WH. Philadelphia: Current Medicine, 1995.)

sitting position that begins in early childhood, usually in the second year of life. The child may 'climb up' his own legs in order to stand, and is often confined to a wheel-chair by the age of 11 years. A child so confined has a lolling head with kyphoscoliosis and exaggerated lumbar lordosis. Death usually occurs by the age of 30 years.

The typical cardiovascular disease is that of a dilated cardiomyopathy. Congestive heart failure may develop. In this disease there is a characteristic ECG (**Fig. 7.9**). The posterolateral wall of the left ventricle shows fibrosis, with loss of myocardial fibers. There may be accompanying mitral regurgitation because of posterior papillary muscle dysfunction. There is relative sparing of the interventricular septum, the right ventricle, and the atria. The ECG thus resembles that of a posterolateral infarction. Cardiac rhythm and conduction disturbances also occur; these may be related to dystrophin deficiency in specialized cardiac tissues, or to small coronary artery disease. Atrial arrhythmias are more common than ventricular arrhythmias.

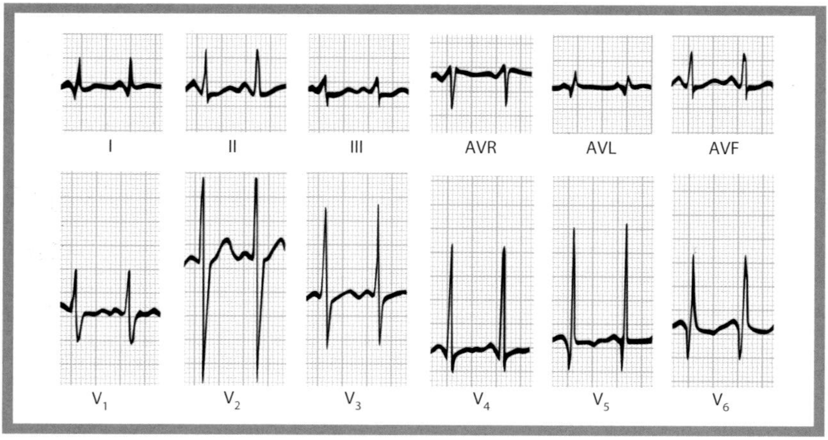

↑ Fig. 7.9
Duchenne muscular dystrophy. This is a typical ECG of a young man in his twenties. There is a prominent Q wave in leads I, AVL, V_5 and V_6; this is due to the posterolateral myocardial fibrosis usually found in the left ventricle of these patients. There is a large R wave in lead V_1, reflecting the loss of posterolateral forces. (With permission from Davies FA, Philadelphia. From Chou TC. *Cardiovascular Clinics* 1973, **5** (3): 199-218.)

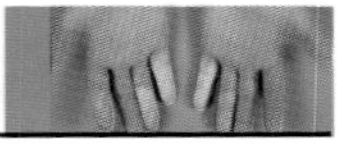

Further Reading

Perloff JK, Henze E, Schelbert HR. Alterations in regional myocardial metabolism, perfusion, and wall motion in Duchenne muscular dystrophy studied by radionuclide imaging. *Circulation* 1984, **69**:33–42.

Cholesterol Emboli (Atheroembolism)

One of the characteristic features of cholesterol emboli is the 'blue toe syndrome' or 'purple toe syndrome' (**Fig. 7.10**). Such cholesterol embolism or atheroembolism typically occurs when an atherosclerotic plaque ruptures in the aorta or the iliac or femoral arteries. This may occur after an angiographic procedure, aortic balloon pumping, or vascular surgery, and may be recognized perhaps weeks or months after an invasive procedure. It also may occur spontaneously. Antecedent anticoagulant therapy may favor cholesterol embolization.

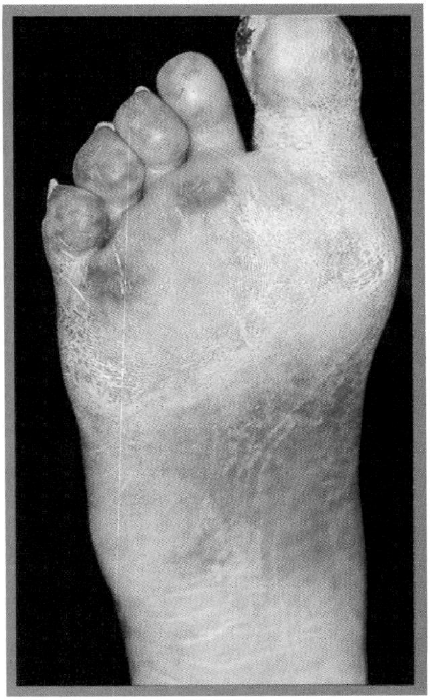

→ Fig. 7.10
Cholesterol emboli (atheroembolism). Characteristic purple toes in a patient with atheroembolism.

The two most common clinical findings are cutaneous lesions, which occur in about 33% of patients, and sudden renal failure, which occurs in about 50%. Skin lesions may be seen on the buttocks, in the genital area, and on the feet. In addition to purpura, livedo reticularis may appear. Other clinical findings in cholesterol embolism include accelerated hypertension, headache, and fever. Transient cerebral ischemic attacks and strokes also may occur. Abdominal pain, melena, nausea and vomiting have been described, and retinal emboli (Hollenhorst plaques) may be seen (see Fig. 3.6).

In patients with atheroemboli, large protruding atherosclerotic plaques may be demonstrated in the aortic arch, descending thoracic aorta, or abdominal aorta. This is best achieved by transesophageal echocardiography. The diagnosis can be confirmed by skin biopsy, but this is usually not necessary. The patient with this disease is usually elderly, and the outlook is poor, with an estimated mortality rate of 72%.

The purple toe syndrome may result from conditions other than atheroembolism. In one study, a non-embolic cause was found in 18 of 80 patients. Also, a cardiac source of embolism, such as infective endocarditis, may be responsible. Hyperviscosity syndromes may cause the purple toe syndrome; these include polycythemia vera, macroglobulinemia, and cryoglobulinemia. Vasculitis resulting from SLE or polyarteritis nodosa may be the cause. Hypercoagulable states, especially cancer, diabetes mellitus, essential thrombocythemia, and antiphospholipid syndrome, may be responsible.

Further Reading

Kronzon I, Tunick PA. Atheromatous disease of the thoracic aorta: pathologic and clinical implications. *Ann Int Med* 1997, **126**:629–637.

O'Keefe ST, Woods BO, Breslin NP, Tsapatsaris NP. Blue toe syndrome: causes and management. *Arch Int Med* 1992, **152**:2197–2202.

Rheumatoid Arthritis

Rheumatoid arthritis (**Figs 7.11–7.14**) has been said to produce pericarditis, myocarditis, valvulitis, aortitis, and coronary arteritis (**Fig. 7.15**). Although the prevalence of abnormalities in rheumatoid arthritis is reported as 30–50% in autopsy studies, clinically detected heart disease is much less common, being found in only 2–10% of patients.

The patient with rheumatoid arthritis shown in Figures 7.11–7.14 had subcutaneous nodules and a large pericardial effusion (**Fig. 7.16**). Pericardial effusion or thickening has been reported in 15–46.6% of patients with rheumatoid arthritis who were studied by echocardiography. Pericardial effusion was found in 44% and 50% of patients with rheumatoid nodules in two studies reported by Mody *et al.*

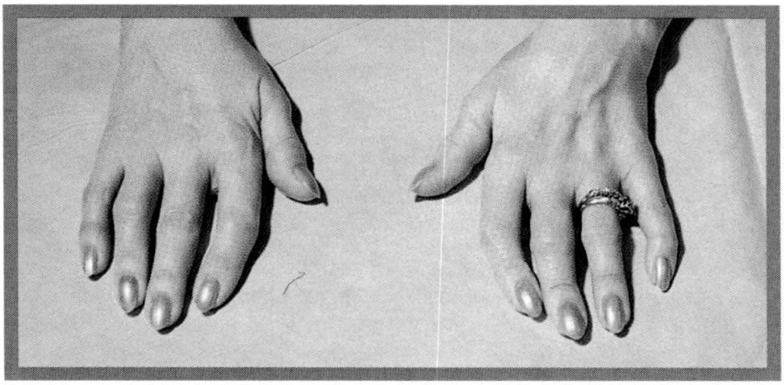

→ Fig. 7.11 Rheumatoid arthritis. Typical deformity of the fingers in a woman with pericardial effusion (see Fig. 7.16). This patient is also pictured in Figures 7.12–7.14.

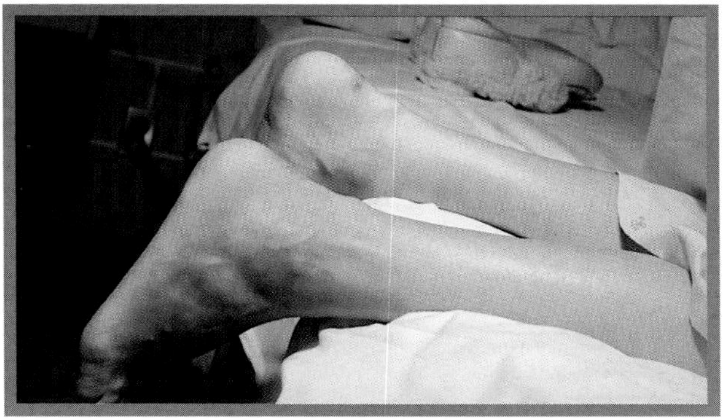

→ Fig. 7.12 Rheumatoid arthritis. Rheumatoid nodules in the Achilles tendons.

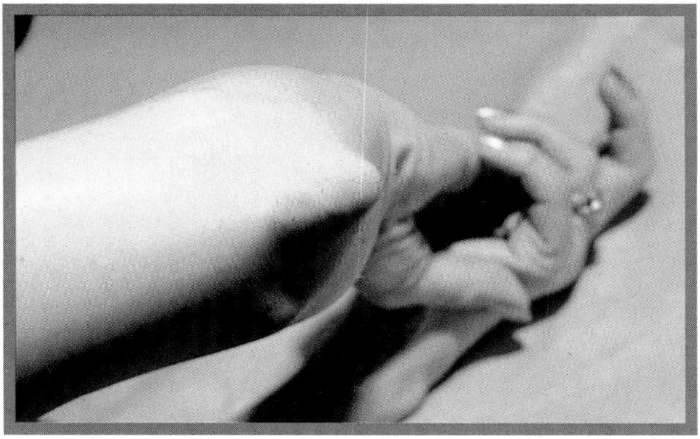

→ Fig. 7.13 Rheumatoid arthritis. Rheumatoid nodule involving the elbow. These nodules must be distinguished from tendinous xanthomas (Fig. 7.3), and the olecranon bursal involvement of gout.

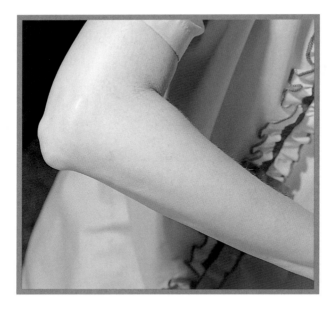

← Fig. 7.14 Rheumatoid arthritis. Rheumatoid nodule involving the elbow.

Cardiovascular features of rheumatoid arthritis
Pericardial disease (up to 50% of patients): fibrosis, effusion, occasional constrictive pericarditis or tamponade
Myocardial fibrosis
Aortic or mitral regurgitation; stenosis rare
Coronary arteritis
Aortitis
Atrioventricular block
Pulmonary hypertension due to fibrosis or vasculitis

← Fig. 7.15 Cardiovascular features of rheumatoid arthritis.

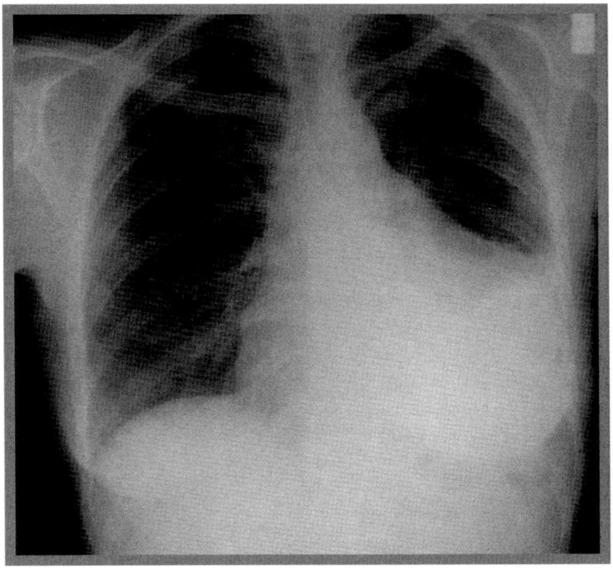

→ Fig. 7.16 Rheumatoid arthritis. Chest radiogram showing pericardial effusion and left pleural effusion, in the patient photographed in Figures 7.11–7.14.

Bonfiglio & Atwater performed an autopsy study of 47 patients with seropositive rheumatoid arthritis, and found evidence of pericarditis in 17. Cardiac hypertrophy, stenotic valvular disease, and myocarditis were no more common than in control individuals. Pulmonary fibrosis was more common, but not significantly so. The authors were unable to conclude that any specific form of rheumatoid valvulitis was present. Deaths of three patients in this series were attributed to myocarditis that might have been due to rheumatoid disease. No definite evidence of coronary vasculitis could be found.

McDonald *et al*. studied 51 outpatients with rheumatoid arthritis, using echocardiography. Thirty-one percent had evidence of pericardial effusion. None had chest pain or signs of tamponade, or constrictive pericarditis. One had evidence of rheumatoid pancarditis with impaired left ventricular function, and 6% had evidence of rheumatic mitral valvular disease. The authors concluded that rheumatoid myocarditis rarely has clinical significance.

Mody *et al.* also used echocardiography to study patients with rheumatoid arthritis. Among 101 patients, except for a decreased E–F slope of the mitral valve in 5% and pericardial effusion in 6%, other cardiac abnormalities were explained by associated disease.

In summary, pericardial effusion is common in patients with rheumatoid arthritis. It is usually asymptomatic, but rarely may lead to constrictive pericarditis. Any cardiac valve may be involved, but this is seldom recognized clinically. Hemodynamically significant mitral valvular disease is found in a small percentage of patients, but is no more common than in control individuals. Aortic valvular disease is even less common (**Fig. 7.17**). Myocarditis and pulmonary fibrosis are uncommon. Coronary vasculitis may occur, but usually does not cause epicardial coronary occlusion.

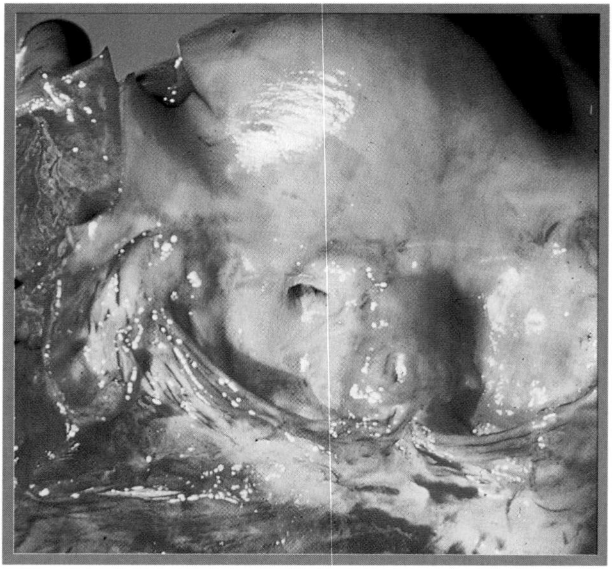

← Fig. 7.17 Rheumatoid arthritis. Involvement of the aortic valve in a patient with rheumatoid arthritis. There is sagging of the aortic valve cusps, leading to aortic insufficiency. Fusion of the commissures is also present. This degree of valvular involvement is unusual in rheumatoid arthritis.

References

Bonfiglio T, Atwater EC. Heart disease in patients with seropositive rheumatoid arthritis. *Arch Int Med* 1969, **124**:714–719.

McDonald WJ, Crawford MH, Klippel JH, Zvaifler NJ, O'Rourke RA. Echocardiographic assessment of cardiac structure and function in patients with rheumatoid arthritis. *Am J Med* 1977, **63**:890–896.

Mody GM, Stevens JE, Meyers OL. The heart in rheumatoid arthritis—a clinical and echocardiographic study. *Q J Med* 1987, **65**:921–928.

8 Skin

Adenoma Sebaceum

The dermatological condition known as adenoma sebaceum is considered pathognomonic for tuberous sclerosis (**Fig. 8.1**). Tuberous sclerosis is a hereditary condition transmitted as an autosomal dominant; the responsible genes have been linked to chromosomes 9 and 16. However, many cases arise without a familial background.

The characteristic lesion is a hamartoma, an overgrowth of normal tissue. The principal areas affected are the skin, kidneys, central nervous system, lungs, and heart. Tuberous sclerosis in the cerebral cortex is often associated with epileptiform seizures beginning in infancy, and about 50% of patients are mentally deficient. Pulmonary lesions may lead to progressive respiratory failure.

Renal involvement takes the form of angiomyolipomas and cysts. Hematuria and chronic renal failure with hypertension may develop, and the prevalence of renal cell carcinoma is increased. About 50% of patients with tuberous sclerosis have the characteristic lesions of adenoma sebaceum.

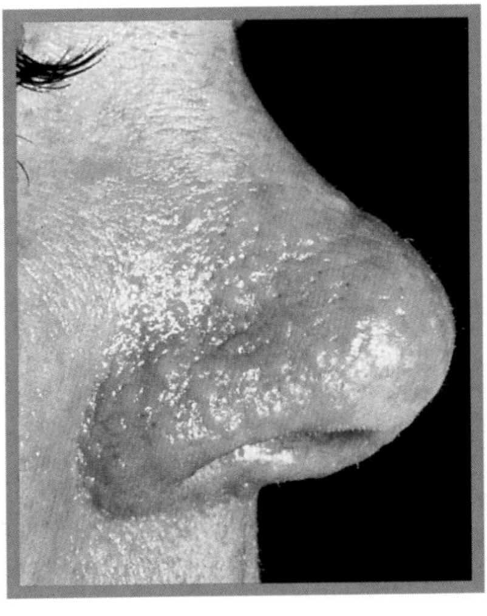

→ Fig. 8.1
Tuberous sclerosis. Characteristic lesions of adenoma sebaceum in a patient with tuberous sclerosis.

Hamartomatous plaques may develop on the back, abdomen, forehead, or in the nailbeds.

The characteristic cardiac lesion is a rhabdomyoma, which is usually present at birth. Echocardiography of 43 children with tuberous sclerosis revealed cardiac rhabdomyomas in 25 (58%). Although ventricular outflow tract obstruction or congestive failure may occur, these complications are uncommon, and most tumors are believed to regress spontaneously.

Patients with tuberous sclerosis have a shortened life expectancy. Death is usually as a result of renal failure, status epilepticus, brain tumor, or pulmonary infection. Shepherd *et al.* reviewed the cause of death of 40 patients with tuberous sclerosis and found that 11 had died of renal disease, 10 died of brain tumors, and four died of pulmonary lymphangiomatosis; 13 died of either status epilepticus or bronchopneumonia. One baby died of heart failure caused by cardiac rhabdomyoma, and one child of ruptured thoracic aortic aneurysm.

Reference

Shepherd CW, Gomez MR, Lie JT, Crowson CS. Causes of death in patients with tuberous sclerosis. Mayo Clin Proc 1991, **66**:792–796.

Further Reading

Accad MF, Fred HL. Gross hematuria in a young woman with seizures and skin lesions. Hosp Pract 1997, **32**:204–208.

Smith HC, Watson GH, Patel RG, Super M. Cardiac rhabdomyomata in tuberous sclerosis: their course and diagnostic value. *Arch Dis Child* 1989, **64**:196–200.

Erythema Marginatum

Erythema marginatum (**Figs 8.2** and **8.3**) is one of the five major manifestations of acute rheumatic fever. The remaining four are carditis, chorea, polyarthritis, and subcutaneous nodules. Two of these five criteria suffice for the diagnosis of rheumatic fever, provided that there is evidence of an antecedent streptococcal infection. Erythema marginatum is most commonly associated with acute rheumatic fever, but is not specific for this disease. It has been found in some 10–15% of patients with acute rheumatic fever. The lesions are predominantly circular macules with a sharp margin of erythema and central pallor. They do not produce itching. They are most common on the trunk, inner arms, and inner thighs. They may appear late in the course of acute rheumatic fever, and may wax and wane while the condition remains active. Some drug-induced rashes may be similar in appearance, but they are usually pruritic. Erythema marginatum has also been described in septicemia, especially staphylococcal septicemia, in glomerulonephritis, and at times with no identifiable etiology. A similar rash may appear in childhood rheumatoid arthritis (Still's disease).

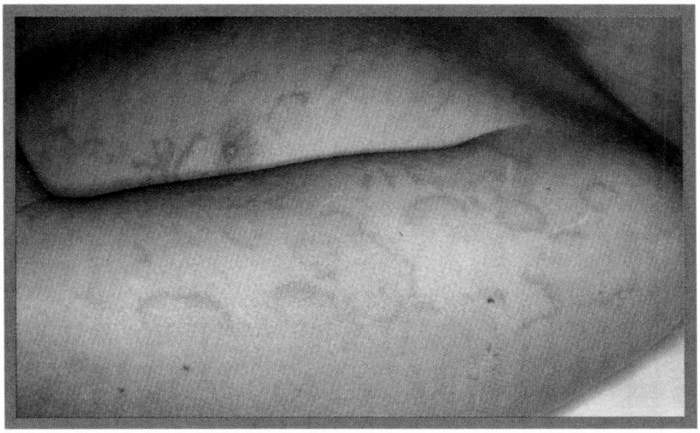

→ Fig. 8.2
Erythema marginatum. Note the erythematous margin and central pallor. Although this is one of the five major manifestations of rheumatic fever, it is not specific for that disease.

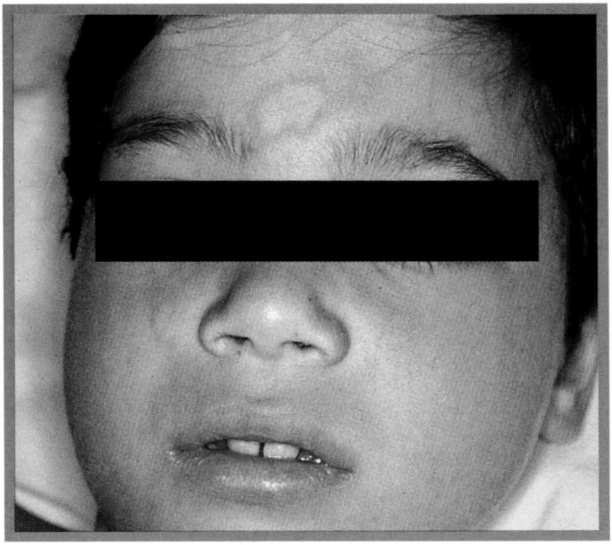

→ Fig. 8.3
Erythema marginatum showing erythematous margin and central pallor.

Further Reading

Massell BF, Fyler DC, Roy SB. The clinical picture of rheumatic fever: diagnosis, immediate prognosis, course, and therapeutic implications. Am J Cardiol 1958, 1:436–439.

Sarcoidosis

Sarcoidosis is a granulomatous disease of unknown cause that chiefly affects the lungs, the eyes, the skin, the bones, the central nervous system, and the heart. However, almost any tissue may be involved. The skin lesions may be the first signs to call attention to the disease (**Fig. 8.4**), but cardiac and other organ involvement often occur in the absence of skin lesions. Cardiac involvement is found in 20–30% of cases at autopsy (**Fig. 8.5**), but clinical evidence of cardiac involvement is found in only about 5% of patients with sarcoidosis (**Fig. 8.5**). Pulmonary involvement may lead to cor pulmonale with right heart failure. The typical pathologic lesion is a non-caseating granuloma (**Fig. 8.6**).

Fleming found the age range of patients with clinical sarcoid heart disease to be 18–88 years, with a peak between 25 and 55 years. Various areas of primary cardiac involvement are recognized (**Fig. 8.7**). Involvement of the interventricular septum may lead to complete A–V block, which may be the most common form of clinical presentation. Paroxysmal atrial and ventricular arrhythmias may lead to syncope or sudden death. Either a dilated or a restrictive cardiomyopathy may occur; papillary muscle involvement may cause mitral regurgitation. Pericardial effusion is not uncommon. Constrictive pericarditis occurs rarely. Myocardial involvement may suggest myocardial infarction on the ECG (**Fig. 8.8**); as a result of such involvement, a ventricular aneurysm may develop (see Fig. 8.7).

The diagnosis of sarcoid heart disease is suggested when there is heart disease with radiograms of the chest that show bilateral hilar adenopathy in the

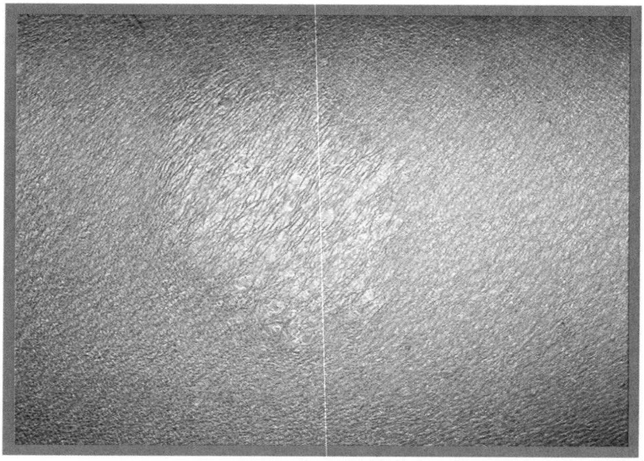

← Fig. 8.4
Sarcoidosis. This characteristic skin lesion suggests the possibility of myocardial sarcoidosis in a patient with known heart disease, but is often absent in the presence of myocardial sarcoidosis.

absence of lymphoma, cancer, tuberculosis, or fungal disease. The characteristic skin lesions also suggest the diagnosis in this setting. Endomyocardial biopsy may be definitive (see Fig. 8.6), but often fails to show the characteristic granuloma, even when sarcoid heart disease is present.

→ Fig. 8.5
General features of sarcoidosis.

General features of sarcoidosis
Non-caseating granulomatus disease
Etiology unknown
Affects lungs, eyes, skin, bones, central nervous system, lymph nodes, heart
Autopsy evidence of heart disease in 20–30%
Clinical cardiac involvement in 5%
Peak age with cardiac involvement – 25 to 55 years

→ Fig. 8.6
Sarcoidosis. Photomicrograph of myocardium at autopsy. There is a non-caseating granuloma (arrows), typical of sarcoidosis. (With permission from Scully RE, Mark EJ, McNeely WF, McNeely BU. Case records of the Massachusetts General Hospital. *N Engl J Med* 1995, **332**:1437.)

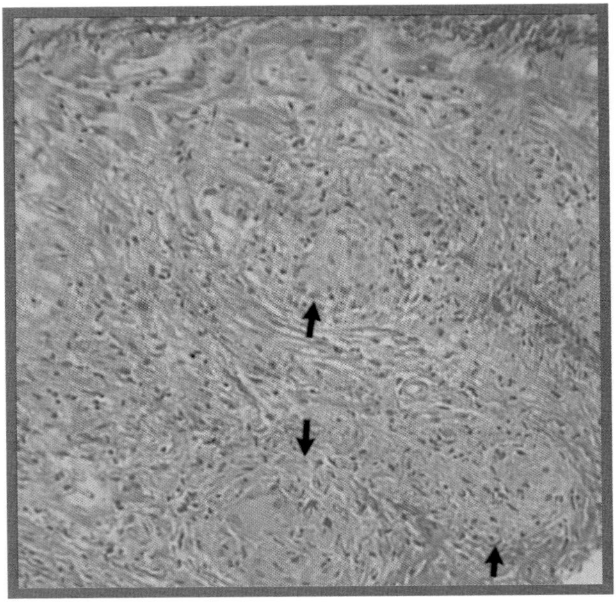

Cardiac involvement in sarcoidosis
Clinical involvement occurs in about 5% of patients with sarcoidosis
Dilated or restrictive cardiomyopathy may result
Atrioventricular block: a cause of complete A–V block in young persons
Pseudoinfarction pattern may be seen on ECG
Pericardial effusion
Constrictive pericarditis (rare)
Cor pulmonale resulting from pulmonary involvement
Paroxysmal atrial or ventricular arrhythmias may occur, leading to syncope or sudden death

← Fig. 8.7
Cardiac involvement in sarcoidosis.

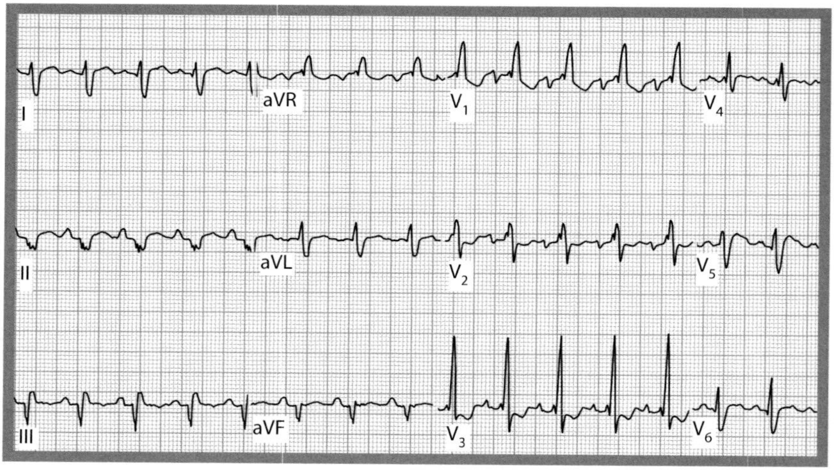

↑ Fig. 8.8
Myocardial sarcoidosis. ECG of a 36-year-old man who had myocardial sarcoidosis. There is a pattern of right bundle branch block and left anterior hemiblock, with abnormal P waves. Note the abnormal Q waves in leads III and aVF. This pseudoinfarction pattern is not uncommon in myocardial sarcoidosis.

Reference

Fleming HA. Sarcoid heart disease (editorial). *BMJ* 1986, **292**:1095–1096.

Further Reading

Lemery R, McGoon MD, Edwards WD. Cardiac sarcoidosis: a potentially treatable form of myocarditis. *Mayo Clin Proc* 1985, **60**:549–554.
Newman LS, Rose CS, Maier LA. Sarcoidosis. *N Engl J Med* 1997, **336**:1224–1234.

Erythromelalgia

Erythromelalgia was first described by Mitchell in 1878 as a syndrome of red congestion and burning pain in the hands and feet; the syndrome has also been called erythermalgia. There are three varieties of erythromelalgia. The most common is that associated with thrombocythemia, which may be isolated or associated with either polycythemia vera or myelofibrosis. The clinical features of this variety are believed to be mediated by platelet-induced arteriolar inflammation and thrombosis. Characteristically, there is burning distress in the feet or hands along with local redness, warmth, and swelling (**Figs 8.9** and **8.10**). Relief is provided by elevation of the limb, and aspirin. The histopathologic findings are those of intimal fibrosis and thrombosis, with occlusion of digital arteries and arterioles. In one series, 30 of 50 patients with thrombocythemia had erythromelalgia.

Primary erythromelalgia, without known cause, is rare. At the time of publication of the paper by Drenth & Michiels in 1990, only 13 cases had been reported in the literature.

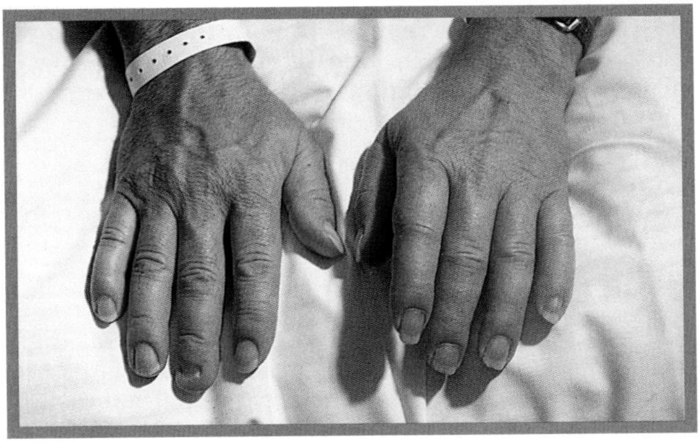

→ Fig. 8.9 Erythromelalgia. Erythema and swelling of the hands in a patient with polycythemia vera (dorsal view).

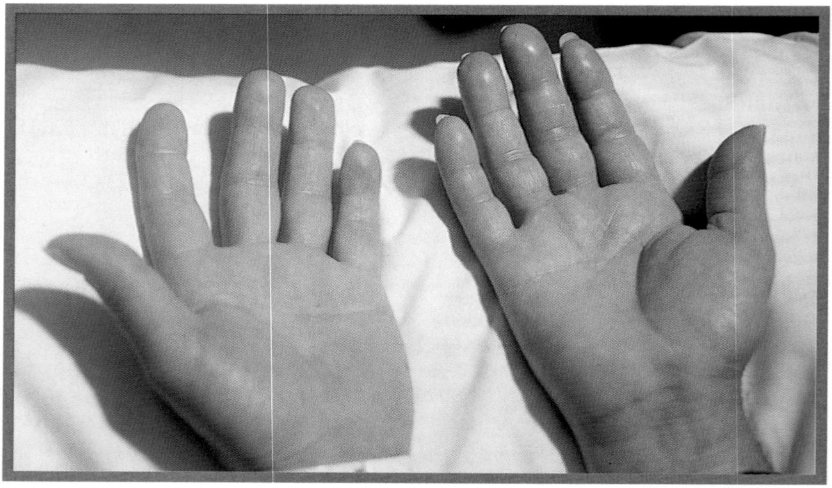

↑ **Fig. 8.10**
Erythromelalgia. Erythema and swelling of the hands in a patient with polycythemia vera (palmar view).

Secondary erythromelalgia represents the third variety of the syndrome. It may occur with connective tissue diseases, thromboangiitis obliterans, cryoglobulinemia, or with various vascular diseases and neurologic disorders. Most importantly, it may occur with the use of certain vasoactive drugs. Causative medications include the calcium channel blocking agents verapamil, nicardipine, and nisoldipine. The ergot derivatives bromocriptine and pergolide may also be responsible.

Reference

Drenth JPH, Michiels JJ. Three types of erythromelalgia. *BMJ* 1990, **301**:454–455.

Malignant Melanoma

Malignant melanoma is the most rapidly increasing form of cancer in the USA, except for lung cancer in women. It is estimated that there are currently 38,300 new cases per year of dermal melanoma in the USA and that, by the year 2000, the lifetime risk for an American of developing malignant melanoma will have increased to 1 in 75. The peak age incidence is between 20 and 50 years, and it is more common in men than in women. Greater recreational exposure to sunlight and depletion of the ozone layer are believed to be important risk factors. Others include a positive family history, a history of basal cell or squamous cell carcinoma of the skin, a state of immunosuppression, and the use of sun-tanning lamps. Caucasians, especially those of light complexion, are more likely to develop melanoma than are blacks in the same geographic area.

Diagnostic features of malignant melanoma of the skin include asymmetry of a pigmented lesion, border irregularity, color variation within the same mole, and diameter greater than 6mm. Although it arises principally in the skin (**Fig. 8.11**), malignant melanoma may also arise in the eye or the meninges.

Malignant melanoma frequently metastasizes to the myocardium or pericardium. Metastatic carcinomas to the heart are most commonly attributable to bronchogenic carcinoma; breast cancer is the second most common cause, and melanoma is third. About 60% of patients with metastatic melanoma have cardiac metastases—so-called charcoal heart (**Fig. 8.12**). Often, melanoma metastatic to the heart produces little or no cardiac dysfunction; however, the patient whose heart is pictured in Figure 8.12 developed congestive heart failure, with a clinical picture of cardiomyopathy.

→ Fig. 8.11 Malignant melanoma. Note the irregular border.

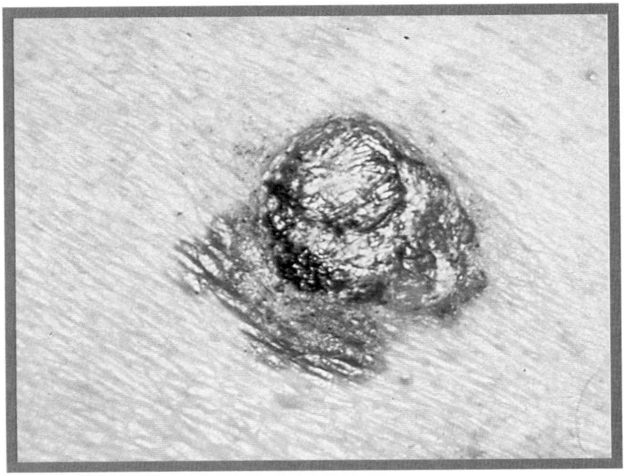

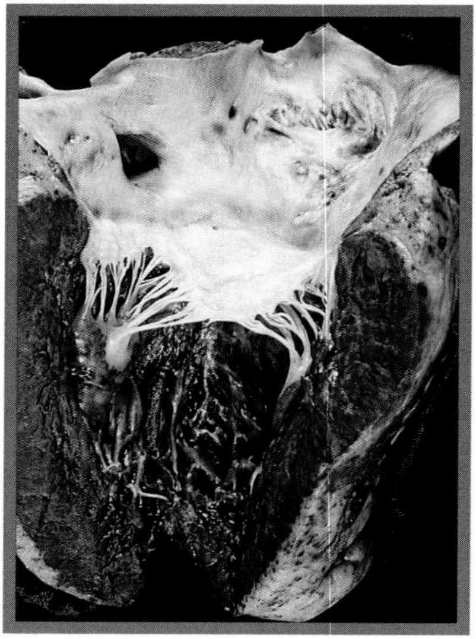

← Fig. 8.12
Malignant melanoma. Photograph of gross cardiac specimen, showing cardiac metastases ('charcoal heart'). The patient had undergone excision of a malignant melanoma several years previously, and presented with the clinical picture of congestive cardiomyopathy.

Reference

Applefield MM, Pollock SH. Cardiac disease in patients who have malignancies. *Curr Probl Cardiol* 1980, **4**:2–37.

Lentigines

Lentigines are flat or slightly raised skin lesions that are brown or brownish black in color (**Fig. 8.13**); they are generally 2–4mm in diameter. They usually appear in childhood and increase in number in early adulthood; later, they may diminish or disappear. These lesions are different from freckles in that they are darker, and are not affected by exposure to sunlight. Unlike freckles, they are not more common in persons of fair complexion.

Lentigines have been linked with a number of clinical syndromes. Carney's complex is an autosomal dominant syndrome, the principal features of which are cardiac myxomas and multiple lentigines (**Figs 8.14–8.17**). The acronym 'LAMB' syndrome (lentigines, atrial myxoma, mucocutaneous myxomas, blue nevi) has been proposed for this association. Lentiginosis has also been associated with hypertrophic cardiomyopathy or 'LEOPARD' syndrome (lentigines, electrocardiographic abnormalities, ocular hypertelorism, pulmonary stenosis, abnormal genitalia, retardation of growth, and deafness).

In addition, a familial syndrome of arterial dissection, multiple lentigines, and cystic medical necrosis was described by Schievink *et al.* In this syndrome, the association of arterial cystic medial necrosis and lentigines was attributed to the common origin of arterial media and melanocytes from neural crest cells.

→ Fig. 8.13
Lentigines. The lesions are larger than freckles and on an area not usually exposed to sunlight.

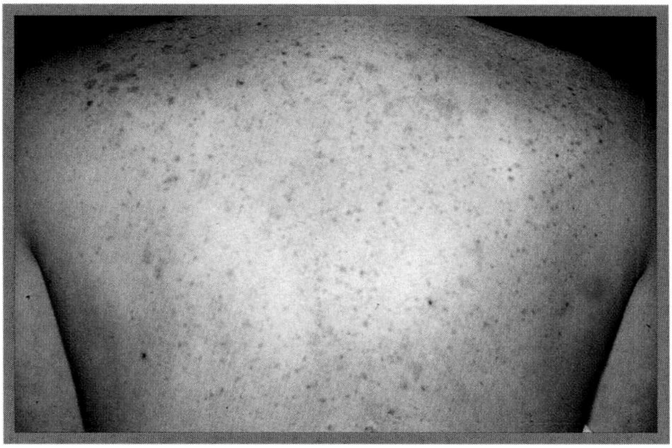

→ Fig. 8.14
Lentigines. Angiocardiogram showing left atrial myxoma (arrows). The tumor extends from the left atrium above, through the mitral valve (broken line) to the left ventricle below.

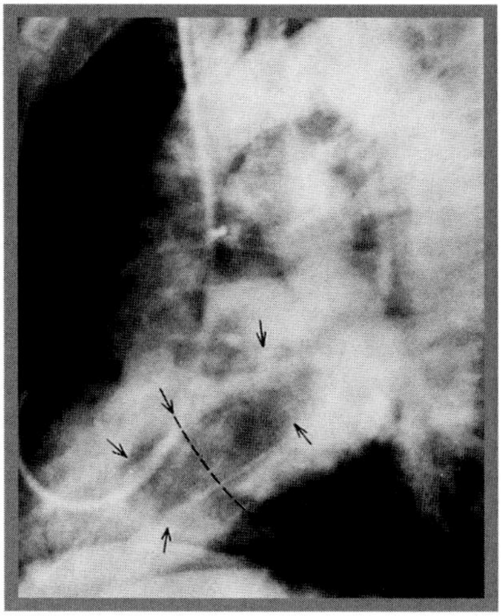

→ Fig. 8.15
Lentigines.
M-mode echocardiogram, showing atrial myxoma inferior to anterior mitral leaflet during diastole.

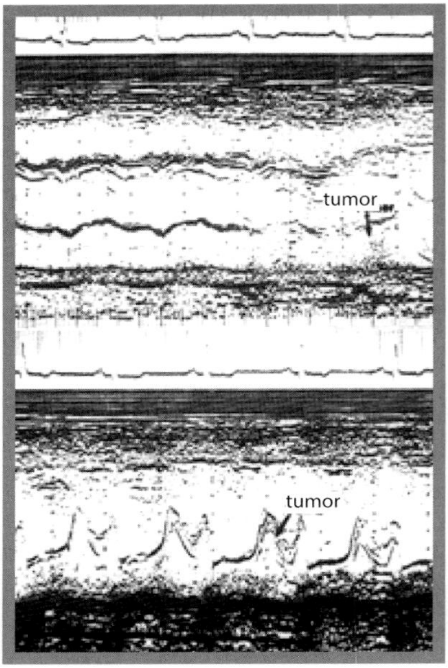

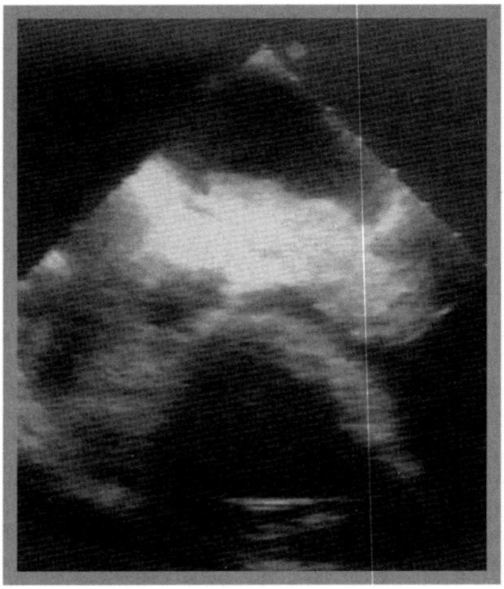

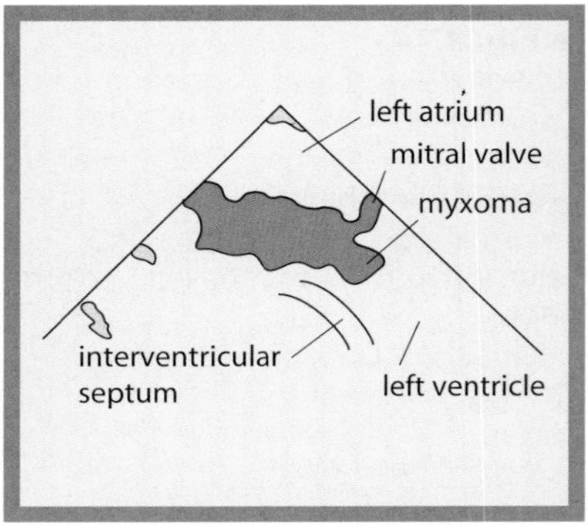

↑ Fig. 8.16a **↑ Fig. 8.16b**
Lentigines. (**a**) Transesophageal echocardiogram showing left atrial myxoma extending from the left atrium through the mitral valve into the left ventricle. See diagram in (**b**)

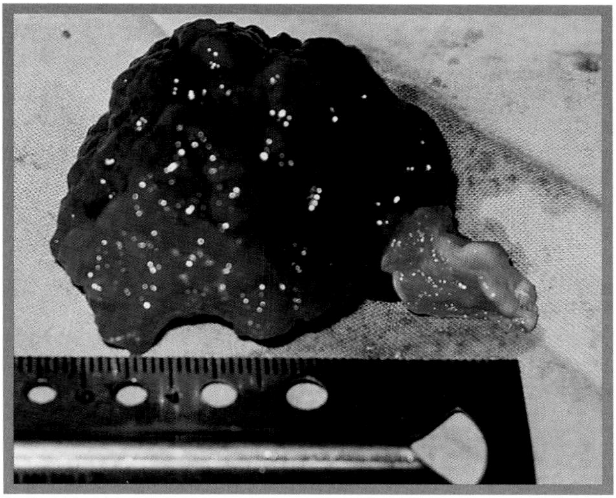

→ Fig. 8.17 Lentigines. Operative specimen of a left atrial myxoma.

Further Reading

Panossian DH, Marais GE, Marais HJ. Familial endocrine myxolentiginosis. *Clin Cardiol* 1995, **18**:675–678.

Reference

Schievink WI, Michels VV, Mokri B, Piepgras DG, Perry HO. Brief report: a familial syndrome of arterial dissections with lentigines. *N Engl J Med* 1995, **332**:576–578.

Neurofibromatosis

Neurofibromatosis (von Recklinghausen's disease) is an autosomal dominant disorder characterized by pigmented skin lesions (café au lait spots and axillary freckles) and neurofibromas of peripheral nerves and the central nervous system (**Fig. 8.18**). This disease may be associated with various tumors and certain circulatory disorders. About 10% of patients develop neurogenic sarcoma. Other neoplasms include gliomas of the brain and optic nerves, acoustic neuromas, meningiomas, and acute leukemia. In addition, 10–20% of adult patients develop interstitial or bullous lung disease.

Circulatory disorders that may develop in this disease include arterial occlusive disease, fibromuscular dysplasia of the renal arteries, and pheochromocytoma. About 10% of patients with neurofibromatosis eventually develop a pheochromocytoma. These tumors are associated with either

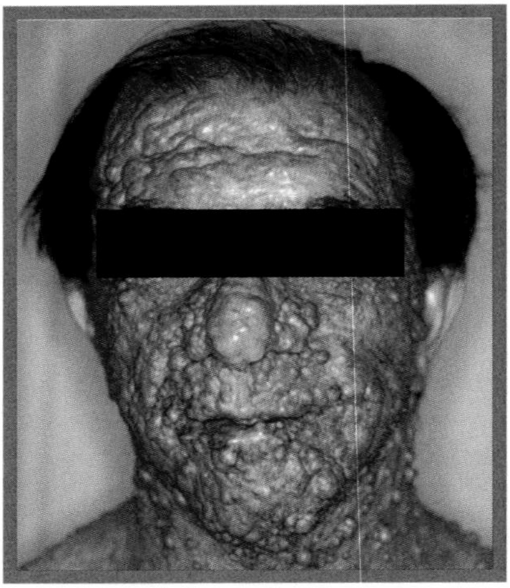

← Fig. 8.18
Neurofibromatosis, showing extensive tumors of the face.

paroxysmal or fixed hypertension and may produce a catecholamine-induced cardiomyopathy. The diagnosis of pheochromocytoma is especially suggested in patients who have paroxysms of hypertension, headache, tachycardia, or sweating, and may be suggested by orthostatic hypotension in a hypertensive patient. Weight loss and impaired glucose tolerance are often present. The diagnosis is confirmed by demonstrating increased 24-hour urinary excretion of catecholamines, vanillylmandelic acid, or metanephrines.

Hereditary Hemorrhagic Telangiectasia

Hereditary hemorrhagic telangiectasia, or Rendu–Osler–Weber syndrome, is a group of autosomal dominant disorders. Its prevalence ranged from 1 in 2351 to 1 in 39,126 persons in various reported populations. Its manifestations are due to abnormalities of vascular structure, consisting of focal dilatations of postcapillary venules, which may connect directly to dilated arterioles (**Fig. 8.19**).

The most common clinical manifestation is recurrent epistaxis, which occurs in the majority of patients, but not all, and begins by the age of 21 years in most. By the age of 40 years, most patients have telangiectases of the lips (**Fig. 8.20**), tongue (**Figs 8.21** and **8.22**), fingertips (**Fig. 8.23**), face (**Fig. 8.24**), conjunctiva, or trunk. Neurologic manifestations may include subarachnoid hemorrhage, intracerebral hemorrhage, or brain abscess. The last may result from pulmonary arteriovenous fistula with right-to-left shunting. Gastrointestinal bleeding does not usually start until the fifth or sixth decade of life. Severe anemia may result, and this may cause a high cardiac output state corrected only by blood transfusion.

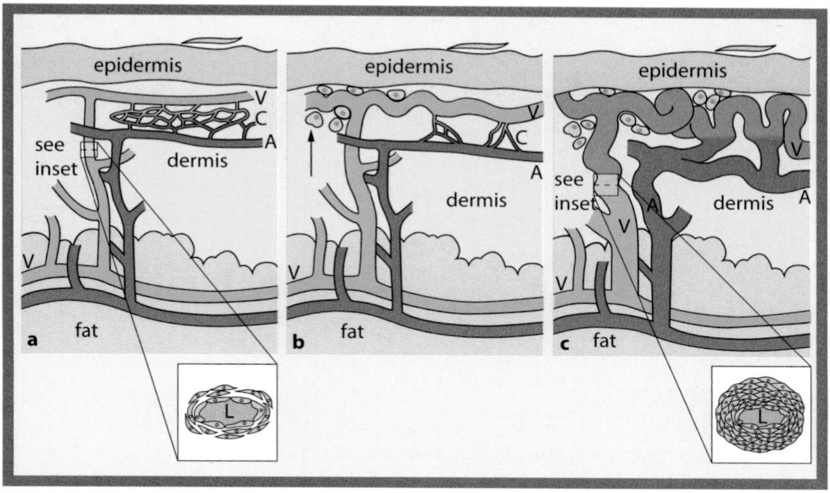

↑ Fig. 8.19
Hereditary hemorrhagic telangiectasia. In normal skin (**a**) arterioles (A) in the papilliary dermis are connected to venules (V) through multiple capillaries (C). These vessels arise from larger arterioles and venules at the junction of the dermis and fat. The ultrastructure of a postcapillary venule (shown in cross-section in the inset) includes the lumen (L), endothelial cells, and two to three layers of surrounding pericytes. In the earliest stages of telangiectasia (**b**), a single venule becomes dilated, but it is still connected to an arteriole through one or more capillaries. A perivascular lymphocytic infiltrate is apparent (arrow). In a fully developed cutaneous telangiectasia (**c**), the venule and its branches have become markedly dilated, elongated, and convoluted throughout the dermis. The connecting arterioles have also become dilated, and communicate directly with the venules without intervening capillaries. The perivascular infiltrate is still present. The thickened wall of the dilated descending limb (shown in cross-section in the inset), contains as many as 11 layers of smooth muscle cells. (Reproduced with permission from Guttmacher AE, *et al. N Engl J Med* 1995, **333**:918–924, Fig 1, p919.)

There are several cardiovascular complications (**Fig. 8.25**). Pulmonary arteriovenous fistula occurs in about 15% of those affected. This condition may produce a continuous murmur heard over the lungs. When the right-to-left shunt is large, cyanosis, digital clubbing, and polycythemia are found. The arterial oxygen tension is decreased, and is not normally increased by breathing 100% oxygen. Paradoxical embolism with brain embolism or ischemic stroke may occur.

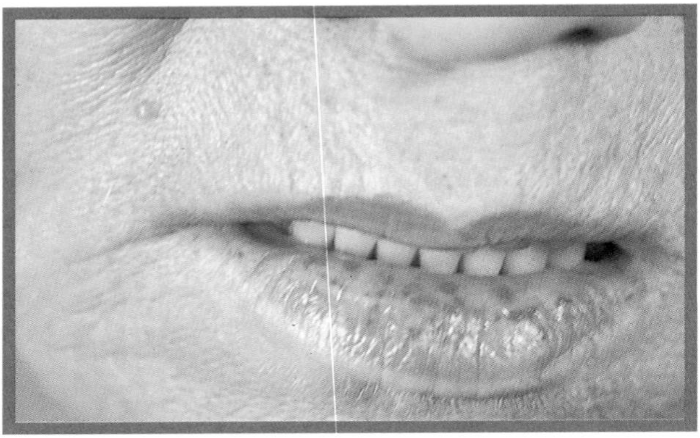

← Fig. 8.20 Hereditary hemorrhagic telangiectasia. Telangiectases of the lips in a patient with pulmonary arterio-venous fistulae.

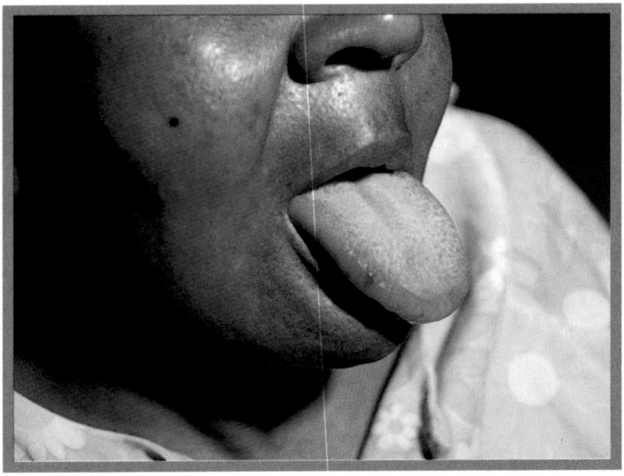

← Fig. 8.21 Hereditary hemorrhagic telangiectasia. Telangiectases of the tongue.

Other complications include pleural or intrapulmonary hemorrhage. Large fistulae may be seen on the chest radiogram, but angiography is more sensitive and more specific (**Fig. 8.26**). Severe pulmonary hypertension may complicate pulmonary arteriovenous fistula (**Fig. 8.27**). Another complication is hepatic arteriovenous fistula. This is suggested by a continuous murmur over the liver and a high cardiac output, at times with congestive failure (**Fig. 8.28 a, b**).

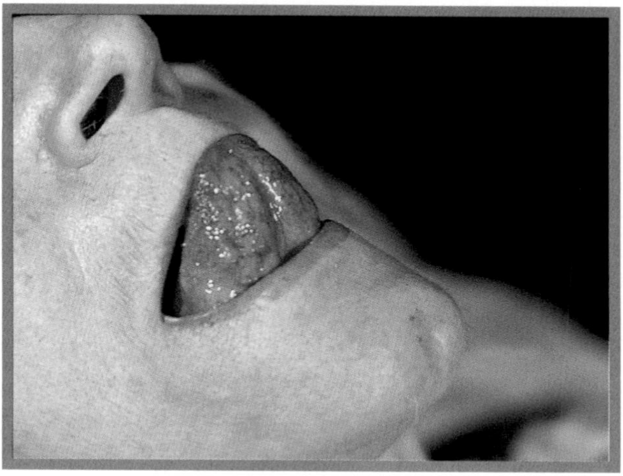

→ Fig. 8.22 Hereditary hemorrhagic telangiectasia. Telangiectases of the tongue in the same patient as in Figure 8.20.

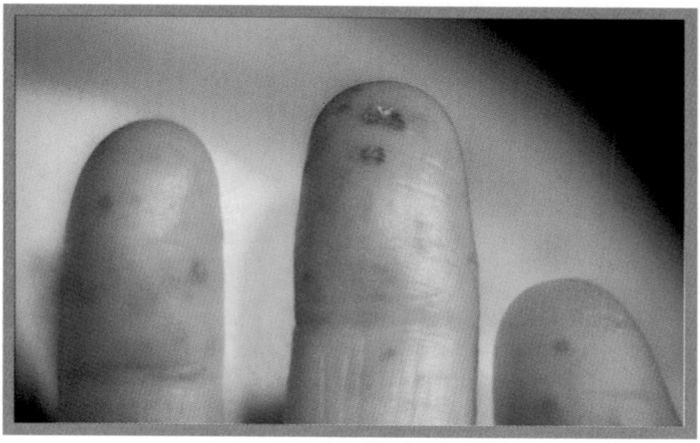

→ Fig. 8.23 Hereditary hemorrhagic telangiectasia. Telangiectases of the fingers.

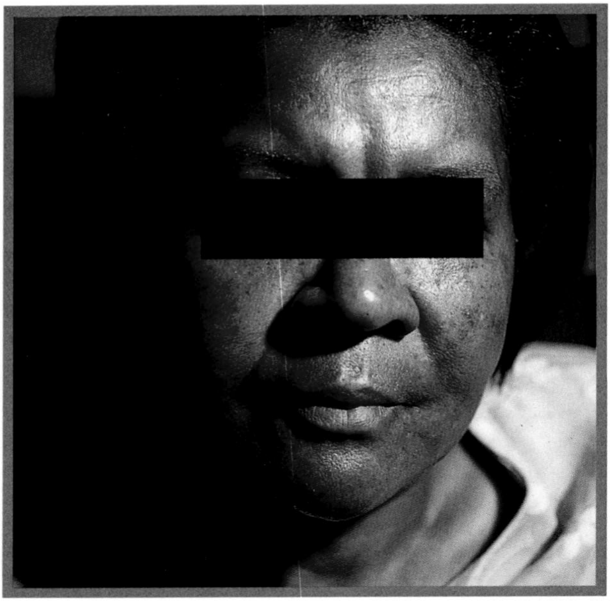

← Fig. 8.24 Hereditary hemorrhagic telangiectasia. Telangiectases of the face.

Characteristics of hereditary hemorrhagic telangiectasia

Autosomal dominant (gene not identified)
(20% no family history)

Telangiectases on tongue, lips, fingertips, nasal mucosae, gastrointestinal tract

Cardiovascular manifestations:
Pulmonary arteriovenous fistulae (15%) with hemoptysis, polycythemia, murmur, cyanosis, clubbing, low arterial Po_2, paradoxical embolism
Hepatic arteriovenous fistula with high cardiac output, right upper quadrant bruit
Pulmonary hypertension
Gastrointestinal bleeding with anemia, high output state
Paradoxical embolism

← Fig. 8.25 Characteristics of hereditary hemorrhagic telangiectasia.

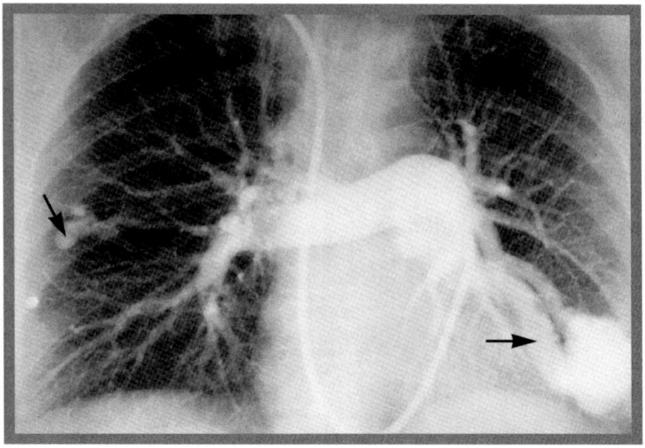

↑ Fig. 8.26
Hereditary hemorrhagic telangiectasia. Pulmonary arteriogram of the patient in Figure 8.20. The arrow on the observer's right indicates the opacified pulmonary vein draining the pulmonary arteriovenous fistula. The opacified vessel just superior to this is the pulmonary artery branch supplying the pulmonary arteriovenous fistula in the patient's left lung. The arrow on the left indicates a small arteriovenous fistula in the right lung. CT scanning may also be used to demonstrate these fistulae. (With permission from Fowler NO. *Diagnosis of heart disease*. Springer–Verlag, 1991.)

→ Fig. 8.27
Hereditary hemorrhagic telangiectasia. Pulmonary arteriogram of a 40-year-old woman with multiple pulmonary arterio-venous fistulae. This patient had severe pulmonary hypertension, with a pulmonary arterial pressure of 94/45mmHg.

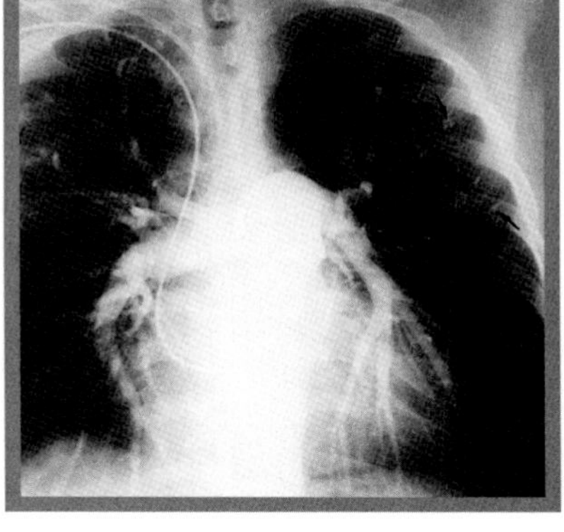

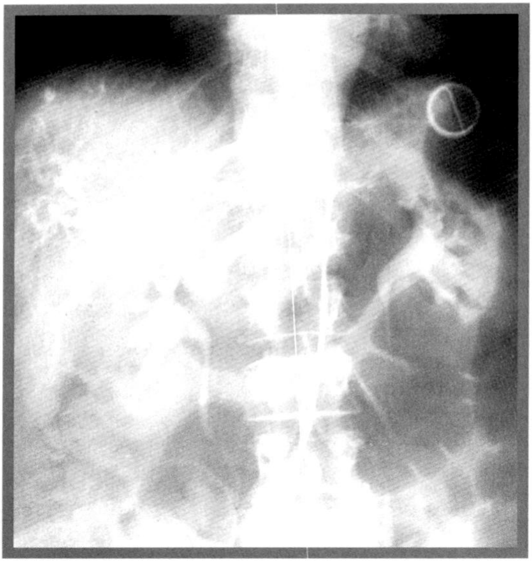

← Fig. 8.28a
Hereditary hemorrhagic telangiectasia. Earlier phase of the hepatic arteriogram showing multiple arteriovenous fistulae in a woman with hereditary hemorrhagic telangiectasia. There was an increased cardiac ouput at rest, and a continuous murmur was heard in the right upper quadrant. Cardiac decompensation was present.

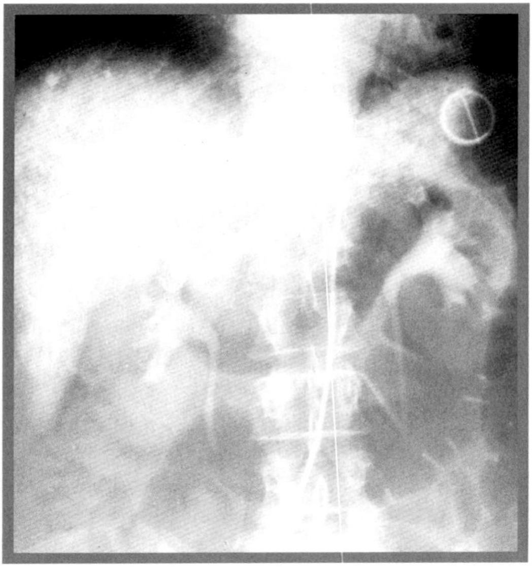

← Fig. 8.28b
Hereditary hemorrhagic telangiectasia. Later phase of the hepatic arteriogram.

Treatment

Lesions of the nasal mucosa may be treated with estrogens, cautery, or laser. Gastrointestinal lesions may be treated by photocoagulation or estrogen-progesterone therapy. Pulmonary arteriovenous fistulae may be treated by surgical resection or transcatheter embolotherapy. Hepatic arteriovenous fistulae may be subjected to segmental embolotherapy, but there is a risk of complications.

Further Reading

Guttmacher AE, Marchuk DA, White RI Jr. Hereditary hemorrhagic telangiectasia. *N Engl J Med* 1995, **333**:918–924.

Peery WH. Clinical spectrum of hereditary hemorrhagic telangiectasia (Osler–Weber–Rendu disease). *Am J Med* 1987, **82**:989–997.

Terry PB, White RI Jr, Barth KH, Kaufman SL, Mitchell SE. Pulmonary arteriovenous malformations. Physiologic observations and result of therapeutic balloon embolization. *N Engl J Med* 1983, **308**:1197–1200.

Pseudoxanthoma Elasticum

Pseudoxanthoma elasticum is a heterogeneous inherited disorder of connective tissue, with considerable variability in clinical manifestations (**Fig. 8.29**). It is inherited in some groups as an autosomal dominant, in others as an

→ Fig. 8.29 Characteristics of pseudoxanthoma elasticum.

Characteristics of pseudoxanthoma elasticum	
Basic:	Fragmentation and calcification of elastic fibers
Skin:	Yellowish papules in flexion areas (neck, axilla, cubital area, groin, popliteal space) Sagging nasolabial folds
Heart:	Coronary artery disease
Blood vessels:	Arterial obstruction (upper extremity, femoral arteries, coronary arteries)
Gastrointestinal:	Hemorrhage due to arterial involvement
Eye:	Angioid streaks (Bruch's membrane)

autosomal recessive. The clinical abnormalities of the disorder are encountered principally in three areas: the skin, the eyes, and the cardiovascular system. Because there is no serologic marker, the diagnosis depends upon the clinical features and the histologic demonstration of abnormal elastic fibers.

The typical skin lesions are yellow macules or papules that can form plaques and redundant folds of skin; they have been likened to plucked chicken skin. The skin lesions are often not recognizable before the second decade of life. Their most common locations are the axillae (**Figs 8.30** and **8.31**), the forearms (**Fig. 8.32**), and the flexural surface of the neck (**Fig. 8.33**). The characteristic histologic features are those of broken elastic fibers and calcification of elastic fibers (**Fig. 8.34**).

Angioid streaks (see Fig. 3.14), caused by breaks in Bruch's membrane (**Fig. 8.35**), represent the characteristic ocular lesion in pseudoxanthoma elasticum. Angioid streaks alone are not diagnostic of the disorder, as they have several other causes (**Fig. 8.36**), but they are highly suggestive of it in the presence of the characteristic skin and vascular lesions. The finding of angioid streaks in a young person with premature vascular disease is, however, very suggestive of pseudoxanthoma elasticum.

The cardiovascular lesions are those of calcification of medium-sized arteries, with progressive occlusion and occasional rupture. Coronary artery disease or

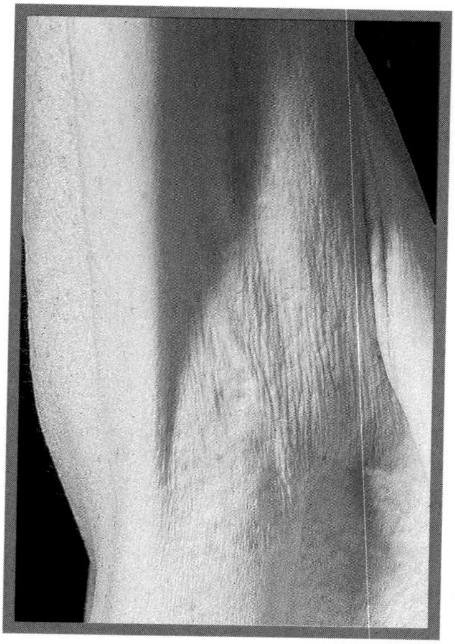

← Fig. 8.30
Pseudoxanthoma elasticum. Characteristic 'plucked chicken' skin appearance. The axilla is one of the most common locations for this lesion.

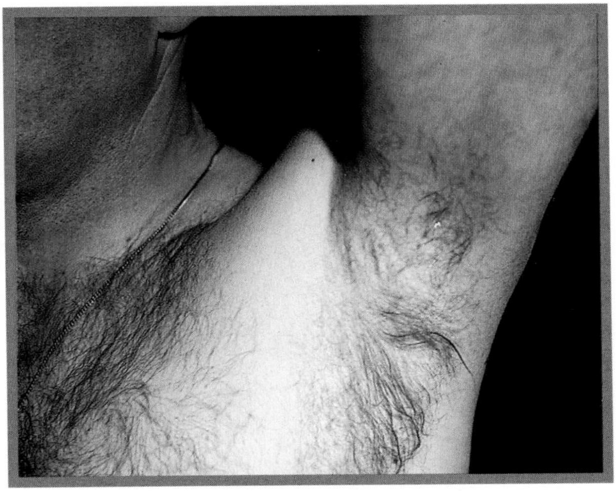

→ **Fig. 8.31**
Pseudoxanthoma elasticum. 'Plucked chicken' appearance of axillary skin.

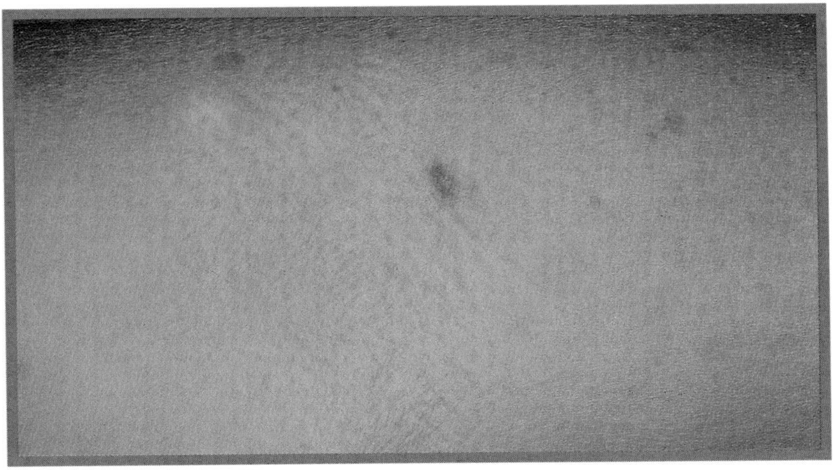

↑ **Fig. 8.32**
Pseudoxanthoma elasticum. Characteristic skin appearance on the flexor surface of the forearm.

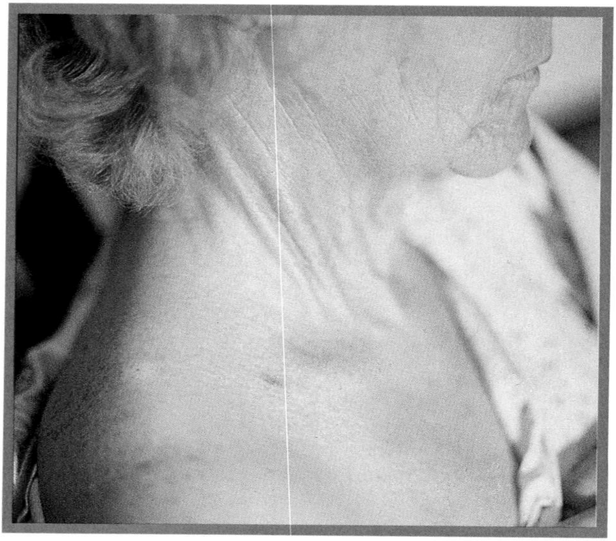

← Fig. 8.33
Pseudoxanthoma elasticum. Skin lesions on the side of the neck—one of the most common locations.

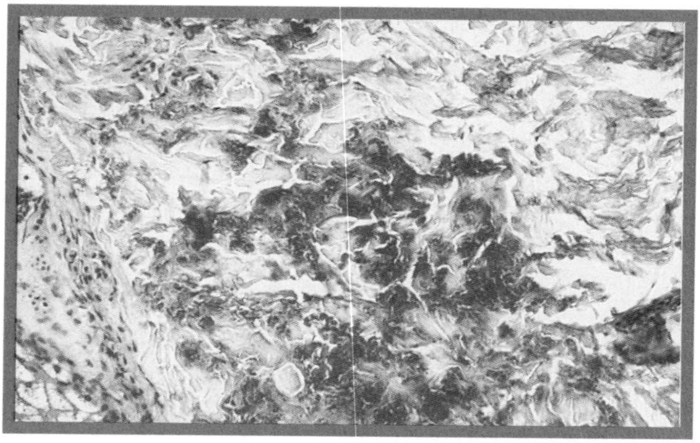

↑ Fig. 8.34
Pseudoxanthoma elasticum. Typical histologic appearance shown in a biopsy specimen of the skin of the neck. There are broken elastic fibers; the reddish purple material is calcium deposited in broken elastic fibers.

→ Fig. 8.35 Bruch's membrane. Diagram of histologic appearance of Bruch's membrane. Tears in this membrane give rise to angioid streaks. S, sclera; C, choroid; RPE, retinal pigment epithelium; R, neural retina. (See Fig. 3.14.) (With permission from D'Amico DJ. *N Engl J Med* 1994, **331**:96.)

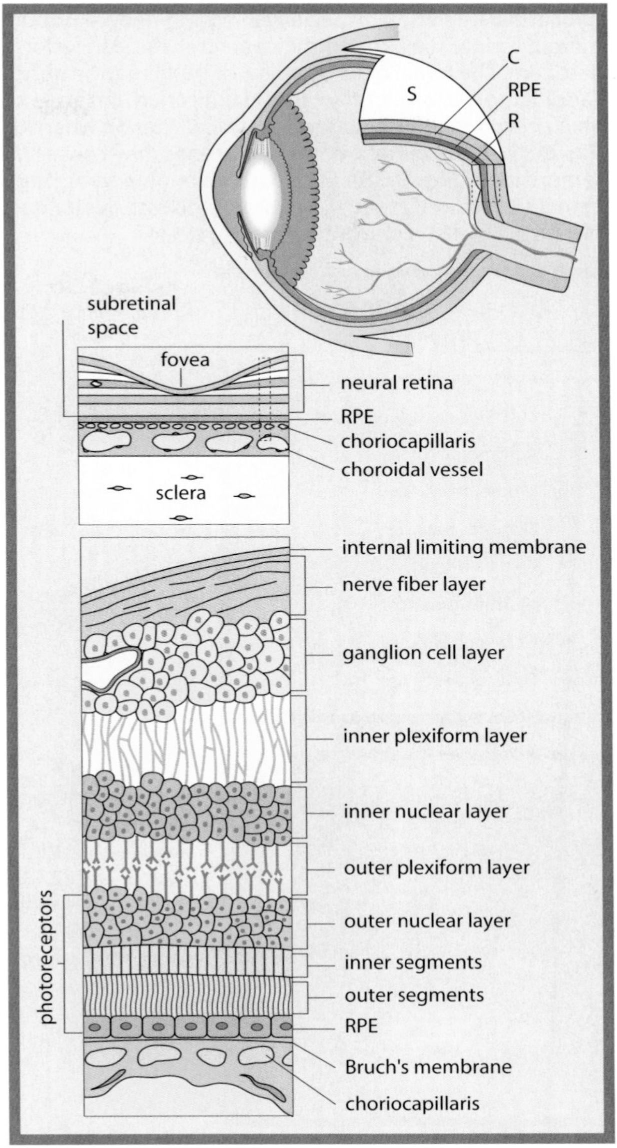

myocardial infarction, especially in young people, should prompt a search for angioid retinal streaks and the characteristic skin lesions of pseudoxanthoma elasticum. The radial or ulnar pulse, or both, may be absent. Involvement of the iliac or femoral arteries may cause claudication and absence of the femoral pulse, which may erroneously suggest aortic coarctation when found in a young person (**Fig. 8.37**). Involvement of cranial arteries may cause strokes or subarachnoid hemorrhage (**Fig. 8.38**). Endocardial involvement may lead to calcification, restrictive cardiomyopathy, or valvular disease. Major gastrointestinal bleeding may be a problem confronting the physician.

Causes of angioid streaks of the retina
Pseudoxanthoma elasticum
Ehlers–Danlos syndrome
Acromegaly
Hemochromatosis
Diabetes mellitus
Paget's disease
Neurofibromatosis
Sickle cell anemia
Tuberous sclerosis

← Fig. 8.36
Causes of angioid streaks of the retina.

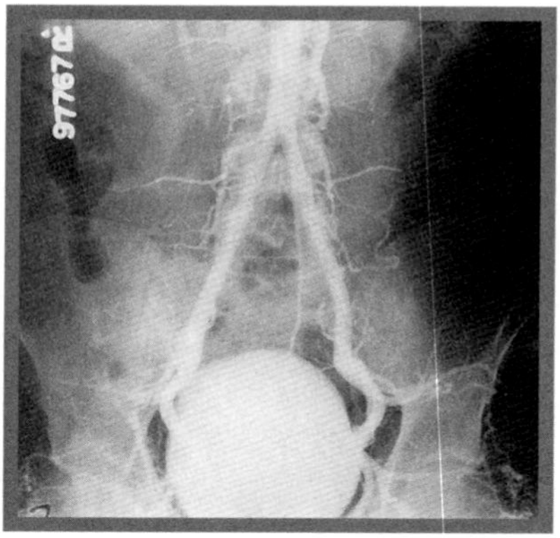

← Fig. 8.37
Pseudoxanthoma elasticum. Aortogram of a 21-year-old man who had retinal angioid streaks. There is narrowing of the external iliac arteries. Femoral pulses were absent, leading to an erroneous initial diagnosis of aortic coarctation.

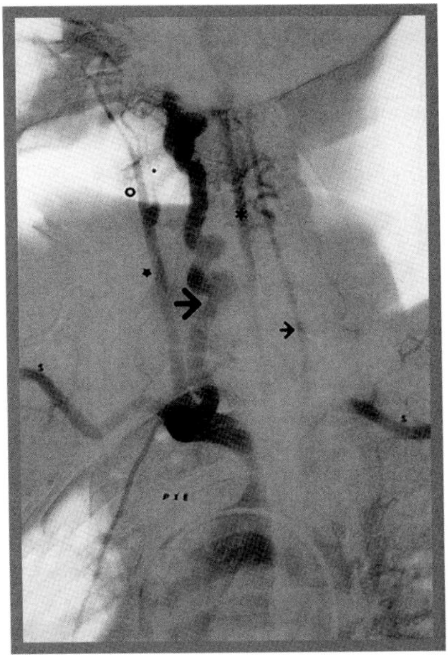

→ Fig. 8.38
Pseudoxanthoma elasticum. Contrast aortographic study of the patient whose skin biopsy histology is shown in Figure 8.34. The large arrow indicates the enlarged, tortuous right vertebral artery. To the left of it is the right common carotid artery (large black star). The small black star indicates the small right internal carotid artery. S, subclavian artery.

Further Reading

Beighton P, ed. *McKusick's heritable disorders of connective tissue, 5th ed.* St Louis: Mosby Yearbook Inc., 1993.

Lebwohl M, Halperin J, Phelps RG. Brief report: occult pseudoxanthoma elasticum in patients with premature vascular disease. *N Engl J Med* 1993, **329**:1237–1239.

Hemochromatosis

Hemochromatosis, also known as bronze diabetes, is the result of a genetic disorder transmitted as an autosomal recessive trait. The responsible gene has been linked to the HLA class I region on chromosome 6. The clinical phenotype of skin pigmentation and organ damage occurs only in homozygotes. In whites, homozygosity occurs with a frequency of 0.005–0.008. There is also a secondary form of the disease, resulting from iron overload. This form usually follows multiple blood transfusions, often of 100 units or more, which may be used in such diseases as aplastic anemia or thalassemia. It may also occur with defects in hemoglobin synthesis or excessive oral intake of iron.

The diagnosis of hemochromatosis is suggested by the clinical clues of hyperpigmented skin, diabetes mellitus, heart failure, hypogonadism, and arthropathy (**Fig. 8.39**). The skin pigmentation (**Fig. 8.40**) is typically generalized, but deeper in areas of sun exposure. The bronze color is caused by melanin; when iron deposition also occurs, the skin color becomes metallic gray. The diagnosis may be strongly suggested by demonstration of an increased serum ferritin concentration and an increased percentage saturation of transferrin (above 50% of capacity). It can be confirmed by biopsy demonstrating iron deposits in the liver.

Cardiac involvement occurs in about 33% of patients. Iron deposits are found in the sarcoplasmic reticulum and in the myocytes; the cardiac conducting system is commonly involved (**Fig. 8.41**). Clinically, there may be no evidence of heart disease, despite extensive myocardial iron deposits. Alternatively, there may be congestive heart failure, with a dilated heart and both systolic and diastolic dysfunction. Supraventricular arrhythmias are common; atrioventricular block and ventricular arrhythmias are less so.

Death usually results from heart failure, hepatic failure or hepatoma, or complications of diabetes.

Clinical features of hemochromatosis

Iron overload may be primary (genetically transmitted autosomal recessive), or secondary to multiple transfusions

Iron deposits in skin (bronzing), liver (cirrhosis, hepatoma), pancreas (diabetes), pituitary (hypopituitarism), heart muscle, and conducting system

Greater than 50% saturation of serum transferrin

Cardiac manifestations (33% of patients)
- Atrial and ventricular arrhythmias
- Atrioventricular block
- Restrictive cardiomyopathy with biventricular enlargement and congestive failure

Clinical cardiac features may be reversible with phlebotomy or chelation therapy

← Fig. 8.39 Clinical features of hemochromatosis

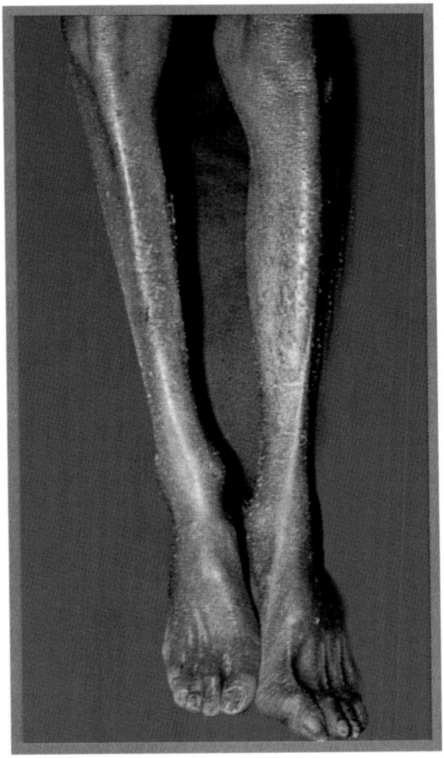

→ Fig. 8.40
Hemochromatosis. Bronzing of the skin of the legs, along with emaciation, in hemochromatosis. (With permission from Hariharan R, Fred HL. *Hosp Pract* 1996, **31**(11):45–49.)

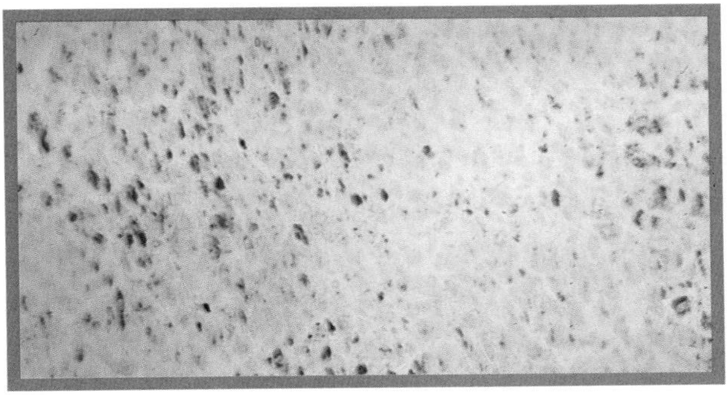

→ Fig. 8.41
Hemochromatosis. Histologic picture. The deep blue staining material represents iron deposited in the myocardium.

Further Reading

Bulaj Z, Griffen LM, Jorde LB, Edwards CQ, Kushner JP. Clinical and biochemical abnormalities in people heterozygous for hemochromatosis. *N Engl J Med* 1996, **335**:1799–1805.

Hariharan R, Fred HL. Diffuse hyperpigmentation in a man with diabetes. *Hosp Pract*, 1996, **31**(11):45–49.

Passen EL, Rodriguez ER, Neumann A, Tan CD, Parillo JE. Images in cardiovascular medicine. Cardiac hemochromatosis. *Circulation* 1996, **94**:2302–2303.

Amyloidosis

Amyloidosis is a disease resulting from tissue deposition of various proteins. Four major clinical varieties of amyloidosis are recognized (**Fig. 8.42**). Primary amyloidosis is caused by deposits of immunoglobulin light chains produced by plasma cells, at times in association with multiple myeloma. The heart is usually involved. Secondary amyloidosis, associated with chronic infections, connective tissue disease, and neoplasms, is produced by proteins that are not immunoglobulins. Clinical cardiac involvement is much less common here, and is found in perhaps 10% of cases. Familial amyloidosis occasionally involves the heart, but late in the course of the disease. Senile amyloidosis commonly involves the heart, but usually does not produce clinical heart disease; however, at times there are large cardiac deposits, resulting in congestive heart failure.

Classification of amyloidosis
Primary amyloidosis. The heart is usually involved
Secondary to chronic disease, e.g. tuberculosis, osteomyelitis, rheumatoid arthritis, ulcerative colitis, connective tissue disease. Cardiac involvement occurs in about 10%
Familial. Occasional cardiac involvement late in the disease
Senile. Commonly involves the heart; clinical heart disease is uncommon

← Fig. 8.42 Classification of amyloidosis.

Primary amyloid disease commonly affects the heart muscle, cardiac valves, and blood vessels, especially in the gums and rectum. Amyloid deposits may lead to a clinical picture of either restrictive cardiomyopathy (**Figs 8.43** and **8.44**),

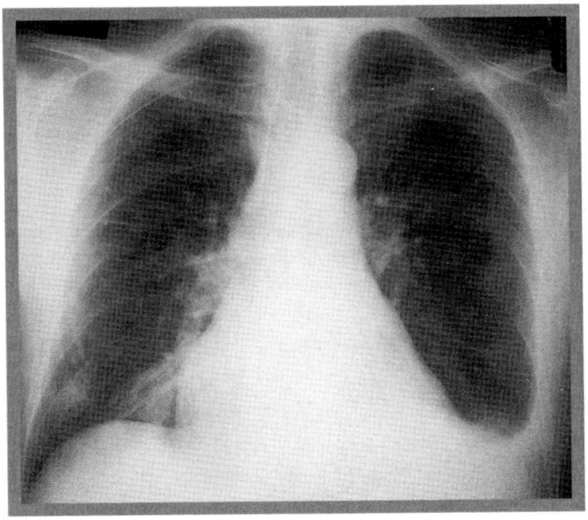

→ Fig. 8.43
Amyloidosis. Chest radiogram of a patient with amyloidosis proved by endomyocardial biopsy. There is cardiac enlargement, accompanied by pulmonary vascular engorgement and left pleural effusion.

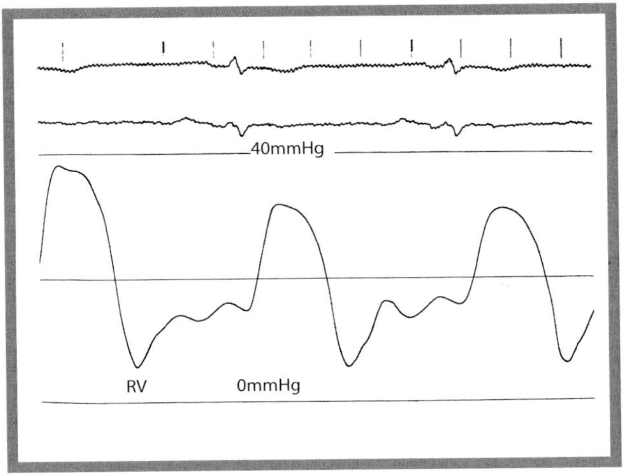

→ Fig. 8.44
Amyloidosis. Right ventricular pressure tracing of the same patient as in Figure 8.43. In this patient, with restrictive cardiomyopathy, the early diastolic dip, followed by a plateau, resembles the pressure tracing of constrictive pericarditis.

or dilated cardiomyopathy with impaired systolic function. Cardiac arrhythmias and A–V block are common. Atrial involvement may cause a sick sinus syndrome; coronary arterial deposits may lead to angina pectoris. The ECG usually shows a reduction in QRS voltage, and often a pseudoinfarction pattern (**Fig. 8.45**). The echocardiogram is characteristic, but not specifically diagnostic. The atria are dilated, and the ventricular walls and interventricular septum are thickened, at times having a characteristic granular, sparkling appearance (**Fig. 8.46**).

The diagnosis of cardiac amyloidosis should be given particular consideration when the pattern of restrictive cardiomyopathy appears in a person older than 70 years, or in a person between 50 and 70 years who has the characteristic ECG and echocardiographic features described above (**Fig. 8.47**). The possibility of

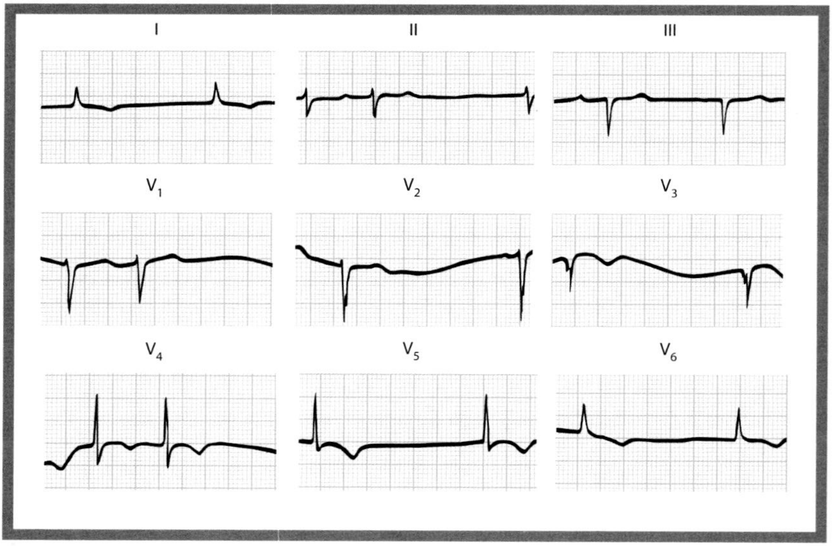

↑ Fig. 8.45
Amyloidosis. The ECG shows A–V junctional rhythm with occasional sinus captures. Lead V_3 shows a pseudoinfarction pattern that is common in amyloidosis, as a result of replacement of cardiac muscle by amyloid deposits. Atrial involvement may lead to loss of normal sinus rhythm, as in this patient. (With permission from Fowler NO. *Diagnosis of heart disease*. Springer–Verlag, 1991.)

→ Fig. 8.46 Echocardiographic features of cardiac amyloidosis. Data from a study of 28 patients. (From Siqueira-Filho AG, *et al.* *Circulation* 1981, **63**:188.)

Echocardiographic features of cardiac amyloidosis

Normal left ventricular dimension

Thickened interventricular septum, right ventricle, left ventricle

Decreased systolic thickening of left ventricle (65%) and interventricular septum (96%)

Global decrease in left ventricular function

Left atrial enlargement (50%)

Pericardial effusion (58%)

Granular, sparkling appearance of cardiac walls in 12 of 13

→ Fig. 8.47 Cardiac amyloidosis.

Cardiac amyloidosis

Appearance of cardiomyopathy in patients >70 years

Appearance of cardiomyopathy in a patient aged 50–70 years
- Low voltage QRS
- Pseudoinfarction ECG pattern
- Heart failure refractory to medical management
- Restrictive hemodynamic pattern
- Features of nephrosis

Familial history of amyloidosis

Causes of secondary amyloidosis: multiple myeloma, neoplasm, rheumatoid disease, tuberculosis, ulcerative colitis, chronic suppuration amyloidosis is increased if the patient has polyneuropathy or orthostatic hypotension, skin lesions (**Fig. 8.48**) or a nephrotic syndrome. The technetium pyrophosphate myocardial scintigram is usually positive. The diagnosis can be confirmed by endomyocardial biopsy (**Fig. 8.49**). Blood vessel deposits can often be demonstrated by biopsy of the gums, rectal mucosa, or bone marrow, and renal biopsy may show amyloid deposits.

The prognosis is poor once heart failure develops, and death usually occurs within 1–2 years. Digitalis is usually ineffective and its use may even be hazardous.

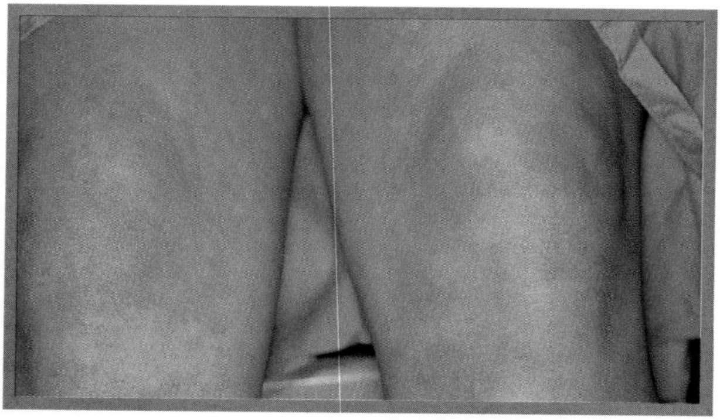

← Fig. 8.48 Amyloidosis. Skin lesions of macular amyloidosis.

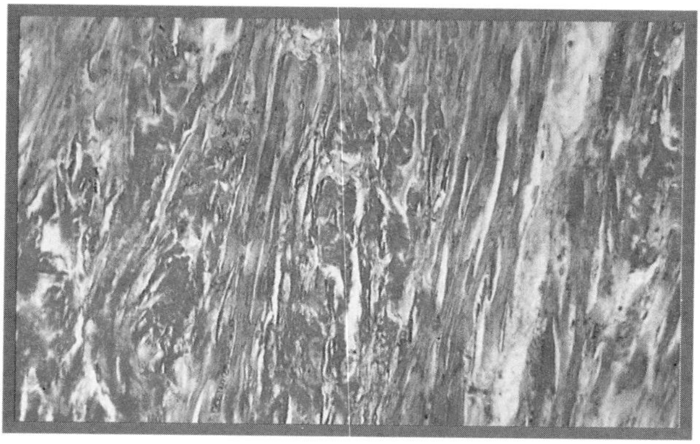

← Fig. 8.49 Amyloidosis. Amyloid deposits in cardiac muscle. Crystal violet stain.

Further Reading

Benson MD. Aging, amyloid, and cardiomyopathy. *N Engl J Med* 1997, **336**:502–504.
Kushwaha SS, Fallon JT, Fuster V. Medical progress. Restrictive cardiomyopathy. *N Engl J Med* 1997, **336**:267–276.

Ehlers–Danlos Syndrome

The Ehlers–Danlos syndromes are a group of heritable connective tissue disorders characterized by skin hyperextensibility (**Fig. 8.50**), articular hypermobility (**Fig. 8.51**), and tissue fragility, together with various cardiovascular features (**Fig. 8.52**).

Although Ehlers–Danlos syndrome has been described principally in Europeans and persons of European descent, it has also been reported in Africans. Its prevalence in southern England has been estimated to be at least 1 in 150,000. As many as 10 forms have been described. Types V–X are rare. Types I, II, III, VII, and VIII are autosomal dominants; type V is X-linked; types VI and X are autosomal recessive. Type IV is associated with a defect in type III collagen and arterial fragility.

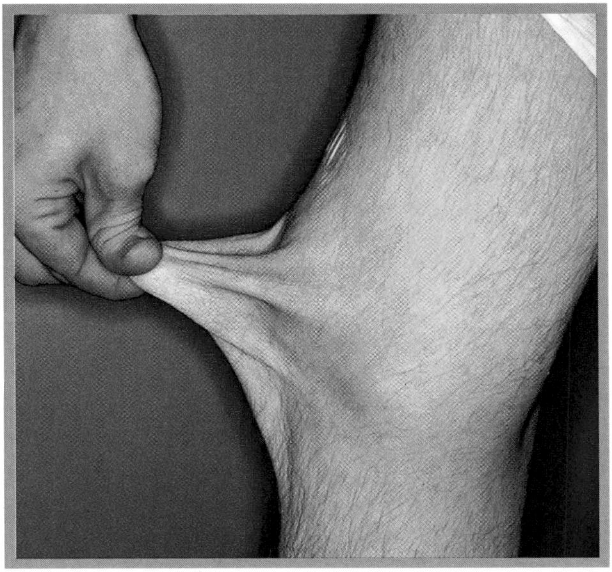

→ Fig. 8.50 Ehlers–Danlos syndrome. Characteristic hyperextensible skin on the knee.

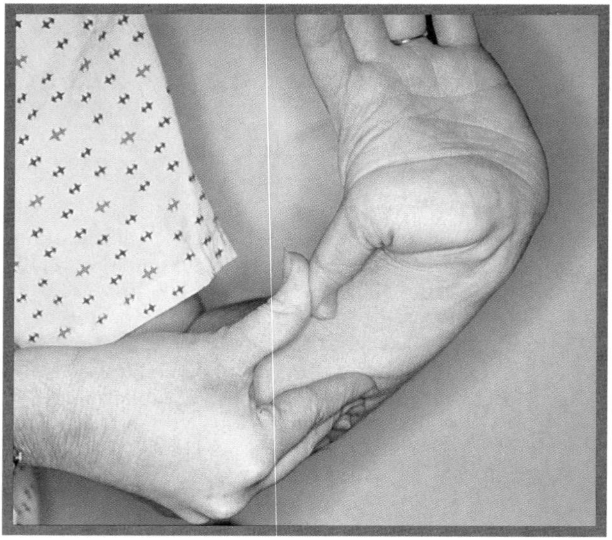

← Fig. 8.51 Ehlers–Danlos syndrome. Hypermobile thumb. Joint hypermobility is one of the major features of the disease. Hyperextensible skin and arterial fragility are also major features.

Clinical features of Ehlers–Danlos syndrome

Abnormal collagen wickerwork

Genetic heterogeneity:
some autosomal dominant;
some X-linked recessive

Diagnostic triad:
- Hyperextensible skin
- Hypermobility of joints
- Connective tissue fragility (easy bruising)

Cardiovascular features:
- Rupture of large arteries
- Aortic rupture or dissection
- Intracranial aneurysm
- Elongated chordae tendineae and mitral prolapse

← Fig. 8.52 Clinical features of Ehlers–Danlos syndrome.

The skin of patients with Ehlers–Danlos syndrome is often velvety, with 'cigaret paper' scars. At times there are localized lax or pendulous regions. Although the skin is easily stretched by pulling, it resumes its normal position when released.

Spontaneous rupture of large arteries is a major cause of death in patients with Ehlers–Danlos syndrome type IV. Patients may rupture the aorta or other large arteries, such as a subclavian artery. Intracranial aneurysms and arteriovenous fistulae are reported. Subarachnoid hemorrhage may be a complication. Aortic dissecting aneurysm and vertebral artery aneurysms may occur.

Serious cardiac difficulties are relatively uncommon. Mitral valve prolapse, mitral regurgitation, and tricuspid regurgitation have been reported. There are infrequent reports of atrial septal defect, tetralogy of Fallot, aortic incompetence, persistent atrioventricular canal, and coronary artery aneurysms.

Reference

Beighton P. *McKusick's heritable disorders of connective tissue, 5th ed.* St Louis: Mosby Yearbook Inc., 1993:189–251.

INDEX

D

E

I

J

K

L